AF581656

Asthma

Asthma: Current Perspectives on Phenotypes, Endotypes, and Treatable Traits

Editor

Nikoletta Rovina

MDPI • Basel • Beijing • Wuhan • Barcelona • Belgrade • Manchester • Tokyo • Cluj • Tianjin

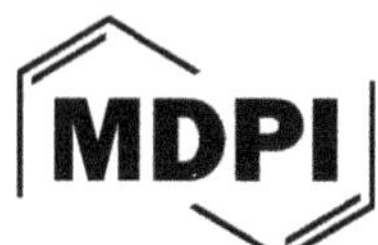

Editor
Nikoletta Rovina
National and Kapodistrian University of Athens
Greece

Editorial Office
MDPI
St. Alban-Anlage 66
4052 Basel, Switzerland

This is a reprint of articles from the Special Issue published online in the open access journal *Journal of Clinical Medicine* (ISSN 2077-0383) (available at: https://www.mdpi.com/journal/jcm/special_issues/Asthma_Pathophysiology).

For citation purposes, cite each article independently as indicated on the article page online and as indicated below:

LastName, A.A.; LastName, B.B.; LastName, C.C. Article Title. *Journal Name* **Year**, *Volume Number*, Page Range.

ISBN 978-3-03943-859-4 (Hbk)
ISBN 978-3-03943-860-0 (PDF)

Contents

About the Editor

Nikoletta Rovina is an Assistant Professor in Pulmonary and Critical Care Medicine at the National and Kapodistrian University of Athens. Her main research interest lies in the investigation of airway inflammation and cellular immunology (mainly in asthma and COPD). She has been a research collaborator of Cellular Immunology Laboratory, Center for Basic Research, Biomedical Research Foundation of the Academy of Athens (BRFAA) since 2019. As an intensivist, her main interest is the research of sepsis through her collaboration with the Hellenic Institute for the Study of Sepsis and the European Sepsis Alliance. In 2020, she has focused on the research of the immunology of SARS-COV2 infection in collaboration with the above-mentioned institutes. She is fully involved in the clinical work of both pulmonology and intensive care (COVID unit). Since 2008, she has run the outpatient clinic of obstructive pulmonary diseases in "Sotiria" hospital, which is the referral hospital for the diseases of the chest in Athens, Greece. Furthermore, she is fully involved in the educational programs of the University for pre- and postgraduate medical students.

Preface to "Asthma: Current Perspectives on Phenotypes, Endotypes, and Treatable Traits"

Asthma is a complex heterogeneous disease with different phenotypes and clinical expressions that greatly affects patients' quality of life. Some aspects of the natural history of the disease are incompletely understood. New insights into the mechanisms that drive the natural history of asthma and the evolution of airway inflammation in preschool age children are discussed. The role of lung microbiome in asthma pathogenesis and its possible manipulation has recently emerged. Likewise, the role of the NLRP3 inflammasome and its targeting as a potential therapeutic approach is of great importance. Particular endotypes of severe asthma such as eosinophilic asthma have gained interest due to the major advances of the novel targeted biological therapies that have changed the treatment landscape of severe asthma. Particular comorbidities such as OSAS in adults and chronic rhinitis in children greatly affect the clinical expression of asthma. In addition to these topics, acid–base disturbances, possible mechanisms, and management of acute severe asthma are also discussed herein.

Nikoletta Rovina
Editor

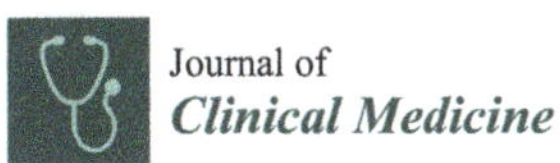
Journal of
Clinical Medicine

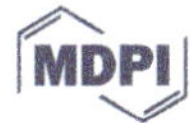

Review

Early Airway Pathological Changes in Children: New Insights into the Natural History of Wheezing

Matteo Bonato †, Mariaenrica Tiné †, Erica Bazzan, Davide Biondini, Marina Saetta *,‡ and Simonetta Baraldo ‡

Department of Cardiac, Thoracic, Vascular Sciences and Public Health, University of Padova, 35128 Padova, Italy
* Correspondence: marina.saetta@unipd.it; Tel.: +39-0498213706
† These authors equally contributed as first authors.
‡ These authors equally contributed as senior authors.

Received: 3 July 2019; Accepted: 4 August 2019; Published: 7 August 2019

Abstract: Asthma is a heterogeneous condition characterized by reversible airflow limitation, with different phenotypes and clinical expressions. Although it is known that asthma is influenced by age, gender, genetic background, and environmental exposure, the natural history of the disease is still incompletely understood. Our current knowledge of the factors determining the evolution from wheezing in early childhood to persistent asthma later in life originates mainly from epidemiological studies. The underlying pathophysiological mechanisms are still poorly understood. The aim of this review is to converge epidemiological and pathological evidence early in the natural history of asthma to gain insight into the mechanisms of disease and their clinical expression.

Keywords: wheezing; bronchial biopsies; symptom persistence; clinical remission

1. Introduction

Asthma is a heterogeneous condition characterized by reversible airflow limitation with different phenotypes and clinical expressions [1,2]. Several studies on lung specimens from adult asthmatic patients have established that asthma is a process involving both the central and peripheral airways. The process includes chronic activation of the inflammatory response as well as structural changes of the airway wall—the latter is collectively called airway remodeling. The inflammatory response in asthma has been demonstrated to have a large heterogeneity and to involve both the innate (i.e., eosinophils, mast cells, innate lymphoid cells) and the acquired immunity (i.e., T-lymphocytes). Airway remodeling consists of shedding of the bronchial epithelium, thickening of the subepithelial reticular basement membrane (RBM) and of the smooth muscle mass, as well as proliferation of bronchial vessels or angiogenesis [3,4]. Although chronic inflammation in asthma is associated with airway remodeling, the mutual relation between the two is still a point of substantial debate.

Although the histopathological features characteristic of asthma have been extensively described since the early 20th century, the molecular mechanisms responsible for the recruitment and activation of inflammatory cells and establishment of the architectural changes typical of airway remodeling are still only partially understood. The majority of studies in this field have considered adult and childhood asthma separately, almost as if they were different disease entities. At present, the evidence on asthma histopathology has been gathered exclusively from studies on adult cohorts, while there is a scarcity of studies on the histopathology of asthma in children. This is due essentially to the difficulty of obtaining bronchial biological samples from children and to the diagnostic dilemma—particularly in infants and preschool children—of discerning true asthma from other wheezing disorders. We suggest that a thorough comprehension of the histopathology of wheezing in children (i.e., at the beginning of the natural history of asthma) and of its interrelationship with the spectrum of clinical phenotypes should be the compass for guiding research into the jungle of inflammatory cells, mediators, and cytokines underlying asthma pathogenesis. Therefore, this review focuses on the major cellular and structural changes present in the airways of children with asthma in relation with the most important clinical phenotypes, in an attempt to integrate these data with those emerging from the longitudinal investigation of outcomes from early childhood to adulthood.

2. Wheezing Disorders and Their Evolution across Developmental Ages

Wheezing is very common in the first 3 years of life. Yet, most preschool children with wheeze will be symptom-free by the time they reach school age, whereas only a minority will remain symptomatic, develop persistent wheeze, and ultimately be diagnosed as asthmatics. The identification of the factors which may predict the future development of asthma in early wheezing children has mainly been addressed by epidemiological studies [5], and is still a matter of vivid debate.

While the great majority of wheezers do not usually progress to asthma in childhood and adolescence, some of them may have relapsing symptoms and be at increased risk of asthma in adulthood, and even of chronic obstructive pulmonary disease (COPD) later on [6]. Furthermore, the adult onset of asthma symptoms may occur in a considerable proportion of asthmatics, especially in women [7]. However, many patients do not completely remember their childhood symptoms, so it is unclear which cases might reflect relapse rather than true new onset.

Phenotypes with documented clinical importance in childhood asthma have been defined in several ways: (i) on the basis of concomitant traits, such as atopy; (ii) on the basis of the temporal pattern of symptoms appearance; (iii) on the basis of the longitudinal evolution of wheezing symptoms. As such, specific wheezing phenotypes that have been investigated in preschool children include: non-atopic and atopic wheezing; episodic and multiple-trigger wheezing; transient, persistent, and late-onset wheezing [2].

Prospective birth cohort studies such as the pioneering Tucson cohort have determined the longitudinal outcome of wheezing and defined specific categories, such as: (i) transient wheeze—children who wheeze during the first years of life, but not after the age of 3; (ii) persistent wheeze—children who start to wheeze before the age of 3 and maintain their symptoms even beyond school age; and (iii) late-onset wheeze—children who start to wheeze after the age of 3 [8]. However, these categories can only be recognized retrospectively, and are of little value in clinical practice [9].

The presence of atopy, and particularly an early sensitization to multiple allergens, is generally considered a fundamental risk factor for the future development of persistent asthma [8,10–13], although the relationship between wheezing and allergic sensitization in the first years of life is still controversial [14]. The predominant role of atopy was so generally accepted that often wheezing was considered by many pediatricians to truly represent asthma only when associated to atopy. Conversely, non-atopic wheezing was thought to be a transient phenotype, mostly triggered by viral infections [1,10–12,14–16]. On the same line, pediatricians proposed a clinical distinction between episodic and multiple-trigger (multitrigger) wheezing. Episodic wheezing is thought to be triggered by viral infections, manifests only in association with coryzal symptoms, and affected children are symptom-free between viral episodes, while multitrigger wheeze is triggered by multiple stimuli (including allergens, viruses, exercise, laughing) and is characterized by the presence of symptoms in between discrete episodes [2]. Multitrigger wheezing is usually considered as the phenotype associated with wheezing persistence over time [8,17]. However, some reports suggest that there is a wide overlap between the two phenotypes, with the wheezing pattern varying over time in many children [9], and that severe viral wheeze is equally associated with a high risk of asthma at school age [18].

Further important determinants of persistent symptoms include prenatal features (preterm birth and low birth weight), pulmonary function deficits and reduced breast feeding in early infancy, as well as indoor and outdoor exposures—particularly to environmental pollutants and cigarette smoking [19]. In the present review we focus mainly on the role of atopy and viral infections, the pathogenetic mechanisms of which are better known.

3. Pathological Changes in Childhood Asthma

Endobronchial biopsy is the main diagnostic technique for evaluating the pathological processes in the bronchial mucosa directly [20,21]: it allows evaluation of the grade and type of inflammation, and provides evidence of the structural changes that may occur during the process of airway remodeling.

Eosinophilic inflammatory infiltrate associated with thickening of the RBM, epithelial shedding, neo-angiogenesis, and smooth muscle enlargement are characteristic changes of asthma that have been widely described in adults [22,23], but scarcely investigated in children.

The first pioneering study that investigated the bronchial histopathology in asthmatic children was by Cutz et al. in 1978, who described a prominent eosinophilic infiltrate and airway remodeling in the specimens of four asthmatic children [24]. After 20 years, Cokuğraş et al. [25] qualitatively examined bronchial biopsy specimens from 10 children with moderate asthma. They described a thickened RBM associated to an inflammatory infiltrate characterized by lymphocytic predominance, and only in one case they identified a prominent eosinophilic infiltrate. Subsequently, Jenkins and colleagues [26] reported a qualitative histopathological analysis of six children with severe asthma. They confirmed a thickened RBM and the presence of lymphocytes in lamina propria, but also recognized eosinophils in the inflammatory infiltrate and smooth muscle enlargement. These studies only performed qualitative analyses on a limited number of cases, and without a proper control group they can be considered as isolated observations. Payne and co-workers were the first to perform a quantitative evaluation of inflammatory and structural changes in a cohort of severe therapy-resistant asthmatic children. In two controlled studies [27,28], they demonstrated that asthmatic children had a thickened RBM in the absence of a prominent eosinophilia, suggesting that structural alterations can even precede inflammation in the natural history of the disease. However, the children examined in these two studies were severe asthmatics, most of them in treatment with maximal inhaled steroid therapy or even oral corticosteroids, which could have influenced the inflammatory process—particularly eosinophils. Conversely, our group has demonstrated in two consecutive studies that eosinophilic inflammation was definitely present in children with milder forms of the disease. Only a minority of children in our cohort were on inhaled corticosteroids (at low dose); the great majority of individuals were on as-needed salbutamol, and therefore free from the potential bias of steroid therapy [29,30]. Of importance, while earlier studies examined populations of school-aged children, our group was the first to assess histopathological changes typical of asthma in preschool children [30]. It is of interest that the early detection of airway eosinophilia in these children was associated with important features of airway remodeling—not only a thickened RBM, but also epithelial shedding and neo-angiogenesis (Figure 1) [30].

The presence of RBM thickening and eosinophilic inflammation was subsequently confirmed in an even younger cohort of children [31] (median age 2.4 years), and was further investigated in several cohorts whose results are summarized in Table 1 [32–38]. Taken together, these studies showed that most of the structural and inflammatory changes typical of asthma are present in asthmatic children, and also in preschool wheezing children, that is, at the beginning of the natural history of the disease. In particular, almost all reports converged on showing a thickened basement membrane, indicating that this is an early event present from 2–3 years of life. Whether RBM thickening is already present in younger infants (1 year of age) is actually a matter of debate, since it was not found in a cohort of 16 infants by Saglani et al. [36], but has been recently reported in a larger cohort of 30 infants by Berankova and coworkers [34]. Some incongruities regarding eosinophilic airway inflammation have been reported, but these could reflect the different treatment levels in different cohorts, rather than true pathogenetic differences as also suggested by other authors [39]. Finally, other aspects of airway remodeling (epithelial loss, angiogenesis, and smooth muscle enlargement have been examined in limited reports [30,33,37,38], and deserve further investigation.

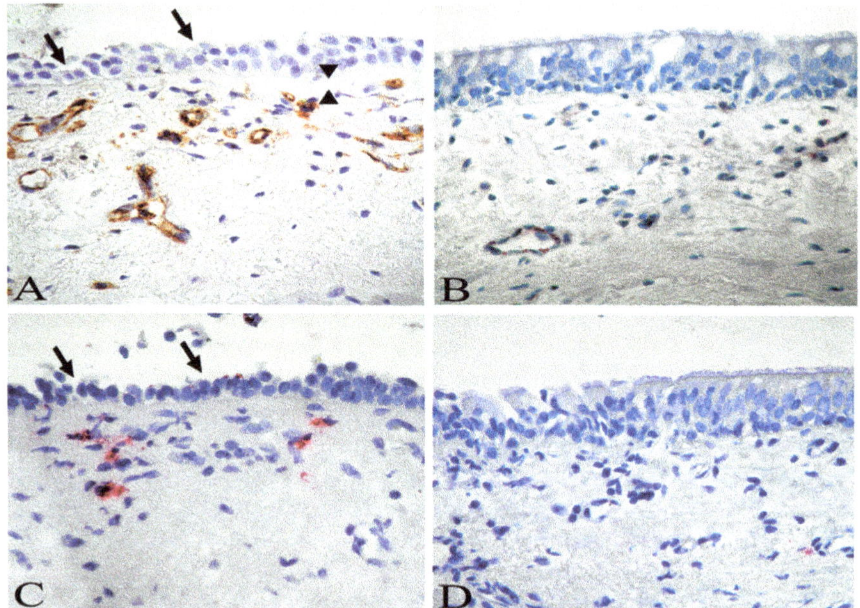

Figure 1. Biopsy sections from a child with asthma (**A**,**C**), and a control child (**B**,**D**). An increased number of subepithelial vessels (**A**, brown) and eosinophils (**C**, red) are demonstrated in the child with asthma. The arrows indicate loss of epithelial cells (**A**,**C**), while the arrowheads indicate reticular basement membrane thickening (**A**). Immunostaining with monoclonal antibody anti-CD31 (**A**,**B**) and anti-EG2 (**C**,**D**). Original magnification ×630. Reprinted with permission of the American Thoracic Society from [30].

Table 1. Histopathologic changes in bronchial biopsies of asthmatic/wheezing children.

	Number of Children	Mean Age (years)	RBM Thickening	Epithelial Loss	SM Enlargement	Submucosal Inflammation	Angiogenesis
Cutz 1978 [24]	4	12 (11–12)	+	0	+	Eos	/
Cokuğraş 2001 [25]	10	9.3 ± 3.8	+	/	/	Ly	/
Jenkins 2003 [26]	6	13.5 (6–17)	+	/	+	Eos Ly	/
Payne 2003 [27]	19	13 (6–16)	+	/	/	0	/
Barbato 2003 [29]	9	8 (4–12)	+	/	/	Eos	/
Payne 2004 [28]	36	13 (6–16)	+	/	/	0	/
Saglani 2005 [36]	16	1 (0.3–2)	0	/	/	0	/
Barbato 2006 [30]	17	5 (2–15)	+	+	/	Eos	+
Saglani 2007 [31]	16	2.4 (0.6–4.75)	+	/	/	Eos	/
Kim 2007 [32]	18	13 ± 1	+	/	/	/	/
Regamey 2008 [37]	24	12.5 (6.7–15.8)	/	/	+	/	/
Zhou 2011 [33]	13	7.2 (1.5–15)	+	+	+	Ly Eos	/
Bossley 2012 [38]	53	12 (9–14)	+	/	+	Eos	/
Berankova 2014 [34]	30	1 (0.3–3.3)	+	/	/	/	/
Van Mastrigt 2015 [35]	107	9.5 ± 4.6	+	/	/	/	/

Age is reported as median (range) or mean ± SD. Definition of abbreviations: Eos: eosinophils; Ly: lymphocytes; RBM: reticular basement membrane; SM: smooth muscle. Presence of the histological feature (+), absence (0), feature not evaluated in the study (/).

In conclusion, these studies conducted in the last twenty years, despite their unquestionable limitations (small cohorts, influence of steroid treatment, and diagnostic wheezing dilemma in preschool children) provide evidence that both inflammation and remodeling are present early in the natural history of the disease, challenging the "classic theory" of asthma pathogenesis which views remodeling as a consequence of a long-lasting chronic inflammation. These observations support the hypothesis that the epithelial–mesenchymal signaling may play a fundamental role in the development of bronchial asthma and its clinical phenotypes. In fact, the chronic damage to the airway epithelium due to a variety of stimuli could activate inflammatory pathways, with the release of damage-related cytokines—especially IL-33, which is hyperexpressed in children and directly correlated to RBM thickness [40], but also IL-25, TSLP, and mitotic/fibrogenic growth factors, thereby promoting angiogenesis as well as thickening of the RBM and smooth muscle [41–43]. The stimuli which have been more extensively investigated are allergens and viral pathogens, and we will now review the evidence in the literature on the activation of these pathogenetic mechanisms in relation to airway histopathological changes in childhood asthma.

4. Atopy and Related Pathological Changes

Atopy is generally considered to be a crucial feature characterizing asthma either in children or in adults, and early onset allergic asthma is considered to be the archetypal phenotype of the disease.

The term atopy (from the Greek "atopos", meaning "out of place") describes the tendency to be hyperallergic, the genetic propensity to mount an IgE response to triggers including pollens, animal dander, and food-based allergens. Allergens are well known triggers of type 2 immunity characterized by the differentiation of naïve T $CD4^+$ cells towards Th2 effector cells, which is typically associated with IgE production, eosinophilia, and mast cell activation. The keystone cytokines in type 2 immune response include IL-4, IL-5, IL-9, and IL-13. IL-4 is crucial for the differentiation of naïve Th0 cells to Th2 cells, which in turn induces isotype switching to IgE production. Specific IgE antibodies bind to their high-affinity FceRI receptors on the surface of basophils or mast cells, leading to the sensitization of those cells. IL-5 and IL-9 are responsible for the activation and recruitment of eosinophils and mast cells, respectively, while IL-13 induces goblet cell hyperplasia, mucus hyper-secretion, and airway hyper-responsiveness [44].

Atopic sensitization, with the resulting activation of the Th2 cascade, has long been considered a key determinant of wheezing persistence and asthma development in childhood. Indeed, it has been reported in several cohorts that children who have either a family history of allergies or who will become sensitized to local aeroallergens are more likely to have wheezing that persists into adulthood, whereas wheezing appears to resolve in adolescence in those children who do not develop atopic sensitization [15]. Based on this evidence, we investigated the hypothesis that a different airway pathology could be present in atopic and non-atopic wheezing children. In a well-characterized cohort of children in whom symptoms of wheezing were those typical of asthma (multitrigger, responsive to bronchodilators), we reported that all the histopathological traits of asthma were observed in both atopic and non-atopic children [45]. These traits included RBM thickening, epithelial desquamation, angiogenesis, and even an eosinophilic inflammatory infiltrate with upregulation of Th2 cytokines IL-4 and IL-5. Further work from our group demonstrated that atopic and non-atopic wheezing children have a similar degree of eosinophilic inflammation even in bronchoalveolar lavage (i.e., eosinophils and eosinophil cationic protein levels) [46]. These data in children complemented the seminal observations by Humbert and co-workers, who showed more similarities than differences in the immunopathology of atopic and non-atopic asthma in adults [47]. In conclusion, studies on bronchial biopsies and BAL demonstrated the similar nature of the histopathological substrate of these two crucial wheezing phenotypes from the beginning of the disease.

5. Viral Infections and Related Pathological Changes

Rhinovirus infections are among the most frequent cause of asthma exacerbations in adults, but even more so in children [48–50]. Indeed, cold-related wheezing is the most common respiratory symptom in preschool children, with up to 40%–50% of children experiencing at least one wheezing episode before the age of three. However, recurrent wheeze in early childhood is not always asthma. Recent techniques with the molecular detection of viral pathogens brought significant advances to understand the relationship between viral infections and asthma inception. Not only viruses are frequently isolated in exacerbations of asthma, but respiratory viral infections in early life—particularly rhinovirus and respiratory syncytial virus (RSV)—are associated with increased risk of asthma later in life [18,51–56].

Defective production of type I and type III interferons (IFNs) upon rhinovirus infection has been documented in adults with asthma, which can lead to impaired viral clearance, thus aggravating the impact of infections on the lung [57,58]. We demonstrated that such impaired immune response by epithelial cells was already present in preschool children with asthma [59]. Of importance, we found that impaired innate lung immunity was associated with structural changes in the airway biopsies (epithelial loss) and to markers of type 2 immunity [59]. We then investigated whether such deranged antiviral response can be considered as a risk for future asthma persistence. After an 8-year follow-up, we showed that children with asthma persisting at adolescence already had deficient IFN production and higher viral replication at preschool age [60]. These findings suggested the hypothesis that the immunologic interactions between viral infections and type 2 immunity predisposes to more severe acute responses to the virus, resulting in chronic insults to the epithelium, and eventually leading to the development of asthma. These observations are also in agreement with findings from the follow-up of large cohorts of children in the Tucson and the COPSAC studies, where children with asthma at school age already exhibited aberrant immune responses in infancy, not only to viruses but also to bacteria [61,62]. Altogether, these observations would support the concept that an aberrant response to infectious pathogens very early in life—mainly driven by the airway epithelium—is a crucial determinant of the evolution toward asthma.

6. Evolution of Asthma Symptoms in Relation to Pathological Changes

The last decades have seen a rapid growth of information on the evolution of asthma-like symptoms in childhood and their determinants. Most infants and young children with wheezing will outgrow their symptoms as their lungs develop, but some will persist in their symptoms over time toward confirmed asthma (Figure 2) [5,63]. Those transient wheezers who do not usually progress to asthma in childhood and adolescence can still have symptoms remittance in adulthood, and can be at increased risk of COPD [6]. Emerging evidence from clinical and epidemiological studies that followed-up children from the care of their pediatrician into adolescence and then into adulthood has helped us to understand the main determinants of symptoms persistence [5]. Early aeroallergen sensitization, respiratory infections in infancy, and cigarette smoking exposure have all been associated with persistent symptoms [19]. Reduced lung function in early infancy (as soon as 1 month of age) is another factor that has been associated with persistent wheezing at 11 years [3]. This has been confirmed by the results of a number of studies [4,10,11,14,15], which have demonstrated that poor airway function shortly after birth (at 2–3 months of age) is a risk factor for asthma in teenagers and young adults (at 11, 16, and 22 years of age). This effect may reflect the variation in genes regulating normal lung growth and airway structure during lung development [64,65]. Furthermore, the association between lung function and symptoms persistence is independent of the effect of airway hyperresponsiveness, atopy, and type 2 allergic inflammation (as measured by blood eosinophil levels) [66]. These findings indirectly suggest that airway structural changes, which start early in life, are crucial determinants of the persistence of asthma symptoms and therefore highlight the need for a better understanding of the pathogenetic mechanisms underlining symptom persistence.

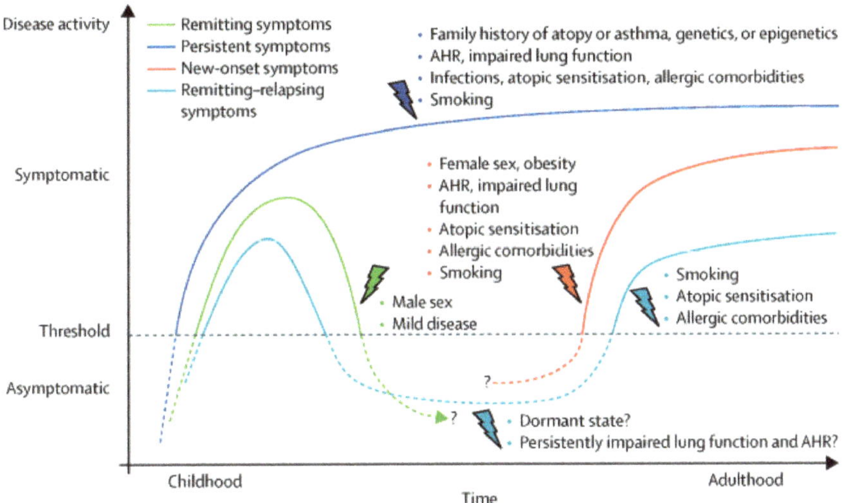

Figure 2. Determinants of disease course across asthma transition and ages. The figure displays putative determinants that affect the disease course of different asthma phenotypes by course and time of onset of symptoms. AHR: airway hyper-responsiveness. Reprinted with permission from Elsevier from [5].

To our knowledge, only four longitudinal studies have investigated the pathological changes able to predict the presence of asthma at follow-up. The first two, by Malmström and co-workers, evaluated a cohort of 53 infants with pathological changes and airway conductance measured at baseline and then re-evaluated them at 3 and 8 years of age. While there was a correlation between RBM thickening and mucosal mast cells with corticosteroid purchase at 3 years (as an indirect index of asthma) [67], the correlations were not present when children were comprehensively reassessed for asthma at 8 years of age [68]. Indeed, no pathologic features at baseline correlated with the presence of confirmed asthma at school age [68]. Then, O'Reilly and co-workers reported a follow-up of a cohort of 47 preschool children with severe recurrent wheezing [69]. RBM thickening and the eosinophilic infiltrate, despite being distinctive features of wheezing children at baseline, were not able to distinguish children who did or did not develop asthma at follow-up. Conversely, airway smooth muscle mass, which was not enlarged at baseline in symptomatic children, was the only histological feature to be associated to the development of asthma at school age. More recently, our group has also completed a clinical follow-up of a cohort of 80 preschool wheezing children (and non-wheezing controls) that had histological parameters assessed at baseline. At variance with previous studies, a thicker RBM and an eosinophilic inflammation in the lamina propria were clearly associated to the persistence of asthma from preschool to school age. When we performed a multivariate analysis, only RBM thickening remained a significant predictor of asthma persistence. Even when we limited our analysis to toddlers only (children under 3 years), RBM thickening at this early age remained a significant predictor of asthma later in life [70].

While the persistence of wheezing from early life to school age is associated with abnormal histological traits, it is also important to know what happens to these traits with the remission of symptoms. Marshall and co-workers compared the lung function and sputum cellularity of children with persistent or transient wheezing after following them through adolescence [71]. They found that airway eosinophilic inflammation and lung function impairment were seen not only in persistent wheezers, but also in children with a transient wheezing phenotype. Similarly, Dutch cohorts that examined young adults in clinical remission from childhood asthma reported persistent airway remodeling despite symptoms disappearance [72,73], suggesting that symptoms remission does not equate remission of the underlying pathology. In support of this hypothesis is the observation that, when assessed with functional tests, the majority of patients in apparent clinical remission still retain impaired lung function and airway hyperresponsiveness [74].

This topic now becomes truly fascinating, since pathological changes in children that predispose them to symptoms persistence are also present in subjects in clinical remission during adolescence/early adulthood. To disentangle this issue, we have created a number of different wheezing phenotypes (atopic/non-atopic, multitrigger/episodic, transient/persistent/late onset, etc.). However, there is no doubt that we are forcing an extensive variety of clinical phenotypes into artificially simple categories—all of them unable to fully capture the real complexity of a disease that is variable by definition. Instead of being distinct pathogenetic entities, these wheezing phenotypes may rather represent different clinical expressions of the same underlying pathology (i.e., different levels of disease severity). Let us imagine the process as a continuum: wheezing children develop airway structural changes very early in life and keep all the pathological hallmarks of asthma also in adolescence, and maybe for their entire life, independently from the clinical "activity" of the disease. To elicit symptoms, a certain threshold of trigger is needed at a given time point; with lower burdens, individuals will remain asymptomatic and this will occur mostly during adolescence/early adulthood when they achieve their maximal levels of pulmonary function. Nonetheless, these subjects, even if in clinical remission, have all the pathological hallmarks of asthma in their airways and will be prone to relapse whenever exposed to a high burden of inflammatory stimuli. The most harmful factor in adolescence is cigarette smoking, against which they should be strongly advised. With the recent widespread use of e-cigarettes in adolescents, whose effects on the lungs are a cause of strong concern, we also need to look carefully at the possible effects of e-cigarette use in these vulnerable children.

The description of the clinical course of asthma and pulmonary function trajectories during the entire human life in relation to airway histopathology is crucial for matching the wide spectrum of asthma phenotypes—from early wheezing in infancy to the late-onset adult forms—with specific pathological traits. We have reviewed here the available data focusing on the early stages of the disease to address the pathology at the onset of asthma symptoms and then investigated its relation with the evolution of symptoms during childhood and adolescence. With the upcoming follow-up of existing cohorts across the whole natural history of asthma, further into adulthood and elder age, we will have a unique opportunity to unravel the mechanisms behind this multifaceted disease.

Funding: University of Padova, Italian Ministry of Education, Universities and Research, Italian Society of Infantile Respiratory Diseases.

Conflicts of Interest: M.S. has received unrestricted research grants from Takeda Ltd, Chiesi Farmaceutici, Laboratori Guidotti Spa, outside this specific study. All others declare no conflicts of interest.

References

1. Martinez, F.D. Development of wheezing disorders and asthma in preschool children. *Pediatrics* **2002**, *109*, 362–367. [PubMed]
2. Brand, P.L.; Baraldi, E.; Bisgaard, H.; Boner, A.L.; Castro-Rodriguez, J.A.; Custovic, A.; de Blic, J.; de Jongste, J.C.; Eber, E.; Everard, M.L.; et al. Definition, assessment and treatment of wheezing disorders in preschool children: An evidence-based approach. *Eur. Respir. J.* **2008**, *32*, 1096–1110. [CrossRef] [PubMed]
3. Turner, S.W.; Palmer, L.J.; Rye, P.J.; Gibson, N.A.; Judge, P.K.; Cox, M.; Young, S.; Goldblatt, J.; Landau, L.I.; Le Souëf, P.N. The relationship between infant airway function, childhood airway responsiveness, and asthma. *Am. J. Respir. Crit. Care Med.* **2004**, *169*, 921–927. [CrossRef] [PubMed]
4. Stern, D.A.; Morgan, W.J.; Wright, A.L.; Guerra, S.; Martinez, F.D. Poor airway function in early infancy and lung function by age 22 years: A non-selective longitudinal cohort study. *Lancet* **2007**, *370*, 758–764. [CrossRef]
5. Fuchs, O.; Bahmer, T.; Rabe, K.F.; von Mutius, E. Asthma transition from childhood into adulthood. *Lancet Respir. Med.* **2017**, *5*, 224–234. [CrossRef]
6. Bush, A. COPD: A pediatric disease. *COPD* **2008**, *5*, 53–67. [CrossRef] [PubMed]

7. Honkamäki, J.; Hisinger-Mölkänen, H.; Ilmarinen, P.; Piirilä, P.; Tuomisto, L.E.; Andersén, H.; Huhtala, H.; Sovijärvi, A.; Backman, H.; Lundbäck, B.; et al. Age and gender-specific incidence of new asthma diagnosis from childhood to late adulthood. *Respir. Med.* **2019**, *154*, 56–62. [CrossRef] [PubMed]
8. Martinez, F.; Wright, A.; Taussing, L.; Holberg, C.; Halonen, M.; Morgan, W. Asthma and wheezing in the first six years of life. *N. Engl. J. Med.* **1995**, *332*, 133–138. [CrossRef] [PubMed]
9. Brand, P.L.; Caudri, D.; Eber, E.; Gaillard, E.A.; Garcia-Marcos, L.; Hedlin, G.; Henderson, J.; Kuehni, C.E.; Merkus, P.J.; Pedersen, S.; et al. Classification and pharmacologica teratment of preschool wheezing: Changes since 2008. *Eur. Respir. J.* **2014**, *43*, 1172–1177. [CrossRef]
10. Guilbert, T.W.; Morgan, W.J.; Zeiger, R.S.; Bacharier, L.B.; Boehmer, S.J.; Krawiec, M.; Larsen, G.; Lemanske, R.F.; Liu, A.; Mauger, D.T.; et al. Atopic characteristics of children with recurrent wheezing at high risk for the development of childhood asthma. *J. Allergy Clin. Immunol.* **2004**, *114*, 1282–1287. [CrossRef]
11. Sears, M.R.; Greene, J.M.; Willan, A.R.; Wiecek, E.M.; Taylor, D.R.; Flannery, E.M.; Cowan, J.O.; Herbison, G.P.; Silva, P.A.; Poulton, R. A longitudinal, population-based cohort study of childhood asthma followed to adulthood. *N. Engl. J. Med.* **2003**, *349*, 1414–1422. [CrossRef] [PubMed]
12. Handerson, J.; Granell, R.; Heron, J.; Sherriff, A.; Simpson, A.; Woodcok, A.; Strachan, D.P.; Shaheen, S.O.; Sterne, J.A.C. Associations of wheezing phenotypes in the first 6 years of life with atopy, lung function and airway responsiveness in mid-childhood. *Thorax* **2008**, *63*, 974–980. [CrossRef] [PubMed]
13. Midozi, W.; Rowe, H.; Majaesic, C.; Saunders, L.; Senthilselvan, A. Predictors for wheezing phenotypes in the first decade of life. *Respirology* **2008**, *13*, 537–545. [CrossRef] [PubMed]
14. Saglani, S.; Bush, A. The early-life origins of asthma. *Curr. Opin. Allergy Clin. Immunol.* **2007**, *7*, 83–90. [PubMed]
15. Stein, R.T.; Martinez, F.D. Asthma phenotypes in childhood: Lessons from an epidemiological approach. *Paediatr. Respir Rev.* **2004**, *5*, 155–161. [CrossRef] [PubMed]
16. Lowe, L.A.; Simpson, A.; Woodcock, A.; Morris, J.; Murray, C.S.; Custovic, A. Wheeze phenotypes and lung function in preschool children. *Am. J. Respir. Crit. Care Med.* **2005**, *171*, 231–237. [CrossRef] [PubMed]
17. Caudri, D.; Wijga, A.; Schipper, M.; Hoekstra, M.; Postma, D.S.; Koppelman, G.H.; Brunekreef, B.; Smit, H.A.; de Jongste, J.C. Predicting the long-term prognosis of children with symptoms suggestive of asthma at preschool age. *J. Allergy Clin. Immunol.* **2009**, *124*, 903–910. [CrossRef] [PubMed]
18. Kappelle, L.; Brand, P.L. Severe episodic viral wheeze in preschool children: High risk of asthma at age 5–10 years. *Eur. J. Pediatr.* **2012**, *171*, 947–954. [CrossRef] [PubMed]
19. Savenije, O.E.M.; Kerkhof, M.; Koppelman, G.H.; Postma, D.S. Predicting who will have asthma at school age among preschool children. *J. Allergy Clin. Immunol.* **2012**, *130*, 325–331. [CrossRef]
20. Regamey, N.; Balfour-Lynn, I.; Rosenthal, M.; Hogg, C.; Bush, A.; Davies, J.C. Time required to obtain endobronchial biopsies in children during fiberoptic bronchoscopy. *Pediatr. Pulmonol.* **2009**, *44*, 76–79. [CrossRef]
21. Payne, D.; McKenzie, S.A.; Stacey, S.; Misra, D.; Haxby, E.; Bush, A. Safety and ethics of bronchoscopy and endobronchial biopsy in difficult asthma. *Arch. Dis. Child.* **2001**, *84*, 423–426. [CrossRef] [PubMed]
22. Saetta, M.; Turato, G. Airway patology in asthma. *Eur. Respir. J.* **2001**, *18*, 18s–23s. [CrossRef]
23. Jeffery, P.K. Remodelling in asthma and chronic obstructive lung disease. *Am. J. Respir. Crit. Care Med.* **2001**, *164*, 28–38. [CrossRef] [PubMed]
24. Cutz, E.; Levison, H.; Cooper, D.M. Ultrastructure in airways in children with asthma. *Hystopatology* **1978**, *2*, 407–421. [CrossRef]
25. Cokuğraş, H.; Akçakaya, N.; Seçkin, I.; Camcioğlu, Y.; Sarimurat, N.; Aksoy, F. Ultrastructural examination of bronchial biopsy specimens from children with moderate asthma. *Thorax* **2001**, *56*, 25–29. [CrossRef] [PubMed]
26. Jenkins, H.; Cool, C.; Szefler, C. Histopatology of severe childhood asthma. *Chest* **2003**, *124*, 32–41. [CrossRef] [PubMed]
27. Payne, D.N.; Rogers, A.V.; Ädelroth, E.; Bandi, V.; Guntupalli, K.K.; Bush, A.; Jeffery, P.K. Early thickening of the reticular basement membrane in children with difficult asthma. *Am. J. Respir. Crit. Care Med.* **2003**, *167*, 78–82. [CrossRef] [PubMed]
28. Payne, D.N.; Qiu, Y.; Zhu, J.; Peachey, L.; Scallan, M.; Bush, A.; Jeffery, P.K. Airway inflammation in children with difficult asthma: Relationships with airflow limitation and persistent symptoms. *Thorax* **2004**, *59*, 862–869. [CrossRef]

29. Barbato, A.; Turato, G.; Baraldo, S.; Bazzan, E.; Calabrese, F.; Tura, M.; Zuin, R.; Beghe, B.; Maestrelli, P.; Fabbri, L.M.; et al. Airway inflammation in childhood asthma. *Am. J. Respir. Crit. Care Med.* **2003**, *168*, 798–803. [CrossRef]
30. Barbato, A.; Turato, G.; Baraldo, S.; Bazzan, E.; Calabrese, F.; Panizzolo, C.; Zanin, M.E.; Zuin, R.; Maestrelli, P.; Fabbri, L.M.; et al. Epithelial damage and angiogenesis in the airways of children with asthma. *Am. J. Respir. Crit. Care Med.* **2006**, *174*, 975–981. [CrossRef]
31. Saglani, S.; Payne, D.N.; Zhu, J.; Wang, Z.; Nicholson, A.G.; Bush, A.; Jeffery, P.K. Early detection of airway wall remodeling and eosinophilic inflammation in preschool wheezers. *Am. J. Respir. Crit. Care Med.* **2007**, *176*, 858–864. [CrossRef]
32. Kim, E.S.; Kim, S.H.; Kim, K.W.; Park, J.W.; Kim, Y.S.; Sohn, M.H.; Kim, K.E. Basement membrane thickening and clinical features of children with asthma. *Allergy* **2007**, *62*, 635–640. [CrossRef]
33. Zhou, C.; Yin, G.; Liu, J.; Liu, X.; Zhao, S. Epithelial apoptosis and loss in airways of children with asthma. *J Asthma* **2011**, *48*, 358–365. [CrossRef]
34. Berankova, K.; Uhlik, J.; Honkova, L.; Pohunek, P. Structural changes in the bronchial mucosa of young children at risk of developing asthma. *Pediatr. Allergy Immunol.* **2014**, *25*, 136–142. [CrossRef]
35. Van Mastrigt, E.; Vanlaeken, L.; Heida, F.; Caudri, D.; de Jongste, J.C.; Timens, W.; Rottier, B.L.; Krijger, R.R.; Pijnenburg, M.W. The clinical utility of reticular basement membrane thickness measurements in asthmatic children. *J Asthma* **2015**, *52*, 926–930. [CrossRef]
36. Saglani, S.; Malmström, K.; Pelkonen, A.S.; Malmberg, L.P.; Lindahl, H.; Kajosaari, M.; Turpeinen, M.; Rogers, A.V.; Payne, D.N.; Bush, A.; et al. Airway remodeling and inflammation in symptomatic infants with reversible airflow obstruction. *Am. J. Respir. Crit. Care Med.* **2005**, *171*, 722–727. [CrossRef]
37. Regamey, N.; Ochs, M.; Hilliard, T.N.; Mühlfeld, C.; Cornish, N.; Fleming, L.; Saglani, S.; Alton, E.W.; Bush, A.; Jeffery, P.K.; et al. Increased airway smooth muscle mass in children with asthma, cystic fibrosis, and non-cystic fibrosis bronchiectasis. *Am. J. Respir. Crit. Care Med.* **2008**, *177*, 837–843. [CrossRef]
38. Bossley, C.J.; Fleming, L.; Gupta, A.; Regamey, N.; Frith, J.; Oates, T.; Tsartsali, L.; Lloyd, C.M.; Bush, A.; Saglani, S. Pediatric severe asthma is characterized by eosinophilia and remodeling without T(H)2 cytokines. *J. Allergy Clin. Immunol.* **2012**, *129*, 974–982. [CrossRef]
39. Castro-Rodriguez, J.A.; Saglani, S.; Rodriguez-Martinez, C.E.; Oyarzun, M.A.; Fleming, L.; Bush, A. The relationship between inflammation and remodeling in childhood asthma: A systematic review. *Pediatr. Pulmonol.* **2018**, *53*, 824–835. [CrossRef]
40. Saglani, S.; Lui, S.; Ullmann, N.; Campbell, G.A.; Sherburn, R.T.; Mathie, S.A.; Denney, L.; Bossley, C.J.; Oates, T.; Walker, S.A.; et al. IL-33 promotes airway remodeling in pediatric patients with severe steroid-resistant asthma. *J. Allergy Clin. Immunol.* **2013**, *132*, 676–685. [CrossRef]
41. Holgate, S.T.; Holloway, J.; Wilson, S.; Bucchieri, F.; Puddicombe, S.; Davies, D.E. Epithelial-mesenchymal communication in the pathogenesis of chronic asthma. *Proc. Am. Thorac. Soc.* **2004**, *1*, 93–98. [CrossRef]
42. Holgate, S.T.; Davies, D.E.; Puddicombe, S.; Richter, A.; Lackie, P.; Lordan, J.; Howarth, P. Mechanisms of aiway epithelial damage epithelial-mesenchymal interactions in the pathogenesis of asthma. *Eur. J. Respir.* **2003**, *22*, S24–S29. [CrossRef]
43. Roan, F.; Obata-Ninomiya, K.; Ziegler, S.F. Epithelial cell-derived cytokines: More than just signaling the alarm. *J. Clin. Invest.* **2019**, *129*, 1441–1445. [CrossRef]
44. Wynn, T.A. Type 2 cytokines: Mechanisms and therapeutic strategies. *Nat. Rev. Immunol.* **2015**, *15*, 271–282. [CrossRef]
45. Turato, G.; Barbato, A.; Baraldo, S.; Zanin, M.E.; Bazzan, E.; Lokar-Oliani, K.; Calabrese, F.; Panizzolo, C.; Snijders, D.; Maestrelli, P.; et al. Non atopic children with multitrigger wheezing have airway pathology comparable to atopic asthma. *Am. J. Respir. Crit. Care Med.* **2008**, *178*, 476–482. [CrossRef]
46. Snijders, D.; Agostini, S.; Bertuola, F.; Panizzolo, C.; Baraldo, S.; Turato, G.; Faggian, D.; Plebani, M.; Saetta, M.; Barbato, A. Markers of eosinophilic and neutrophilic inflammation in bronchoalveolar lavage of asthmatic and atopic children. *Allergy* **2010**, *65*, 978–985. [CrossRef]
47. Humbert, M.; Menz, G.; Ying, S.; Corrigan, C.J.; Robinson, D.S.; Durham, S.R.; Kay, A.B. The immunopathology of extrinsic (atopic) and intrinsic (non-atopic) asthma: More similarities than differences. *Immunol. Today* **1999**, *20*, 528–533. [CrossRef]

48. Corne, J.M.; Marshall, C.; Smith, S.; Schreiber, J.; Sanderson, G.; Holgate, S.T.; Johnston, S.L. Frequency, severity, and duration of rhinovirus infections in asthmatic and non-asthmatic individuals: A longitudinal cohort study. *Lancet* **2002**, *359*, 831–834. [CrossRef]
49. Johnston, S.L.; Pattemore, P.K.; Sanderson, G.; Smith, S.; Lampe, F.; Josephs, L.; Symington, P.; O'Toole, S.; Myint, S.H.; Tyrrell, D.A. Community study of role of viral infections in exacerbations of asthma in 9–11 year old children. *BMJ* **1995**, *310*, 1225–1229. [CrossRef]
50. Jackson, D.J.; Gern, J.E.; Lemanske, R.F., Jr. The contributions of allergic sensitization and respiratory pathogens to asthma inception. *J. Allergy Clin. Immunol.* **2016**, *137*, 659–665. [CrossRef]
51. Sigurs, N.; Bjarnason, R.; Sigurbergsson, F.; Kjellman, B. Respiratory syncytial virus bronchiolitis in infancy is an important risk factor for asthma and allergy at age 7. *Am. J. Respir. Crit. Care Med.* **2000**, *161*, 1501–1507. [CrossRef]
52. Lemanske, R.F.; Jackson, D.J.; Gangnon, R.E.; Evans, M.D.; Li, Z.H.; Shult, P.A.; Kirk, C.J.; Reisdorf, E.; Roberg, K.A.; Anderson, E.; et al. Rhinovirus illnesses during infancy predict subsequent childhood wheezing. *J. Allergy Clin. Immunol.* **2005**, *116*, 571–577. [CrossRef]
53. Kusel, M.M.; de Klerk, N.H.; Kebadze, T.; Vohma, V.; Holt, P.G.; Johnston, S.L.; Sly, P.D. Early-life respiratory viral infections, atopic sensitization, and risk of subsequent development of persistent asthma. *J. Allergy Clin. Immunol.* **2007**, *119*, 1105–1110. [CrossRef]
54. Jackson, D.J.; Gangnon, R.E.; Evans, M.D.; Roberg, K.A.; Anderson, E.L.; Pappas, T.E.; Printz, M.C.; Lee, W.M.; Shult, P.A.; Reisdorf, E.; et al. Wheezing rhinovirus illnesses in early life predict asthma development in high-risk children. *Am. J. Respir. Crit. Care Med.* **2008**, *178*, 667–672. [CrossRef]
55. Rubner, F.J.; Jackson, D.J.; Evans, M.D.; Gangnon, R.E.; Tisler, C.J.; Pappas, T.E.; Gern, J.E.; Lemanske, R.F., Jr. Early life rhinovirus wheezing, allergic sensitization, and asthma risk at adolescence. *J. Allergy Clin. Immunol.* **2017**, *139*, 501–507. [CrossRef]
56. Martinez, F.D. Respiratory syncytial virus bronchiolitis and the pathogenesis of childhood asthma. *Pediatr. Infect Dis. J.* **2003**, *22*, S76–S82. [CrossRef]
57. Papadopoulos, N.; Stanciu, L.; Papi, A.; Holgate, S.; Johnston, S. A defective type 1 response to rhinovirus in atopic asthma. *Thorax* **2002**, *57*, 328–332. [CrossRef]
58. Contoli, M.; Message, S.D.; Laza-Stanca, V.; Edwards, M.R.; Wark, P.A.; Bartlett, N.W.; Kebadze, T.; Mallia, P.; Stanciu, L.A.; Parker, H.L. Role of deficient type III interferon-lambda production in asthma exacerbations. *Nat. Med.* **2006**, *12*, 1023–1026. [CrossRef]
59. Baraldo, S.; Contoli, M.; Bazzan, E.; Turato, G.; Padovani, A.; Marku, B.; Calabrese, F.; Caramori, G.; Ballarin, A.; Snijders, D.; et al. Deficient antiviral immune responses in childhood: Distinct roles of atopy and asthma. *J. Allergy Clin. Immunol.* **2012**, *130*, 1307–1314. [CrossRef]
60. Baraldo, S.; Contoli, M.; Bonato, M.; Snijders, D.; Biondini, D.; Bazzan, E.; Cosio, M.G.; Barbato, A.; Papi, A.; Saetta, M. Deficient immune response to viral infections in children predicts later asthma persistence. *Am. J. Respir. Crit. Care Med.* **2018**, *197*, 673–675. [CrossRef]
61. Stern, D.A.; Guerra, S.; Halonen, M.; Wright, A.L.; Martinez, F.D. Low IFN-gamma production in the first year of life as a predictor of wheeze during childhood. *J. Allergy Clin. Immunol.* **2007**, *120*, 835–841. [CrossRef]
62. Madura-Larsen, J.; Brix, S.; Thysen, A.H.; Birch, S.; Rasmussen, M.A.; Bisgaard, H. Children with asthma by school age display aberrant immune responses to pathogenic airway bacteria as infants. *J. Allergy Clin. Immunol.* **2014**, *133*, 1008–1013. [CrossRef]
63. Strachan, D.P.; Butland, B.K.; Anderson, H.R. Incidence and prognosis of asthma and wheezing illness from early childhood to age 33 in a national British cohort. *BMJ* **1996**, *312*, 1195–1199. [CrossRef]
64. Malmström, K.; Pelkonen, A.S.; Mäkelä, M.J. Remodeling, inflammation and airway responsiveness in early childhood asthma. *Curr. Opin. Allergy Clin. Immunol.* **2013**, *13*, 203–210. [CrossRef]
65. Moffatt, M.F.; Gut, I.G.; Demenais, F.; Strachan, D.P.; Bouzigon, E.; Heath, S.; von Mutius, E.; Farrall, M.; Lathrop, M.; Cookson, W.O.C.M.; et al. A large-scale, consortium-based genomewide association study of asthma. *N. Engl. J. Med.* **2010**, *363*, 1211–1221. [CrossRef]
66. Wang, A.L.; Datta, S.P.; Weiss, S.T.; Tantisira, K.G. Remission of persistent childhood asthma: Early predictors of adult outcomes. *J. Allergy Clin. Immunol.* **2019**, *143*, 1752–1759. [CrossRef]
67. Malmström, K.; Pelkonen, A.S.; Malmberg, L.P.; Sarna, S.; Lindahl, H.; Kajosaari, M.; Turpeinen, M.; Saglani, S.; Bush, A.; Haahtela, T.; et al. Lung function, airway remodelling and inflammation in symptomatic infants: Outcome at 3 years. *Thorax* **2011**, *66*, 157–162. [CrossRef]

68. Malmström, K.; Malmberg, L.P.; O'Reilly, R.; Lindahl, H.; Kajosaari, M.; Saarinen, K.M.; Saglani, S.; Jahnsen, F.L.; Bush, A.; Haahtela, T.; et al. Lung function, airway remodeling, and inflammation in infants: Outcome at 8 years. *Ann. Allergy Asthma Immunol.* **2015**, *114*, 90–96. [CrossRef]
69. O'Reilly, R.; Ullmann, N.; Irving, S.; Bossley, C.; Sonnappa, S.; Zhe, J.; Oates, T.; Banya, W.; Heffery, P.; Bush, A.; et al. Increased airway smooth muscle in preschool wheezers who have asthma at school age. *J. Allergy Clin. Immunol.* **2013**, *131*, 1024–1032. [CrossRef]
70. Bonato, M.; Bazzan, E.; Snijders, D.; Tiné, M.E.; Biondini, D.; Turato, G.; Balestro, E.; Papi, A.; Cosio, M.G.; Barbato, A.; et al. Clinical and pathologic factors predicting future asthma in wheezing children. *Am. J. Respir. Cell Mol. Biol.* **2018**, *59*, 458–466. [CrossRef]
71. Marshall, L.; Beardsmore, C.S.; Pescatore, A.M.; Kuehni, C.E.; Gaillard, E.A. Airway eosinophils in older teenagers with outgrown preschool wheeze: A pilot study. *Eur. Respir. J.* **2015**, *46*, 1486–1489. [CrossRef]
72. Van den Toorn, L.M.; Overbeek, S.E.; de Jongste, J.C.; Leman, K.; Hoogsteden, H.C.; Prins, J.B. Airway inflammation is present during clinical remission of atopic asthma. *Am. J. Respir. Crit. Care Med.* **2001**, *164*, 2107–2113. [CrossRef]
73. Broekema, M.; Timens, W.; Vonk, J.M.; Volbeda, F.; Lodewijk, M.E.; Hylkema, M.N.; Ten Hacken, N.H.; Postma, D.S. Persisting remodeling and less airway wall eosinophil activation in complete remission of asthma. *Am. J. Respir. Crit. Care Med.* **2011**, *183*, 310–316. [CrossRef]
74. Vonk, J.M.; Postma, D.S.; Boezen, H.M.; Grol, M.H.; Schouten, J.P.; Koëter, G.H.; Gerritsen, J. Childhood factors associated with asthma remission after 30 year follow up. *Thorax* **2004**, *59*, 925–929. [CrossRef]

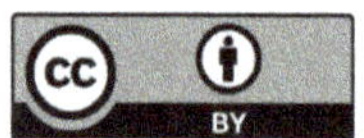

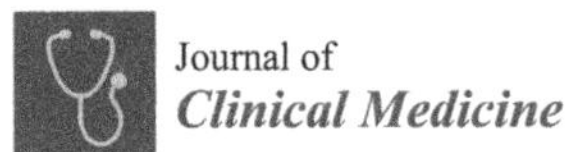

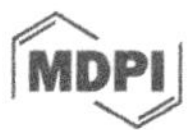

Article

Evolution of Airway Inflammation in Preschoolers with Asthma—Results of a Two-Year Longitudinal Study

Paraskevi Xepapadaki [1,*,†], Paraskevi Korovessi [1,†], Claus Bachert [2], Susetta Finotto [3], Tuomas Jartti [4], John Lakoumentas [1], Marek L. Kowalski [5], Anna Lewandowska-Polak [6], Heikki Lukkarinen [4], Nan Zhang [2], Theodor Zimmermann [7] and Nikolaos G. Papadopoulos [1,8]

1 Allergy Department, 2nd Pediatric Clinic, National and Kapodistrian University of Athens, 11527 Athens, Greece; vkorovessi@gmail.com (P.K.); john.lakoo@gmail.com (J.L.); ngpallergy@gmail.com (N.G.P.)
2 Upper Airways Research Laboratory, Ghent University Hospital, 9000 Ghent, Belgium; Claus.Bachert@ugent.be (C.B.); Nan.Zhang@UGent.be (N.Z.)
3 Department of Molecular Pneumology, Friedrich-Alexander-Universität Erlangen-Nürnberg, Universitätsklinikum Erlangen, 91054 Erlangen, Germany; Susetta.Neurath-Finotto@uk-erlangen.de
4 Department of Paediatrics and Adolescent Medicine, Turku University Hospital and University of Turku, 20520 Turku, Finland; hepelu@utu.fi (H.L.); tuomas.jartti@utu.fi (T.J.)
5 Department of Immunology, Rheumatology and Allergy, Medical University of Lodz, 92213 Lodz, Poland; marek.kowalski@umed.lodz.pl
6 Department of Rheumatology, Medical University of Lodz, 92213 Lodz, Poland; anna.lewandowska-polak@umed.lodz.pl
7 Department of Pediatrics and Adolescent Medicine, Dept of Allergy and Pneumology, Children's Hospital, Friedrich-Alexander-Universität Erlangen-Nürnberg, Universitätsklinikum Erlangen, 91054 Erlangen, Germany; Theodor.Zimmermann@uk-erlangen.de
8 Division of Infection, Immunity & Respiratory Medicine, University of Manchester, Manchester M13 9PL, UK
* Correspondence: vickyxepapadaki@gmail.com; Tel.: +30 213 200 9160; Fax: +30 213 777 6964
† Equally contributing authors.

Received: 26 November 2019; Accepted: 6 January 2020; Published: 9 January 2020

Abstract: Fractional exhaled nitric oxide (FeNO) is a non-invasive marker for eosinophilic airway inflammation and has been used for monitoring asthma. Here, we assess the characteristics of FeNO from preschool to school age, in parallel with asthma activity. A total of 167 asthmatic children and 66 healthy, age-matched controls were included in the 2-year prospective PreDicta study evaluating wheeze/asthma persistence in preschool-aged children. Information on asthma/rhinitis activity, infections and atopy was recorded at baseline. Follow-up visits were performed at 6-month intervals, as well as upon exacerbation/cold and 4–6 weeks later in the asthmatic group. We obtained 539 FeNO measurements from asthmatics and 42 from controls. At baseline, FeNO values did not differ between the two groups (median: 3.0 ppb vs. 2.0 ppb, respectively). FeNO values at 6, 12, 18 and 24 months (4.0, CI: 0.0–8.6; 6.0, CI: 2.8–12.0; 8.0, CI: 4.0–14.0; 8.5, CI: 4.4–14.5 ppb, respectively) increased with age (correlation $p \leq 0.001$) and atopy ($p = 0.03$). FeNO was non-significantly increased from baseline to the symptomatic visit, while it decreased after convalescence ($p = 0.007$). Markers of disease activity, such as wheezing episodes and days with asthma were associated with increased FeNO values during the study ($p < 0.05$ for all). Age, atopy and disease activity were found to be important FeNO determinants in preschool children. Longitudinal and individualized FeNO assessment may be valuable in monitoring asthmatic children with recurrent wheezing or mild asthma.

Keywords: asthma; PreDicta; preschool; FeNO; spirometry

---

1. Introduction

The use of objective measurements, including the measurement of lung function and airway inflammation by means of fractional exhaled nitric oxide (FeNO) is currently becoming reinforced in most official recommendations for children with asthma, even though there are not always clear correlations between the two. Moreover, associations between disease activity and airway inflammation are frequently inconclusive or negative, probably because they have mostly been assessed cross-sectionally or for limited time periods [1,2].

As defined by the Global Initiative for Asthma (GINA), FeNO measurements are associated with clinical asthma control indices in school-aged children and adults [3]. However, the preschool-age group is of particular interest because preschool age is often a milestone whereby wheezing disease is expected to transform by either resolving or becoming persistent in a significant number of patients. Few studies, however, have evaluated how inflammation progresses or correlates with symptoms in asthmatic preschoolers [4–6]. A limited number of cross-sectional studies have shown that preschool children with increased wheezing morbidity, as assessed by symptom frequency and persistence, present higher levels of FeNO, which suggests that FeNO levels might correlate with current and/or subsequent asthma diagnosis [7,8]. Moreover, fluctuations in airway inflammation have not been extensively studied in young children with asthma-associated symptoms, either due to difficulties in obtaining acceptable and repeatable maneuvers or to the potential impact of viral respiratory infections, use of inhaled corticosteroids and atopy per se [9].

In order to understand wheeze/asthma in preschoolers and how it relates to asthma later in life, we need to understand the main characteristics of obstructive airway disease over time, particularly bronchoconstriction, inflammation and hyper-responsiveness. The PreDicta pediatric longitudinal cohort, within "PreDicta", a European Commission-funded project under the 7th Framework Program for Research and Technological Development (FP7), was designed as a 2-year prospective study with the aim of evaluating wheeze/asthma persistence in preschool- to school-age children [10]. Herein, we evaluate the evolution of airway inflammation from preschool to school age, in parallel with disease activity.

2. Methods

2.1. Study Population

The PreDicta cohort study was conducted across five major cultural and climatic regions of Europe: Greece, Germany, Belgium, Poland and Finland. Children 4–6 years of age with an asthma diagnosis of mild to moderate severity according to GINA [11] confirmed by a doctor from one of the participating study centers within the last 2 years were invited to participate as cases. Moreover, healthy, age-matched children with no reported history of wheeze/asthma served as cross-sectional controls at the beginning of the 2-year follow-up period. The eligibility and exclusion criteria, study design and baseline characteristics of the cohort have been described previously [10]. The study was approved by all participants' institutional ethics committees and written informed consent was obtained from parents.

2.2. Study Design

At baseline, children were required to be asymptomatic, without a cold or an exacerbation for at least 4 weeks. A questionnaire including detailed information on asthma and rhinitis activity and severity and infection history was filled in by all participants, while the presence of atopy was assessed by skin prick tests (SPTs) to common aeroallergens [10].

Follow-up visits were performed at 6-month intervals for two years in the asthmatic group. At regular follow-up visits, a questionnaire with information regarding asthma and rhinitis activity and infections during the previous period was obtained. Moreover, children were assessed in the clinic during symptomatic periods on the basis of their daily symptom score or their parent's perception and were reassessed 4–6 weeks later at convalescence, through a questionnaire and clinical examination. At all of the time points, airway inflammation was determined with FeNO measurements in parts per billion (ppb), using the Bedfont NObreath equipment (Bedfont Ltd., UK) [12]. Data were available from the four follow-up visits for 146, 125, 121 and 140 subjects, respectively. Measurements were also performed during 75 symptomatic visits and 56 of the respective convalescent visits.

2.3. FeNO Measurements

FeNO values were measured at visits using the Bedfont NObreath equipment (Bedfont Ltd., Maidstone, UK), in parts per billion (ppb). According to the 2005 American Thoracic and European Respiratory Society's guidelines [12] and the Bedfont NObreath specifications, for a correct FeNO measurement, a single breath sample was instantly analyzed after the subject inhaled to total lung capacity through a NO-scrubbing filter to avoid contamination with ambient NO. All exhalations were performed with an exhalation pressure of 10 to 20 cm H_2O to maintain a fixed flow rate of 50 ± 5 mL/s (<6 attempts per visit). The pressure is necessary to ensure closure of the soft palate, to avoid contamination of the FeNO with gas from the nasopharynx where NO concentrations are very high. In addition, the targeted constant-flow exhalation rate consists of a washout phase followed by a 2-s NO plateau. It is generally considered that this plateau represents NO derived primarily from the lower respiratory tract. A ball moving within frames was used to help young children blow at the right pressure during the exhalation. Whenever possible, the two most consistent attempts (i.e., lasting 6–10 s and/or agree within 10%) were recorded. Children had not eaten or drunk anything for at least 2 h before and avoided nitrate-rich meals for at least 20 h before the measurements. Directions were given according to these dietary recommendations for regular visits. Exacerbation visits were arranged according to the last meal or snack. FeNO analysis was performed before spirometry because spirometric maneuvers have been shown to transiently reduce airway inflammation measurements.

The following algorithm was used in order to calculate FeNO values at different time points: (a) if at least one value was 0 or 1 ppb, the maximum value was recorded; (b) if both values were greater than 1, then ($b._1$) if the absolute difference was ≤10 ppb, we calculated the average value, or ($b._2$) in case the absolute difference was >10 ppb, the maximum value was recorded. Personal best FeNO was defined as the minimum value recorded in all visits, baseline and follow-up for all cases.

2.4. Predictors of FeNO Measurements

Disease activity markers were derived from the questionnaires obtained at baseline and during symptomatic/convalescent periods. These were selected from the following guidelines (a) the GINA guidelines for determining asthma control and severity level, on the basis of criteria such as frequency of day and night asthma symptoms, night-time awakenings due to asthma, limitation of activities, need for reliever and controller medication and hospitalizations for asthma; (b) the PRACTALL consensus for asthma phenotyping [13]; and (c) the Allergic Rhinitis and its Impact on Asthma (ARIA) initiative for assessing the frequency and severity of rhinitis symptoms [14]. Moreover, history of infections including the frequency and duration of upper and lower respiratory infections, the use of antibiotics and family history of atopy-associated diseases were included as predictors. Symptoms recorded in diary cards during symptomatic and convalescent visits were used for comparisons. All the predictors that were assessed are depicted in the Supplementary Materials, Table S1.

2.5. Statistical Analysis

All variables assessed were non-parametric, according to the Shapiro-Wilk test for composite normality; thus, descriptive statistics are presented as medians (25–75 percentiles—IQRs). In order to identify dependencies between FeNO and other variables, non-parametric tests were applied: the Wilcoxon rank-sum test was used for qualitative variables and Kendall's correlation was used for quantitative variables (such as the subjects' age).

The Friedman test was used in order to compare values at three consecutive visits (baseline or follow-up, symptomatic and convalescent) for each patient. Post-hoc analysis was carried out using the Wilcoxon paired signed-rank test, along with the Bonferroni correction.

All tests were considered two-sided and statistical significance was defined as $p < 0.05$. Statistical analysis was performed with the R software for statistical computing, along with the RStudio interface (both open-source products).

3. Results

A total of 167 cases (102 males, 61%, mean age: 5.2 ± 0.7) and 66 controls (30 males, 45%, mean age: 5.1 ± 0.8) were recruited from the five participating centers. The demographic characteristics of the two groups at inclusion have been reported elsewhere [10]. FeNO measurements were available for 131 (79.6%) asthmatic children (median: 3.0, CI: 0.0–6.7 ppb) and 35 (53%) healthy controls (median: 2.0, CI: 0.0–7.2 ppb, $p = 0.37$).

Baseline characteristics regarding disease activity and atopic history of the asthmatic children are depicted in Table 1.

Table 1. Baseline characteristics regarding disease activity and atopic history of the asthmatic children.

Atopic History Disease Activity	Baseline Characteristics	*n*
Atopic history	Family history of atopic disease (yes), *n* (%)	94 (91)
	Family history of asthma/rhinitis (yes), *n* (%)	89 (86)
	Any positive skin prick test (yes), *n* (%)	70 (56)
Upper Respiratory Symptoms	Rhinitis symptoms are present	
	<4 days/week, *n* (%)	61 (47)
	Rhinitis duration	
	<4 consecutive weeks, *n* (%)	67 (51)
	Are rhinitis symptoms associated with … ?	
	Sleep disturbance (yes), *n* (%)	65 (89)
	School impairment (yes), *n* (%)	17 (24)
	Leisure—sport (yes), *n* (%)	35 (49)
	Visual analogue scale, median (CIs)	5 (3–6)
	Number of medication courses for rhinitis in the last 12 months, median (CIs)	1 (0–5)
Lower Respiratory Symptoms	Days with symptoms in the last 3 months	
	<1/week, *n* (%)	83 (64)
	>1/week but <1/day, *n* (%)	37 (28)
	daily, *n* (%)	11 (8)
	Nights with symptoms in the last 3 months	
	≤2 times/month, *n* (%)	81 (62)
	>2 times/month, *n* (%)	15 (12)
	>1/week, *n* (%)	24 (18)
	daily, *n* (%)	11 (8)
	Cough, wheeze or difficulty in breathing during or after exercise in the last 12 months (yes), *n* (%)	84 (64)
	Limitation of activities limited by asthma symptoms (yes), *n* (%)	46 (35)
	Child completely well between symptomatic periods (yes), *n* (%)	92 (70)
	Number of episodes of wheezing/asthma/cough in the last 3 months, median (25–75 percentiles)	1 (1–2)
	Number of episodes of wheezing/asthma/cough in the last 12 months, median (CIs)	5 (3–8)
	Inhaled corticosteroids as prophylactic treatment (yes), *n* (%)	107 (82%)

Atopic asthmatics presented increased FeNO levels compared to non-atopic asthmatics, however, the results were not statistically significant either when assessed in terms of the occurrence of any positive SPT (median: 3.0, CI: 0.0–6.9 vs. 2.0, CI: 0.0–5.2, respectively, $p = 0.47$) or by quantifying, i.e., by summation of positive SPTs (descriptive: 4.8, $p = 0.48$). Reported personal and family history of atopy-related diseases was not associated with increased FeNO levels at baseline.

3.1. FeNO Evolution during the Two-Year Follow-Up

During the visits we obtained a total of 42 FeNO measurements from controls (35 at baseline) and 539 from cases. FeNO was measured in 67.8% of children at 6 months of follow-up (median: 4, CI: 0.0–8.6 ppb), 74.4% at 12 months (median: 6.0, CI: 2.8–12.0 ppb), 83.5% at month 18 (median: 8.0, CI: 4.0–14.0 ppb) and 72.1% at the final visit (median: 8.5, CI: 4.4–14.5 ppb), suggesting an increasing trend with time/age in asthmatics.

Kendall's correlation reveals a correlation of 16.4% between FeNO value and age in controls ($p = 0.14$) and a correlation of 19.3% ($p < 0.001$) in children with asthma (Figure 1a). Post-hoc power analysis yielded powers of 18% and 99%, respectively, for the above outcomes at the significance level of 0.05; however, the slopes of the corresponding linear fits do not differ significantly between cases and controls ($p = 0.8$). With regards to atopy, children with at least one positive SPT presented a significantly increased FeNO trajectory compared to non-atopics ($p = 0.03$, Figure 1b).

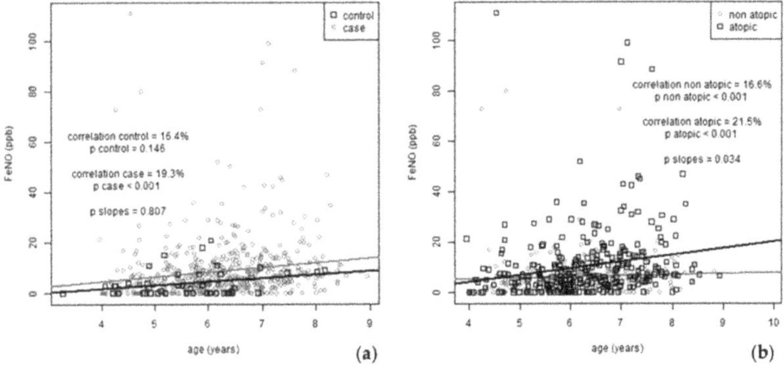

Figure 1. (**a**) Non-parametric correlation between subjects' fractional exhaled nitric oxide (FeNO) and age, separately assessed in controls and cases. "P slopes" denote the p-value of the comparison between the slopes of the two separate trend lines, i.e., controls (black line) vs. cases (gray line). (**b**) FeNO progression slopes in preschool asthmatics for atopics (black line) and non-atopics (gray line), at baseline and during the 2-year follow-up.

At all time points, no differences were noted in FeNO values in respect to sex when assessed cross-sectionally in asthmatics.

3.2. FeNO and Seasonality

The FeNO values, either as absolute or % change from baseline values, were independent of the season when they were assessed, at all visits; nevertheless, the number of symptomatic visits (either due to a cold or an exacerbation) significantly increased during "cold months" (autumn = 26, winter = 27, spring = 16, summer = 8).

3.3. Variation in FeNO Values from Healthy State (Asymptomatic) to Exacerbation and Convalescent Visit

In order to evaluate the variation in FeNO levels in asthmatic children during periods of different health status, a comparison was performed at three distinct time points: (a) either at baseline or during the last follow-up visit before a symptomatic visit, when the child was still asymptomatic; (b) at the subsequent symptomatic visit; and (c) at the respective convalescent visit. Forty-nine children (65.3%) were able to perform FeNO measurements upon exacerbation and forty-two (75%) at convalescence. In total, 28 measurements were available for comparison for all three time points. A post-hoc power analysis yielded a power of 66% for the following outcomes at the significance level of 0.05. There was an increase in absolute FeNO values from the baseline to the symptomatic visit, although there was no significant difference (baseline median: 3.5, CI: 0.7–9.1 ppb vs. symptomatic median: 4.5, CI: 1.7–13.2, respectively, $p = 0.32$).A significant drop was observed between the symptomatic and the convalescent visit (median: 2.0, CI: 0.0–5.0, $p = 0.007$), (Figure 2A). The % FeNO differences were also significant from symptomatic and convalescent visits (symptomatic visits: median 100, CI: −38.6–504.1, convalescent: median 0.0, CI: −62.8–87.5, $p = 0.005$) (Figure 2B). The differences from symptomatic to convalescent visits in absolute ($p = 0.007$) and % FeNO values ($p = 0.005$) are depicted in Figure 3A,B. The effect of inhaled corticosteroids (ICS) could not be assessed since most asthmatic children were on prophylactic treatment at all three time points (baseline: 80.7, symptomatic: 76.7, convalescent: 81.6).

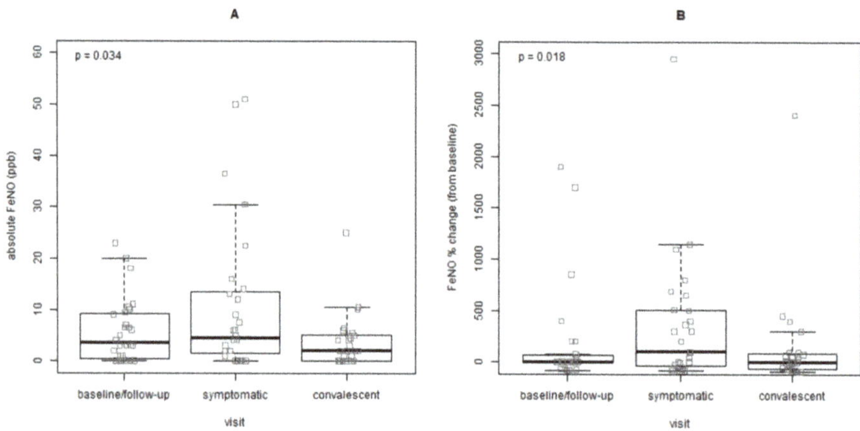

Figure 2. Variations in FeNO measurements from healthy state (baseline/follow-up) to the subsequent exacerbation and convalescence periods in preschool-aged children with recurrent wheeze/asthma. (**A**) Comparison of absolute FeNO values, (**B**) Comparison of FeNO % change.

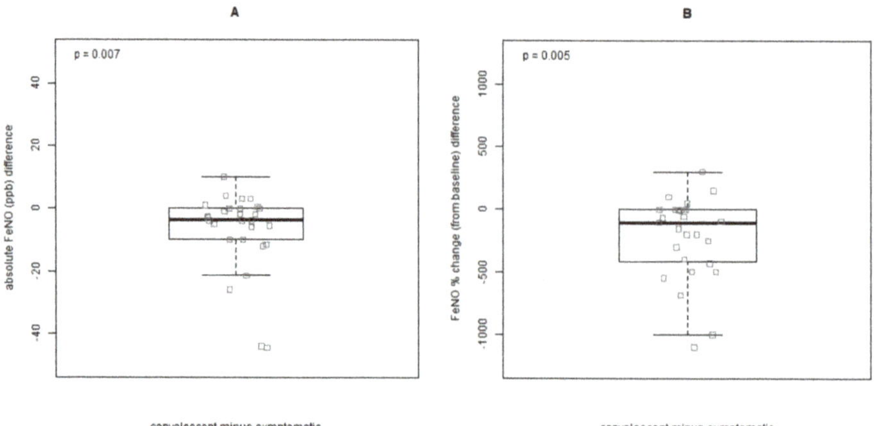

Figure 3. Difference in FeNO values of preschoolers with asthma during exacerbations and at their respective convalescent visits (**A**) in absolute values, (**B**) in FeNO % change (from baseline).

3.4. Predictors of FeNO Measurements at Baseline and during the Two-Year Follow-Up

Predictors derived from the questionnaires obtained at all-time points were assessed in respect to FeNO values (Supplementary Materials, Table S1). FeNO measurements at baseline were significantly correlated with the number of reported asthma episodes in the preceding 12 months (correlation coefficient: 13.7, $p = 0.03$), while wheezing episodes and the number of days with asthma symptoms were positively associated with increased FeNO values at the end of the 2-year follow-up (median: 19.5, IQR: 15.75–46.25 and correlation coefficient: 16.1, $p = 0.04$, respectively).

4. Discussion

In our cohort, FeNO levels did not differ significantly between "asthmatic"/recurrent wheezers when asymptomatic (at baseline) and healthy preschool children. A gradual and significant increase in airway inflammation was noted in asthmatics in respect to time/age when prospectively assessed; however, slopes between asthmatics and controls did not differ. In the presence of atopy, as assessed by SPTs, asthmatics presented significant increases in airway inflammation during the study. Moreover, FeNO values were significantly associated with markers of asthma activity such as the number of days with asthma symptoms reported in the preceding 12 months and the number of asthma exacerbations during the 2-year follow-up period.

FeNO levels, in both asthmatic and healthy children, were within normal limits, as indicated by international guidelines [12] and in line with previous studies, suggesting that FeNO values in preschoolers are less than 10 ppb [15]. Increased FeNO values have been reported previously in preschoolers with recurrent or persistent asthma-associated symptoms compared to healthy controls [16]; however, this was not the case in our cohort, which is probably due to mild to moderate disease severity [10] or to the fact that measurements were performed during asymptomatic periods at baseline. The lack of difference between the groups with regard to the increase in the FeNO slopes in the 2-year follow-up might suggest that, potentially, FeNO increases are age-dependent, as noted in previous studies [15], and independent of disease activity in this age group, although the impact of small size on controls cannot be excluded. Nevertheless, atopy per se was a significant risk factor for the increased FeNO trajectory in asthmatics, which is in line with reports supporting a strong association between FeNO and allergic sensitization [17].

During episodic periods, FeNO levels significantly increased, while 4–6 weeks later, the values recorded were even lower than their respective "baseline" ones. High levels of FeNO are typically considered a marker of airway eosinophilic inflammation and are associated with deterioration in asthma control [18]. FeNO levels increase during virus-induced asthma exacerbations, which are mainly attributed to rhinoviruses, and reflect epithelial host-defense responses [19]. In our cohort, viral respiratory infections, mostly by rhinoviruses, were the most commonly identified triggers for asthma worsening (manuscript in preparation). It is plausible that the intermittent inflammatory airway response that follows an episode accounts for the brief increase in FeNO levels. It is well-established that FeNO levels are affected by the intake of corticosteroids, either oral or inhaled, to the extent that the use of FeNO has been proposed as a marker for glucocorticoid response, or alternatively for adjusting ICS dosing. The vast majority of asthmatic preschoolers in our cohort (95%) were on prophylactic treatment at baseline, as described elsewhere [10]; thus, this may account for the low FeNO values noted at inclusion. Moreover, treatment with increased doses of inhaled corticosteroids, which is frequently recommended as an add-on therapy to b2-agonists during exacerbations [20], may explain the lower FeNO levels noted at convalescence [21]. This further suggests that treatment may improve airway inflammation, even if children appear asymptomatic.

We recorded FeNO values in 75.5% of all scheduled visits on average, and in 65% of visits during episodes in asthmatics, indicating that FeNO determination is feasible in most, but not all preschoolers, following proper training. Reliable FeNO measurements can be obtained in a standardized way from the age of 4 years. Reports have shown that the NObreath equipment provides results that are comparable with other techniques [22]. In addition, FeNO measurements were performed during morning hours, thus excluding the possibility of bias due to circadian fluctuations [23].

Our data support the monitoring of asthma with objective measurements, even in preschoolers. FeNO personalized monitoring (±bronchodilator reversibility) was reported to be dominate over other diagnostic tests, while an economic analysis indicated that FeNO monitoring could have value as such a strategy [24]; thus, most recent guidelines suggest the incorporation of FeNO into the asthma management algorithm [25]. Recently, an increasing number of reports have emerged that utilize the measurement of FeNO at multiple expiratory flows and mathematical modeling of pulmonary NO dynamics in order to estimate different components of FeNO, i.e., alveolar or acinar; nevertheless, only a few publications have reported values in children with asthma and no data are available for preschoolers. [26–28]. Future research is needed in order to establish the usefulness of the aforementioned FeNO technique in clinical practice, especially in the pediatric population.

All in all, we were able to demonstrate significant fluctuations in airway inflammation, depending on the activity and severity of the disease, which indicates that an individualized approach, i.e., using the personal best as a reference value, may be preferable for this age group. Nevertheless, the age- and atopy-dependent increase needs to be taken into account, suggesting that regular baseline measurement may be necessary. FeNO changes, at least in preschoolers, should be longitudinally and individually assessed, in order to efficiently aid disease management.

The major strength of our study is its multinational character and longitudinal design. Diagnosis and disease assessment were made by specialists, while airway inflammation and atopy were quantified via objective standardized measures. We have previously shown that our cohort is powered to prospectively evaluate the role of infection on asthma persistence and it is representative of preschool asthma, with well-balanced demographic and atopy-related characteristics [10]. Children were assessed for an extended time period at regular follow-up visits and during symptomatic and convalescence periods. We obtained a significant number of FeNO measurements at baseline and regular follow-up visits (561) in the cohort. Although the available number of measurements for comparison during symptomatic periods and convalescence was small, the statistical power obtained was moderate, due to the moderate effect size (significant differences in the compared distributions' median values) that was present.

However, a weakness of this study is that several parameters, including asthma activity, severity and medication use were assessed based on parental reports, which are subject to recall bias, although previous studies have proven that short-term parental reports can be accurate.

5. Conclusions

This study clearly shows that indices of asthma and rhinitis activity and the presence of atopy in preschool-aged children with asthma are significantly correlated with airway inflammation as assessed by longitudinal follow-up. Airway inflammation increases during acute events, then values return to better than the "personal normal" values 4–6 weeks later, suggesting a treatment effect. Thus, longitudinal assessment of FeNO measurements can be valuable for monitoring preschool children with recurrent wheeze/asthma. However, estimations can only be based on personalized, rather than reference values.

Supplementary Materials: The following are available online at http://www.mdpi.com/2077-0383/9/1/187/s1, Table S1: Disease activity predictors during baseline and 2-year follow-up.

Author Contributions: Conceptualization: N.G.P.; Data curation: J.L.; Formal analysis: J.L.; Investigation: C.B., S.F., T.J., M.L.K., A.L.-P., H.L., N.Z. and T.Z.; Resources: C.B., S.F., T.J., M.L.K., A.L.-P., H.L., N.Z., and T.Z.; Writing—original draft: P.K.; Writing—review & editing: P.X. and N.G.P. All authors have read and agreed to the published version of the manuscript.

Funding: This work was supported by the European Commission's Seventh Framework program under grant agreement N° 260895 (PREDICTA).

Conflicts of Interest: The authors declare no conflict of interest.

References

1. Debley, J.S.; Stamey, D.C.; Cochrane, E.S.; Gama, K.L.; Redding, G.J. Exhaled nitric oxide, lung function, and exacerbations in wheezy infants and toddlers. *J. Allergy Clin. Immunol.* **2010**, *125*, 1228–1234. [CrossRef] [PubMed]
2. Konstantinou, G.N.; Xepapadaki, P.; Manousakis, E.; Makrinioti, H.; Kouloufakou-Gratsia, K.; Saxoni-Papageorgiou, P.; Papadopoulos, N.G. Assessment of airflow limitation, airway inflammation, and symptoms during virus-induced wheezing episodes in 4 to 6-year-old children. *J. Allergy Clin. Immunol.* **2013**, *131*, 87–93. [CrossRef] [PubMed]
3. Moeller, A.; Carlsen, K.H.; Sly, P.D.; Baraldi, E.; Piacentini, G.; Pavord, I.; Lex, C.; Saglani, S. Monitoring asthma in childhood: Lung function, bronchial responsiveness and inflammation. *Eur. Respir. Rev.* **2015**, *24*, 204–215. [CrossRef] [PubMed]
4. Lee, J.W.; Shim, J.Y.; Kwon, J.W.; Kim, H.Y.; Seo, J.H.; Kim, B.J.; Kim, H.B.; Lee, S.Y.; Jang, G.C.; Song, D.J.; et al. Exhaled nitric oxide as a better diagnostic indicator for evaluating wheeze and airway hyperresponsiveness in preschool children. *J. Asthma* **2015**, *52*, 1054–1059. [CrossRef] [PubMed]
5. Soh, J.E.; Kim, K.M.; Kwon, J.W.; Kim, H.Y.; Seo, J.H.; Kim, H.B.; Lee, S.Y.; Jang, G.C.; Song, D.J.; Kim, W.K.; et al. Recurrent wheeze and its relationship with lung function and airway inflammation in preschool children: A cross-sectional study in South Korea. *BMJ Open* **2017**, *7*, e018010. [CrossRef] [PubMed]
6. De Abreu, F.C.; da Silva Júnior, J.L.R.; Rabahi, M.F. The Fraction Exhaled Nitric Oxide as a Biomarker of Asthma Control. *Biomark. Insights* **2019**, *14*, 1177271919826550. [CrossRef] [PubMed]
7. Castro-Rodriguez, J.A.; Sardón, O.; Pérez-Yarza, E.G.; Korta, J.; Aldasoro, A.; Corcuera, P.; Mintegui, J. Young infants with recurrent wheezing and positive asthma predictive index have higher levels of exhaled nitric oxide. *J. Asthma* **2013**, *50*, 162–165. [CrossRef]
8. Vilmann, L.; Buchvald, F.; Green, K.; Nielsen, K.G. Fractional exhaled nitric oxide and multiple breath nitrogen washout in preschool healthy and asthmatic children. *Respir. Med.* **2017**, *133*, 42–47. [CrossRef] [PubMed]
9. Baptist, A.P.; Li, L.; Dichiaro, C.A. The importance of atopy on exhaled nitric oxide levels in African American children. *Ann. Allergy Asthma Immunol.* **2015**, *114*, 399–403. [CrossRef]
10. Xepapadaki, P.; Bachert, C.; Finotto, S.; Jartti, T.; Konstantinou, G.N.; Kiefer, A.; Kowalski, M.; Lewandowska-Polak, A.; Lukkarinen, H.; Roumpedaki, E.; et al. Contribution of repeated infections in asthma persistence from preschool to school age: Design and characteristics of the PreDicta cohort. *Pediatric Allergy Immunol.* **2018**, *29*, 383–393. [CrossRef]
11. GGIfARP. Available online: https://ginasthma.org/wp-content/uploads/2019/04/GINA-2019-main-Pocket-Guide-wms.pdf (accessed on 22 June 2019).
12. American Thoracic Society; European Respiratory Society. ATS/ERS recommendations for standardized procedures for the online and offline measurement of exhaled lower respiratory nitric oxide and nasal nitric oxide, 2005. *Am. J. Respir. Crit. Care Med.* **2005**, *171*, 912–930. [CrossRef]
13. Bacharier, L.B.; Boner, A.; Carlsen, K.H.; Eigenmann, P.A.; Frischer, T.; Gotz, M.; Helms, P.J.; Hunt, J.; Liu, A.; Papadopoulos, N.; et al. Diagnosis and treatment of asthma in childhood: A PRACTALL consensus report. *Allergy* **2008**, *63*, 5–34. [CrossRef] [PubMed]
14. Brożek, J.L.; Bousquet, J.; Agache, I.; Agarwal, A.; Bachert, C.; Bosnic-Anticevich, S.; Brignardello-Petersen, R.; Canonica, G.W.; Casale, T.; Chavannes, N.H.; et al. Allergic Rhinitis and its Impact on Asthma (ARIA) guidelines-2016 revision. *J. Allergy Clin. Immunol.* **2017**, *140*, 950–958. [CrossRef] [PubMed]
15. Buchvald, F.; Baraldi, E.; Carraro, S.; Gaston, B.; De Jongste, J.; Pijnenburg, M.W.; Silkoff, P.E.; Bisgaard, H. Measurements of exhaled nitric oxide in healthy subjects age 4 to 17 years. *J. Allergy Clin. Immunol.* **2005**, *115*, 1130–1136. [CrossRef] [PubMed]
16. Baraldi, E.; Dario, C.; Ongaro, R.; Scollo, M.; Azzolin, N.M.; Panza, N.; Paganini, N.; Zacchello, F. Exhaled nitric oxide concentrations during treatment of wheezing exacerbation in infants and young children. *Am. J. Respir. Crit. Care Med.* **1999**, *159*, 1284–1288. [CrossRef]
17. Scott, M.; Raza, A.; Karmaus, W.; Mitchell, F.; Grundy, J.; Kurukulaaratchy, R.J.; Arshad, S.H.; Roberts, G. Influence of atopy and asthma on exhaled nitric oxide in an unselected birth cohort study. *Thorax* **2010**, *65*, 258–262. [CrossRef] [PubMed]

18. Hoyte, F.C.L.; Gross, L.M.; Katial, R.K. Exhaled Nitric Oxide: An Update. *Immunol. Allergy Clin. North Am.* **2018**, *38*, 573–585. [CrossRef] [PubMed]
19. De Gouw, H.W.; Grünberg, K.; Schot, R.; Kroes, A.C.; Dick, E.C.; Sterk, P.J. Relationship between exhaled nitric oxide and airway hyperresponsiveness following experimental rhinovirus infection in asthmatic subjects. *Eur. Respir. J.* **1998**, *11*, 126–132. [CrossRef] [PubMed]
20. Kalayci, O.; Abdelateef, H.; Pozo Beltrán, C.F.; El-Sayed, Z.A.; Gomez, R.M.; Hossny, E.; Morais-Almeida, M.; Nieto, A.; Phipatanakul, W.; Pitrez, P.; et al. Challenges and choices in the pharmacological treatment of non-severe pediatric asthma: A commentary for the practicing physician. *World Allergy Organ. J.* **2019**, *12*, 100054. [CrossRef] [PubMed]
21. Kharitonov, S.A.; Barnes, P.J. Effects of corticosteroids on noninvasive biomarkers of inflammation in asthma and chronic obstructive pulmonary disease. *Proc. Am. Thorac. Soc.* **2004**, *1*, 191–199. [CrossRef]
22. Yune, S.; Lee, J.Y.; Choi, D.C.; Lee, B.J. Fractional exhaled nitric oxide: Comparison between portable devices and correlation with sputum eosinophils. *Allergy Asthma Immunol. Res.* **2015**, *7*, 404–408. [CrossRef] [PubMed]
23. Wilkinson, M.; Maidstone, R.; Loudon, A.; Blaikley, J.; White, I.R.; Singh, D.; Ray, D.W.; Goodacre, R.; Fowler, S.J.; Durrington, H.J. Circadian rhythm of exhaled biomarkers in health and asthma. *Eur. Respir. J.* **2019**, *54*, 1901068. [CrossRef]
24. Harnan, S.E.; Tappenden, P.; Essat, M.; Gomersall, T.; Minton, J.; Wong, R.; Pavord, I.; Everard, M.; Lawson, R. Measurement of exhaled nitric oxide concentration in asthma: A systematic review and economic evaluation of NIOX MINO, NIOX VERO and NObreath. *Health Technol. Assess.* **2015**, *19*, 1–330. [CrossRef] [PubMed]
25. Ferraro, V.; Carraro, S.; Bozzetto, S.; Zanconato, S.; Baraldi, E. Exhaled biomarkers in childhood asthma: Old and new approaches. *Asthma Res. Pract.* **2018**, *4*, 9. [CrossRef] [PubMed]
26. Paraskakis, E.; Brindicci, C.; Fleming, L.; Krol, R.; Kharitonov, S.A.; Wilson, N.M.; Barnes, P.J.; Bush, A. Measurement of bronchial and alveolar nitric oxide production in normal children and children with asthma. *Am. J. Respir. Crit. Care Med.* **2006**, *174*, 260–267. [CrossRef] [PubMed]
27. Cameli, P.; Bargagli, E.; Bergantini, L.; Refini, R.M.; Pieroni, M.; Sestini, P.; Rottoli, P. Evaluation of multiple-flows exhaled nitric oxide in idiopathic and non-idiopathic interstitial lung disease. *J. Breath Res.* **2019**, *13*, 026008. [CrossRef]
28. Chinellato, I.; Piazza, M.; Peroni, D.; Sandri, M.; Chiorazzo, F.; Boner, A.L.; Piacentini, G. Bronchial and alveolar nitric oxide in exercise-induced bronchoconstriction in asthmatic children. *Clin. Exp. Allergy* **2012**, *42*, 1190–1196. [CrossRef]

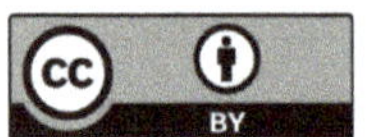

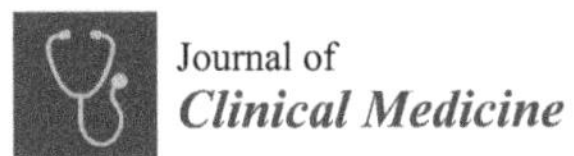
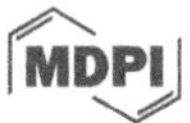

Article

Virus-Induced Asthma/Wheeze in Preschool Children: Longitudinal Assessment of Airflow Limitation Using Impulse Oscillometry

George N Konstantinou [1,2,*], Nikolaos G Papadopoulos [2,3], Emmanouel Manousakis [2] and Paraskevi Xepapadaki [2]

1 424 General Military Training Hospital, 56429 Thessaloniki, Greece
2 Allergy Department, 2nd Pediatric Clinic, National and Kapodistrian University of Athens, 11527 Athens, Greece
3 Division of Infection, Immunity & Respiratory Medicine, University of Manchester, Manchester M13 9PL, UK
* Correspondence: gnkonstantinou@gmail.com

Received: 8 August 2019; Accepted: 11 September 2019; Published: 16 September 2019

Abstract: Several researchers have assessed the utility of Impulse Oscillometry System (IOS) in diagnosing and evaluating the severity of respiratory diseases in childhood, but none has investigated the impact of the fluctuations of IOS parameters in an individualized manner. In this two-year prospective study, we aimed to longitudinally evaluate changes in airflow limitation and bronchodilator responsiveness in steroid-naïve four- to six-year-old children during a virus-induced wheezing episode, with IOS pulmonary resistance parameters set at 5 (R5) and 20 (R20) Hz. Moreover, feasibility and reproducibility, in addition to the diagnostic properties of these parameters were examined. Lung function was assessed every six weeks (baseline), within the first 48 h following an acute wheezing episode (Day 0), after 10, and after 30 days. Forty-three out of 93 recruited children (4.5 ± 0.4 years old) experienced a wheezing episode during the study period. All children were able to perform the IOS effort in an acceptable and highly reproducible manner. R5 and R20 fluctuated independently of atopy, age, height, and weight. On Day 0, R5 values were significantly lower than the respective baseline values and returned to individual baseline levels within 10 days. Post-bronchodilation R5 values were similar to the baseline ones, reflecting a reversible airway obstruction on Day 0. Response to bronchodilation (ΔR5) was significantly more pronounced on Day 0. ΔR5 values lower than -20.5% had a sensitivity of 70% and a specificity of 76% and could accurately identify up to 75% of the examined preschoolers. This study provides evidence in favor of the objective utility of IOS as an easy, highly reproducible, and sensitive technique to assess clinically significant fluctuations and bronchodilation responses suggestive of airflow limitation. Reference values although necessary are suboptimal, utilizing the personal best values as personal reference is useful and reliable.

Keywords: lung function; bronchodilation; resistance; obstruction; reproducible; inflammation; spirometry

---

1. Introduction

Asthma is the most common chronic lower respiratory disease in childhood throughout the world. Current guidelines are highly in favor of documenting reversible airflow obstruction as a cardinal characteristic of asthma, both for the diagnosis and the subsequent monitoring of asthma, preferably prior to controller treatment, in all age groups [1]. The most widely used pulmonary function test is spirometry, which estimates lung volumes by rapid and maximal inspiratory and expiratory maneuvers that are often difficult to perform even in older children.

In contrast, the Forced Oscillation Technique (FOT) superimposes small air pressure perturbations on the natural breathing of a subject to measure the mechanical properties of the lungs [2]. The Impulse Oscillometry System (IOS), based on the aforementioned technique, measures the resistance and reactance of the respiratory system, thus providing an indirect analysis of lung function through the use of short pulses (impulses) of acoustic waves—most commonly over a range of frequencies (5Hz to 20Hz)—applied at the mouth, during spontaneous, quiet breathing [3]. IOS has been used to distinctively quantify the airflow limitation in the central and peripheral airways [4,5]. Low oscillation frequencies like 5 Hz can penetrate the periphery of the bronchial tree (diameter <2 mm) and, therefore, resistance of the respiratory system at 5 Hz (R5) reflects obstruction in both the peripheral and the central airways. On the contrary, higher frequencies cannot be transmitted distally. Thus, resistance of the respiratory system at 20 Hz (R20) reflects the proximal airways resistance. The change in resistance from low to high-frequency ranges (e.g., R5 minus R20, R(5–20)) has been identified as an index of the peripheral airways resistance only, and has been used as a potential marker of small airways obstruction [6].

IOS has been developed as a patient-friendly lung function test that minimizes demands on the patient and requires only passive cooperation with normal breathing through the mouth. It has been successfully used for assessing lung function and asthma control in healthy and asthmatic children [5,6], including preschoolers, and in patients who recently underwent surgery or are unable to perform spirometry, both as an adjunct or even alternative to standard spirometry [4,7,8].

Pediatric reference values and positive bronchodilation responses indicating peripheral air trapping have been standardized and published [9]. R5 is the main parameter to assess bronchodilation. However, no consensus has been reached on the optimal cutoff values that could discriminate patients from healthy individuals. These values vary between 20 and 50% and have been used to diagnose and evaluate the severity of chronic respiratory diseases in childhood or compare to a number of techniques routinely used to assess lung function [10–14]. Nevertheless, none of the studies has prospectively followed either baseline fluctuations of IOS parameters or fluctuations in the course of virus-induced wheeze episodes in preschool children.

In this prospective study, we aimed to longitudinally evaluate changes in airflow limitation and bronchodilator responsiveness by means of the main IOS resistance parameters, in steroid-naïve four- to six-year-old children during the course of a virus-induced wheezing episode. Moreover, IOS feasibility and reproducibility, in addition to the diagnostic properties of the main IOS resistance parameters were examined.

2. Methods

2.1. Study Population

Children four to six years of age from the outpatient clinics of the Allergy Department in the Second Pediatric Clinic of the National and Kapodistrian University of Athens with a previous diagnosis of "episodic viral wheeze" according to the European Respiratory Society Task Force [15] or "virus-induced asthma" according to the Practical Allergy (PRACTALL) Consensus Report [16] were invited to participate. Patients were eligible if they (1) had been given this diagnosis within the 12 months preceding the index visit, (2) had at least one mild wheezing episode (based on reference [16]) in the 12 months preceding the index visit, and (3) if—according to their medical records—there were prescribed inhaled β-agonists, inhaled corticosteroids or montelukast, but did not require hospitalization. Patients receiving inhaled corticosteroids or montelukast on a regular or episodic basis were recruited after a minimum 14-week wash-out period. For the present study, children were required to be able to perform acceptable and repeatable IOS maneuvers after proper training. Since the protocol per se included both spirometric and IOS pulmonary function testing, children were required to be able to perform a technically acceptable maximal expiratory flow/volume effort with a forced expiratory time (FET) of 0.5 s or greater [17]. The study was approved by the institutional ethics committee, and written informed consent was obtained from all parents. The outcomes of additional methods and the baseline characteristics of the study population recruited have been previously described [18].

2.2. Study Design

Upper and lower airway symptoms and medication use were recorded daily by the parents on diary cards. Parents were advised to contact the study physicians to arrange an appointment within 48 h after the child started wheezing or coughing, had difficulty breathing or nighttime awakening due to breathing difficulties. The children were followed up at regular six-week intervals, until either they had a wheezing episode or reached their sixth birthday. Study physicians were responsible to evaluate the diary cards and to perform all IOS maneuvers at baseline, during the first 48 h following a physician-diagnosed wheezing exacerbation (day 0), and then 10 (day 10) and 30 (day 30) days following the initiation of the episode. During the episodes, children were added as a study observation if they could be controlled with 200–400 µg of salbutamol, 3–4 times a day and as needed.

2.3. Allergic Sensitization

Levels of serum-specific IgE (ImmunoCAP; Phadia AB, Uppsala, Sweden) to a panel of locally relevant common aeroallergens (*Dermatophagoides pteronyssinus*, *Dermatophagoides farinae*, cat dander, dog epithelium, grass pollen, *Cladosporium* species, *Aspergillus* species, *Alternaria* species, olive, cypress, and wall pellitory pollen), and food allergens (hen's egg, cow's milk, nuts, and peanut) were measured either after the wheezing episode or at the age of six years for those children without a wheezing episode during the study. A patient was classified as atopic if at least one allergen-specific IgE was greater than 0.7 IU/mL.

2.4. Lung Function Test Maneuvers

IOS was performed using MasterScreen IOS (Jaeger, Würzburg, Germany), applying a standardized protocol based on manufacturer's instructions. The system was calibrated through several full strokes of a single volume (3 L) of air at different flow rates, which were verified with a reference resistance device (2.0 cm H_2O/L/sec) supplied by the manufacturer. Children withheld the use of short-acting bronchodilators at least 6–8 h prior to testing, which was performed and analyzed in accordance with European Respiratory Society (ERS)/American Thoracic Society (ATS) guidelines [17,19]. IOS testing was performed before the spirometry in order to prevent potential bronchoconstriction [7]. Prior to testing, the child was familiarized with the procedure and was placed in a relaxed standing position, with the head in a neutral or slightly extended position. Subsequently, the patient was instructed to breathe normally during the test, making a tight seal with their lips around the mouthpiece. A nasal clip was also used, while the cheeks were firmly supported. After a short sampling period to ensure compliance, three to five efforts lasting 20–60 s were recorded. The 20–60 s period provides the min-max limits of an effort to record an artifact-free maneuver. In case there was no evidence of coughing, swallowing, vocalization or breath-holding causing artifacts during this period, the trial was saved. Pulmonary resistance (R) at frequencies of 5 Hz (R5) and 20 Hz (R20) were calculated with the pre-installed software and assessed by researchers. Each visit-observation consisted of an optimum of three reproducible maneuvers. Reproducibility was defined as R5 within 10% of highest obtained value. R5 and R20 measurements from the three saved reproducible efforts for each IOS parameter were averaged. Calculations of the R(5−20) were assessed with an algorithm based on the equation R5 − R20.

Spirometry was performed with the children in the standing position by using a nose clip and an incentive animation. Results were reported only if at least two technically acceptable curves (<8 maneuvers per visit), as determined according to standard criteria [17], with a FET ≥0.5 s, were obtained.

In order to assess airway reversibility, a short-acting bronchodilator was administered (four puffs of albuterol, 100 µg each) using a spacer. After 15 min, IOS was repeated. Predicted values for R5 and

R20 were based on gender and height according to the equipment's default normal reference values, as recommended by the manufacturer, based on existing reference values [20,21].

2.5. Statistical Analysis

Since all the analyzed parameters were normally distributed, descriptive statistics for continuous variables are presented as means ± standard deviation (SD). Student's t-tests were used to compare binary outcomes at the same time point. Student's paired t-tests were used for between-time point comparisons of the same variable. Associations between categorical data were assessed using the Pearson χ^2 test. Analyses across these time points were performed with generalized estimating equations (GEE) after adjusting for known confounders, such as height, age, and atopy. For the period from day 0 to day 30, all variables were treated as time-dependent, except age, sex, atopy, and height.

A logistic regression analysis was performed among the binary outcome "having" or "not having" a symptomatic wheezing episode, the resistance parameter of interest, and the above-mentioned potential confounders. The same analysis was performed either by using the data from the cohort of patients with a wheezing episode alone or after pooling data from both the children with and without a wheezing episode. Between and within individuals, variability was taken into account in the analysis of the pooled data. Predictor levels corresponding to "having a wheezing episode" with a probability of ≥95% (95% predictive decision points) were identified, and so were their performance characteristics (sensitivity, specificity, positive and negative predictive values calculated). Receiver operating characteristic (ROC) analyses and curves were fitted to identify "optimal decision points," and the area under the curve (AUC) was calculated to compare the accuracy of each analyzed resistance parameter. Additional information can be found in this article's supplementary data.

3. Results

All 98 consecutively examined children were able to perform an acceptable IOS effort and consent to be included in the study. Five of them were unable to achieve an acceptable spirometric maneuver with FET ≥0.5 s, even after three visits of continuous training efforts, and were excluded. All 93 finally recruited children (mean age 4.5 ± 0.4 years) were able to perform an IOS effort both at baseline and during the wheezing episodes. None of the children needed more than three demonstrations and an equal number of efforts during their initial visit to accomplish a technically correct IOS maneuver. Among them, 49 (52.7%) were able to perform a correct spirometric maneuver during the first visit, 32 (34.4%) needed two visits, and the remaining 12 (12.9%) needed three visits to be trained well enough to perform an acceptable and repeatable spirometric maneuver. Two out of these 12 were not able to perform spirometry and an acceptable IOS effort during their first wheezing episode.

Regular follow-up visits occurred every 40 ± 4 days. Four children were lost to follow-up. Among the remaining 89 children, 43 had at least one wheezing episode 0.6 ± 0.3 years after recruitment. This corresponds to a median of five visits for each patient. According to the study protocol, among these regular visits, the very last one was considered the baseline.

Following initial assessment at the beginning of an episode (day 0), the children were re-evaluated 10 ± 1 days (day 10) and 30 ± 3 days (day 30) later. None of the children reported wheezing unrelated to an apparent respiratory tract infection.

There was no significant seasonality for the wheezing episodes except the period from early May until late September (fewer episodes).

The variability of R5 and R20 among different visits was also estimated. Measurements at regular visits and during the course of a wheezing episode were examined. Pre- and post-bronchodilation R5 variability ranged from 2.9% to 33.7% (median: 15%, upper 95% percentile: 32.3%) and 1% to 27.7% (median 10.2%, upper 95% percentile 23.4%), respectively. Pre- and post-bronchodilation R20 variability ranged from 3% to 19.2% (median 8%, upper 95% percentile: 18.5%) and 1.7% to 25% (median 7%, upper 95% percentile: 16.5%).

The baseline demographic and somatometric characteristics and IOS measurements were similar between atopic children, non-atopic children, and children completing the study without any wheezing episode. Bronchodilation responses assessed by R5 and R20 did not differ either (Table 1 and Supplementary Table S1).

Table 1. Baseline characteristics of children experiencing a wheezing episode during the study period, and children without a wheezing episode during the study period.

	Children with Wheezing Episode * (n = 43)	Children with no Episode † (n = 46)
Age (years)	5 ± 0.5	5 ± 0.7
Male, n (%)	23 (54%)	20 (44%)
Height (m)	1.15 ± 0.08	1.14 ± 0.08
Weight (kg)	22.9 ± 3.9	21.9 ± 4.3
Atopic	25 (58%)	21 (46%)
Baseline pre-bronchodilation R5Hz (kPa/lt/sec)	0.943 ± 0.269	0.980 ± 0.222
Baseline post-bronchodilation R5Hz (kPa/lt/sec)	0.817 ± 0.227	0.809 ± 0.186
ΔR5Hz	−12% ± 13.5%	−15.8% ± 15.4%
Baseline pre-bronchodilation R20Hz (kPa/lt/sec)	0.757 ± 0.191	0.764 ± 0.173
Baseline post-bronchodilation R20Hz (kPa/lt/sec)	0.669 ± 0.157	0.675 ± 0.153
ΔR20Hz	−10.1% ± 13.9%	−11.5% ± 17.2%
Previously treated with Bronchodilators alone §	32 (74.4%)	32 (69.6%)

Values presented as mean ± (standard deviation) SD. All comparisons are non-significantly different. * baseline values obtained eight weeks prior to the recorded wheezing episode; † baseline values obtained at recruitment and atopic status at the age of six years old; § the rest of the children had been treated prior to enrolment with inhaled corticosteroids and/or montelukast; Pulmonary resistance (R) at 5 Hz (R5) and 20 Hz (R20); $\Delta Rx = (Rx_{post\text{-}bronchodilation} - Rx_{pre\text{-}bronchodilation})/Rx_{pre\text{-}bronchodilation}$.

During the first 48 h from the beginning of a wheezing episode (day 0), pre-bronchodilation R5 values were significantly higher than their respective baseline values (1.114 ± 0.280 kPa/lt/sec vs 0.943 ± 0.269 kPa/lt/sec, $p < 0.001$). The aforementioned measurements returned to baseline levels within 10 days from the initiation of the episode (Figure 1). There were no significant differences in respect to the atopic status at all time points (Supplementary Table S2).

A similar fluctuation pattern, independent of the atopic status, was recorded for R(5–20) values, namely day 0 vs baseline: 0.314 ± 0.163 kPa/lt/sec vs 0.186 ± 0.115 kPa/lt/sec, respectively, $p < 0.001$. In respect to the R20, a small but significant increase was noted on day 0 compared to baseline, namely 0.801 ± 0.162 kPa/lt/sec vs 0.757 ± 0.191 kPa/lt/sec, respectively, $p = 0.048$.

R5 and R20 were not found to be significantly related to age, gender, and somatometric measures (cross-sectional logistic regression models at each time point and longitudinal GEE models). Gender and height, however, are used by the predicted equations to estimate the equipment's default normal reference values. Pairwise correlation coefficients, although statistically significant, did not indicate strong correlations between reference/predicted values and actual values for both pre-bronchodilation R5 and R20 with Pearson's correlation coefficients 0.522 vs 0.415 respectively, $p < 0.001$ (Supplementary Figures S1 and S2). The same applied for the post-bronchodilation values with Pearson's correlation coefficients 0.496 and 0.308, respectively, $p < 0.001$ (Supplementary Figures S3 and S4). Independence of age, height and weight and suboptimal reference/predicted values suggested that, at least for the examined ages (four to six years of age), the personal best baseline measurement (lowest values) should be the reference values for each individual. Therefore, the reference/predicted values were not taken into consideration in any of the performed calculations. Additional information can be found in this article's supplementary data.

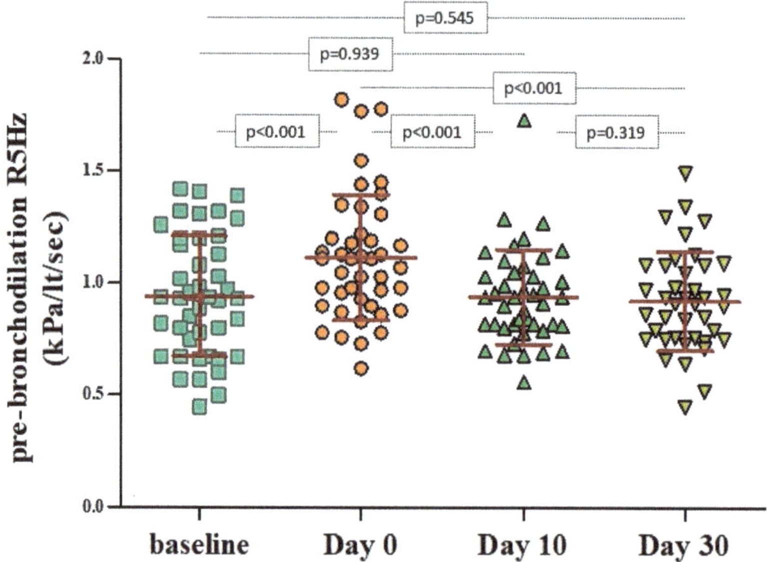

Figure 1. Pairwise comparisons of R5Hz values at baseline, on day 0 (beginning of the wheezing episode), and 10 and 30 days after. The bars and in-between lines represent the mean and standard deviation (SD). All pairwise comparisons are presented with *p*-values that have been estimated with paired Student's t-test.; Pulmonary resistance (R) at 5 Hz (R5).

All post-bronchodilation values were significantly different in relation to the respective pre-bronchodilation at all time points for both R5 and R20 (Table 2). Post-bronchodilation R5 values on day 0 were similar to the baseline pre-bronchodilation values, reflecting the reversible airway obstruction occurring at the beginning of a wheezing episode both in atopic and non-atopic children (Table 2).

Table 2. Mean R5Hz pre- and post-bronchodilation in atopic and non-atopic children and percentage of response to bronchodilation: baseline and day 0, 10, and 30 from the beginning of the wheezing episode.

	Atopics			Non-Atopics		
	R5Hz Bronchodilation (kPa/lt/sec)		Mean ΔR5Hz%*	R5Hz Bronchodilation (kPa/lt/sec)		Mean ΔR5Hz%*
Time	Pre	Post		Pre	Post	
Baseline	0.930 ± 0.273	0.798 ± 0.230	−12.8% ± 14.9%	0.961 ± 0.271	0.844 ± 0.227	−10.8% ± 11.6%
Day 0	1.106 ± 0.279	0.847 ± 0.218 †	−22.5 ± 12.8% ‡	1.125 ± 0.289	0.818 ± 0.171 †	−25.8% ± 11.1% ‡
Day 10	0.959 ± 0.225 †	0.831 ± 0.218 †	−12.9% ± 13.5%	0.914 ± 0.192	0.803 ± 0.155 †	−11.2% ± 11.3%
Day 30	0.905 ± 0.248 †	0.792 ± 0.159 †	18.6% ± 10.7%	0.947 ± 0.179	0.772 ± 0.191 †	−10.3% ± 12.6%

All bronchodilation responses are significantly different at all time points. $\Delta R5 = (R5_{post\text{-}bronchodilation} - R5_{pre\text{-}bronchodilation}) / R5_{pre\text{-}bronchodilation}$; † non-significant results compared with the respective (atopics, non-atopics) baseline pre-bronchodilation values; ‡ Significant bronchodilation differences when compared with the respective (atopics, non-atopics) baseline ΔR5Hz (*p*-value= 0.008 and *p*-value <0.001 respectively). All other comparisons with baseline ΔR5Hz are not significant, irrespectively of atopic status.

In particular, bronchodilation responses assessed by ΔR5 were significantly more pronounced only during the first 48 h from the initiation of the wheezing episode (day 0: −23.9% ± 12.1% versus baseline: −12% ± 13.5%, $p < 0.001$), irrespectively of atopic status (Table 2 and Figure 2). The same applied for the ΔR(5–20), as depicted in Figure 3. Bronchodilation responses measured with ΔR20 values on day 0 did not differ from the responses recorded at baseline or on days 10 and 30 (Figure 4), therefore excluding any potential diagnostic value of ΔR20 to classify wheezing episodes correctly.

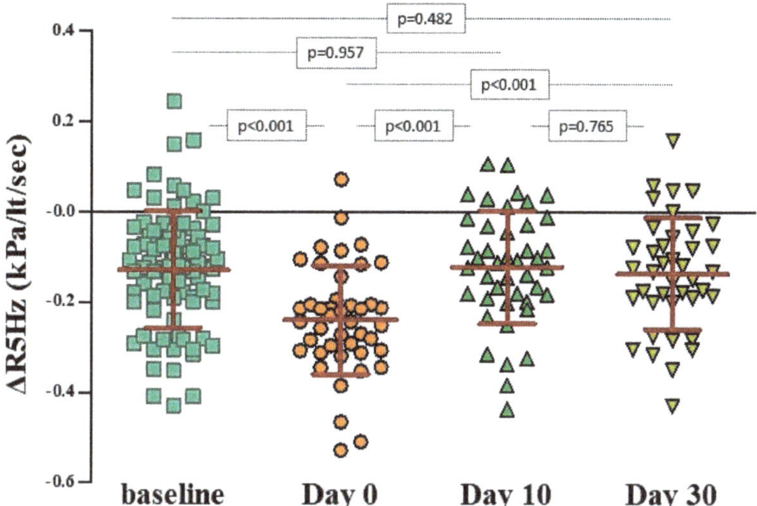

Figure 2. Pairwise comparisons of ΔR5Hz values at baseline, on day 0 (beginning of the wheezing episode), and 10 and 30 days after. The bars and in-between lines represent the mean and SD. All pairwise comparisons are presented with *p*-values that have been estimated with paired Student's *t*-test.; Pulmonary resistance (R) at 5 Hz (R5); $\Delta R5Hz = (R5Hz_{\text{post-bronchodilation}} - R5Hz_{\text{pre-bronchodilation}}) / R5Hz_{\text{pre-bronchodilation}}$

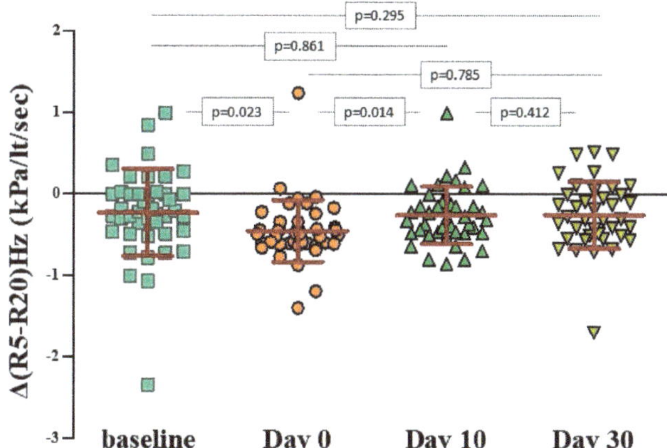

Figure 3. Pairwise comparisons of Δ(R5Hz−R20Hz) values at baseline, on day 0 (beginning of the wheezing episode), and 10 and 30 days after. The bars and in-between lines represent the mean and SD. All pairwise comparisons are presented with *p*-values that have been estimated with paired Student's t-test. Pulmonary resistance (R) at 5 Hz (R5) and 20 Hz (R20); $\Delta R(5-20)Hz = ((R5Hz-R20Hz)_{\text{post-bronchodilation}} - (R5Hz-R20Hz)_{\text{pre-bronchodilation}}) / (R5Hz-R20Hz)_{\text{pre-bronchodilation}}$.

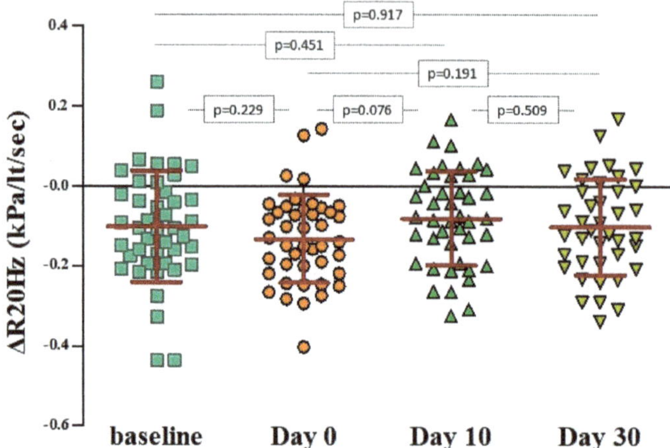

Figure 4. Pairwise comparisons of ΔR20Hz values at baseline, on day 0 (beginning of the wheezing episode), and 10 and 30 days after. The bars and in-between lines represent the mean and SD. All pairwise comparisons are presented with *p*-values that have been estimated with paired Student's t-test. Pulmonary resistance (R) at 20 Hz (R20); $\Delta R20Hz = (R20Hz_{post\text{-}bronchodilation} - R20Hz_{pre\text{-}bronchodilation}) / R20Hz_{pre\text{-}bronchodilation}$.

ΔR5 and ΔR(5–20) were additionally examined as potential diagnostic markers of clinically significant increase in peripheral resistance (assessed during a wheezing episode) in comparison with measures during asymptomatic periods (baseline, day 10, and day 30). For this reason, a ROC analysis was performed. The models examined were unadjusted since none of the other parameters was found to be significant.

The AUCs were 0.725 and 0.671 for ΔR5 and ΔR(5–20) (p = 0.118). Although the AUCs were not significantly different, the higher number for the ΔR5Hz and the simplicity of its calculation render it preferable.

In the ROC analysis, a value of ΔR5 ≤−46.4% accurately classified 80.6% of the wheezing episodes, while values ≤−35.1% correctly identified 77.3% of them (Supplementary Figure S5). Selected cutoff values for ΔR5 and their respective sensitivity, specificity, positive predictive value (PPV) and negative predictive value (NPV), are presented in Table 3.

Table 3. Positive and negative predicted values, sensitivity and specificity between selected ΔR5Hz values, and their ability to correctly classify wheezing episodes (or increase in peripheral resistance as it is assessed during a wheezing episode).

ΔR5Hz (%)	PPV	NPV	Sensitivity	Specificity	Accuracy
−46.4%	100.00%	80.38%	4.65%	100.00%	80.57%
−35.1%	30.77%	80.30%	9.30%	94.64%	77.25%
−31.3%	32.00%	81.18%	18.60%	89.88%	75.36%
−20.5%	42.25%	90.71%	69.77%	75.60%	74.41%
−12.4%	28.57%	90.22%	79.07%	49.40%	55.45%
−8.3%	26.03%	92.31%	88.37%	35.71%	46.45%
−7.1%	25.16%	94.23%	93.02%	29.17%	42.18%

Data are given as percentages. PPV = Positive predictive value of having a wheezing episode if ΔR5Hz is lower than or equal to that specified in the first column; NPV = negative predictive value of not having a wheezing episode if ΔR5Hz is higher than or equal to that specified in the first column.

4. Discussion

To our knowledge, this is the first study to prospectively assess IOS indices in virus-induced wheezing illnesses, suggesting that this method could be used in this age group, where spirometry might not be feasible for a substantial proportion of the children.

The IOS technique is easy to perform in preschoolers. All recruited children were trained within a few minutes, and more importantly, none of them experienced difficulties in cooperating during the episode. On the contrary, during the recruitment period, 44 out of 93 children (47.3%) needed more than a regular (according to the study protocol) visit to be properly trained in order to perform a correct spirometric effort, while two of them did not achieve a technically acceptable spirometric maneuver during the episode. Taking into consideration the fact that measurements were performed in a research setting, it is rather self-explanatory that, in everyday clinical practice, spirometry might be quite time-consuming for the medical personnel, thus indisputably supporting the IOS's superiority in this age group. Since there is an unmet need for objective measures in preschoolers with asthma-related symptoms, seeing that the documentation of reversibility using spirometry is often problematic due to effort dependency, IOS merits the consideration of being included in the diagnostic and therapeutic algorithm.

In particular, we showed that, in preschool children with virus-induced wheeze, IOS indices mainly reflecting peripheral airways, such as R5, are indicative of airflow limitation during an asthma-associated episode. R5 values increased significantly, while bronchodilation responses were more pronounced upon the initiation of the wheezing illness than at baseline. Fluctuations of the IOS resistance parameters resemble the correspondent fluctuations of symptoms (noisy breathing, cough, and shortness of breath), airway inflammation (FeNO) and spirometric parameters (such as $FEV_{0.5}$)—as shown in our previously published study, indicating that these episodes share common characteristics with the well-defined asthma exacerbations in older children [18].

In general, the within- and between-visit variability of R5 and R20 is estimated to be up to 10%. This variability indicates acceptable repeatability among multiple efforts performed by the same subject [22]. In children, this variability is expected to be higher and has been estimated to be up to 16% for measurements within the same day or up to 30% among several weeks [7,10,19,23,24]. When assessing post-bronchodilation values, their variability is expected to vary even more, with coefficients of variation twice the amount of these reported for measurements before bronchodilation [19]. This was also the case in our cohort. The median variability ranged from 7% to 15% after taking into consideration pre- and post- bronchodilation measurements for R5 and R20 at regular visits and during the course of a wheezing episode. The variability did not differ significantly before and after bronchodilation and, on both occasions, it was within the acceptable extent, suggesting excellent repeatability and reliability in recorded measurements at different time points.

In our cohort, moderate to low correlations (ranging from 0.308 to 0.522) were found between predicted and recorded values for both R5 and R20, before and after bronchodilation. Moreover, neither pre- nor post-bronchodilation R5 and R20 values were found to be correlated with either age, gender, or somatometric parameters. Predicted values for R5 and R20 were based on gender- and height-adjusted existing reference values from a Swedish and a Polish study, as recommended by the manufacturer [20,21]. In the Swedish study by Denker et al. [20], 350 children, 2.1 to 11.1 years old with height 90–160 cm were examined. The investigators found significant correlations with height but weak with weight for both R5 and R20. No significant gender-related difference was found for respiratory resistance. The investigators stated that there were more observations in the height interval 130–145 cm (vs. 107–121 cm in our study population). They do not provide information about the number of children between the 4–6 year of age but based on the height information, it is clear that the predicted equations are weighted for older and higher children and are not representative for preschoolers. In the Polish study by Nowowiejska et al. [21], 626 children, 3.1–18.9 years old (mean age for boys 10.6 years and for girls 10.9 years), with height 95–193 cm (mean height for boys 144.8 cm and for girls 141.9 cm) were examined. Similar correlations with the Swedish study were found for both R5 and R20. Again, the predicted equations were weighted over older and higher children.

In general, young children exhibit higher pulmonary resistance than older children and adults, and, therefore, airway resistance is inversely proportional to age, especially at lower frequencies [25]. In a recent meta-analysis, a correlation with anthropometric variables has been suggested too [26]. The lack of similar correlations in our study could be explained by the narrow range of height and weight in the sample of 4- to 6-year-old children examined. The Polish and Swedish studies provide predicted equations with anthropometric data based mainly on older and higher children, with values over a wide spectrum. Thus, extrapolating data in younger and smaller children appears to provide suboptimal reference values. Additionally, it should be underscored that the differences in ethnicity might also influence the estimated reference values which do not seem to be appropriate at least for the Greek children.

Nevertheless, based on the low variability and excellent repeatability in our study, measures up to six months apart (based on this study average observational period until a wheezing episode occurred), even during different seasons, could be considered stable and independent of known confounders like gender, height or weight. For these reasons, at least in this age-group, reference values are not recommended, until appropriate studies are conducted. An individualized approach using the personal best value, recorded either when the child is asymptomatic or at least 10 days after a mild wheezing episode occurs, is recommended. These values can be used up to at least six months apart to follow-up mild wheezers.

Atopy does not seem to affect the resistance baseline measurements or the bronchodilation responses either when these parameters are assessed cross-sectionally or longitudinally. This finding has also been shown in spirometry and FE_{NO} in preschoolers [18]. This independence could be explained by the intermittent, short-lasting inflammatory responses during mild wheezing episodes in our cases. It remains to be shown [27] whether the probably new, atopy-related inflammation could predispose patients to a more chronic inflammatory process since multiple relapses could lead to alterations in the peripheral resistance measures and bronchodilation responses in atopics.

R5 and R(5–20) values, as indicators of bronchial obstruction, increased significantly during wheezing episodes and spontaneously returned to baseline within 10 days. Post-bronchodilation R5 values on day 0 were similar to the pre-bronchodilation baseline values, reflecting a reversible airway obstruction at the beginning of a wheezing episode, independently of atopic status as has previously been shown for $FEV_{0.5}$ [18].

Mean bronchodilation responses were significantly higher at the beginning of the episode compared to the respective changes at baseline or on day 10 and 30 for ΔR5 (representing the total airway resistance) and ΔR(5–20) (representing peripheral resistance) but not for ΔR20 (representing the resistance of the large airways). Considering the resistance that each of these variables reflects, this is to be expected. In particular, the bronchodilation responses assessed by ΔR5 were more pronounced within the first 48 h from the initiation of the wheezing episode than the responses assessed by ΔR(5–20). When both ΔR5 and ΔR(5–20) were examined for their potential diagnostic value in discriminating clinically significant increase in peripheral resistance during the first days of a wheezing episode (day 0, day 10 and day 30), compared to measurements during asymptomatic periods (baseline) their AUCs were not significantly different (0.725 vs 0.671, respectively). Nevertheless, the higher absolute magnitude of $AUC_{\Delta R5}$ renders this parameter preferable for analyzing performance characteristics with a ROC analysis.

Indeed, the ROC analysis provided specific diagnostic cutoff values. Based on the analysis of this cohort, the optimal cutoff point with the highest sensitivity and specificity was found to be −20.5% (Table 3). Taking into account that the cutoff values have been calculated in patients using measurements even during a wheezing episode, the bronchodilation magnitude is expected to be overestimated in healthy individuals of similar age, and, hence, the proposed cutoff values are expected to be of greater diagnostic value.

The major strength of this study is the steroid-naïve cohort that has been longitudinally examined, providing robust data. To our knowledge, this is the first study to assess airflow limitation in preschool children experiencing wheezing episodes with such study design, that is, by utilizing the IOS technique, and it is also the first time cutoff values have been calculated based on longitudinal measures during and outside an episode for a short period, to adjust for intra- and inter-variability. Considering the fact that the two most likely sources to rely on for the calculation of cutoffs are either population surveys—using only non-wheezers—or studies comparing wheezers with non-wheezers during asymptomatic periods, the data of this study are expected to be more reliable.

A weakness of the study is the lack of a healthy control group because of ethical considerations regarding salbutamol administration to healthy children [28]. This issue has been overcome by assessing the value of a personalized approach and proving that the personal best value is reliable enough to follow up with such patients. Moreover, the sample was small, although the multiple measurements per studied child provided robust longitudinal analyses. Last but not least, it is not known if the inferences could be applied in children with severe viral-induced wheezing episodes.

In summary, we have shown that IOS is an easy, highly reproducible, and sensitive technique that can be successfully performed to assess airflow limitation objectively in preschool children with virus-induced wheezing illnesses. The study design supports the superiority of the longitudinal approach of such data, suggesting, that reference or predicted values, although necessary, are suboptimal, and that an individualized approach utilizing the personal best values as the personal reference is useful and reliable. Among the commonly measured parameters, the R5 seems to be the best to assess clinically significant fluctuations and bronchodilation responses suggestive of airflow limitation. Cutoff values do have diagnostic properties that can help identify significant bronchodilation responses. Considering the difficulties in examining preschoolers using spirometry and the time required to train them and perform an acceptable spirometric maneuver, IOS could be suggested as the future gold standard to examine airflow limitation in children even in everyday clinical practice. Further studies with similar design are needed for children with persistent or moderate to severe symptoms.

Supplementary Materials: The following are available online at http://www.mdpi.com/2077-0383/8/9/1475/s1, Figure S1: Pairwise correlation between reference/predicted values and actual values for pre-bronchodilation R5, Figure S2: Pairwise correlation between reference/predicted values and actual values for pre-bronchodilation R20, Pairwise correlation between reference/predicted values and actual values for post-bronchodilation R5, Figure S4: Pairwise correlation between reference/predicted values and actual values for post-bronchodilation R20, Figure S5: Receiver operating characteristic (ROC) curve, Table S1. Baseline characteristics of atopic and non-atopic children with a wheezing episode and children without a wheezing episode during the study period, Table S2. Pre-bronchodilation R5Hz measurements: reference (baseline), on day 0, 10th (day 10), and 30th (day 30) from the beginning of the wheezing episode.

Author Contributions: Conceptualization, K.N.G. and P.G.N.; Data curation, K.N.G. and X.P.; Formal analysis, K.N.G.; Funding acquisition, P.G.N.; Investigation, K.N.G., P.G.N., M.E., and X.P.; Methodology, K.N.G., P.G.N., and X.P.; Project administration, K.N.G. and P.G.N.; Resources, K.N.G., M.E., and X.P.; Software, K.N.G.; Supervision, P.G.N.; Validation, K.N.G.; Visualization, K.N.G.; Writing—original draft, K.N.G. and X.P.; Writing—review & editing, K.N.G., P.G.N., M.E., and X.P.

Funding: The APC was funded by GlaxoSmithKline S.A., Greece. The funders had no role in the design of the study; in the collection, analyses, or interpretation of data; in the writing of the manuscript, or in the decision to publish the results.

Conflicts of Interest: The authors declare no conflict of interest.

References

1. Global Initiative for Asthma. Global Strategy for Asthma Management and Prevention. 2019. Available online: www.ginasthma.org (accessed on 1 June 2019).
2. Bickel, S.; Popler, J.; Lesnick, B.; Eid, N. Impulse oscillometry: Interpretation and practical applications. *Chest* **2014**, *146*, 841–847. [CrossRef] [PubMed]

3. Meraz, E.G.; Nazeran, H.; Ramos, C.D.; Nava, P.; Diong, B.; Goldman, M.D.; Goldman, C.A. Analysis of impulse oscillometric measures of lung function and respiratory system model parameters in small airway-impaired and healthy children over a 2-year period. *Biomed. Eng. Online* **2011**, *10*, 21. [CrossRef] [PubMed]
4. Song, T.W.; Kim, K.W.; Kim, E.S.; Park, J.W.; Sohn, M.H.; Kim, K.E. Utility of impulse oscillometry in young children with asthma. *Pediatric Allergy Immunol. Off. Publ. Eur. Soc. Pediatric Allergy Immunol.* **2008**, *19*, 763–768. [CrossRef] [PubMed]
5. Shi, Y.; Aledia, A.S.; Tatavoosian, A.V.; Vijayalakshmi, S.; Galant, S.P.; George, S.C. Relating small airways to asthma control by using impulse oscillometry in children. *J. Allergy Clin. Immunol.* **2012**, *129*, 671–678. [CrossRef] [PubMed]
6. Shi, Y.; Aledia, A.S.; Galant, S.P.; George, S.C. Peripheral airway impairment measured by oscillometry predicts loss of asthma control in children. *J. Allergy Clin. Immunol.* **2013**, *131*, 718–723. [CrossRef] [PubMed]
7. Komarow, H.D.; Skinner, J.; Young, M.; Gaskins, D.; Nelson, C.; Gergen, P.J.; Metcalfe, D.D. A study of the use of impulse oscillometry in the evaluation of children with asthma: analysis of lung parameters, order effect, and utility compared with spirometry. *Pediatric Pulmonol.* **2012**, *47*, 18–26. [CrossRef] [PubMed]
8. Dos Santos, K.; Fausto, L.L.; Camargos, P.A.M.; Kviecinski, M.R.; da Silva, J. Impulse oscillometry in the assessment of asthmatic children and adolescents: From a narrative to a systematic review. *Paediatr. Respir. Rev.* **2017**, *23*, 61–67. [CrossRef] [PubMed]
9. Frei, J.; Jutla, J.; Kramer, G.; Hatzakis, G.E.; Ducharme, F.M.; Davis, G.M. Impulse oscillometry: Reference values in children 100 to 150 cm in height and 3 to 10 years of age. *Chest* **2005**, *128*, 1266–1273. [CrossRef] [PubMed]
10. Klug, B.; Bisgaard, H. Specific airway resistance, interrupter resistance, and respiratory impedance in healthy children aged 2–7 years. *Pediatric Pulmonol.* **1998**, *25*, 322–331. [CrossRef]
11. Hellinckx, J.; De Boeck, K.; Bande-Knops, J.; van der Poel, M.; Demedts, M. Bronchodilator response in 3–6.5 years old healthy and stable asthmatic children. *Eur. Respir. J.* **1998**, *12*, 438–443. [CrossRef]
12. Thamrin, C.; Gangell, C.L.; Udomittipong, K.; Kusel, M.M.; Patterson, H.; Fukushima, T.; Schultz, A.; Hall, G.L.; Stick, S.M.; Sly, P.D. Assessment of bronchodilator responsiveness in preschool children using forced oscillations. *Thorax* **2007**, *62*, 814–819. [CrossRef]
13. Mansur, A.H.; Manney, S.; Ayres, J.G. Methacholine-induced asthma symptoms correlate with impulse oscillometry but not spirometry. *Respir. Med.* **2008**, *102*, 42–49. [CrossRef]
14. Kalliola, S.; Malmberg, L.P.; Kajosaari, M.; Mattila, P.S.; Pelkonen, A.S.; Mäkelä, M.J. Assessing direct and indirect airway hyperresponsiveness in children using impulse oscillometry. *Ann. Allergy Asthma Immunol. Off. Publ. Am. Coll. Allergy Asthma Immunol.* **2014**, *113*, 166–172. [CrossRef] [PubMed]
15. Brand, P.L.; Baraldi, E.; Bisgaard, H.; Boner, A.L.; Castro-Rodriguez, J.A.; Custovic, A.; de Blic, J.; de Jongste, J.C.; Eber, E.; Everard, M.L.; et al. Definition, assessment and treatment of wheezing disorders in preschool children: An evidence-based approach. *Eur. Respir. J.* **2008**, *32*, 1096–1110. [CrossRef]
16. Bacharier, L.B.; Boner, A.; Carlsen, K.H.; Eigenmann, P.A.; Frischer, T.; Götz, M.; Helms, P.J.; Hunt, J.; Liu, A.; Papadopoulos, N.; et al. Diagnosis and treatment of asthma in childhood: A PRACTALL consensus report. *Allergy* **2008**, *63*, 5–34. [CrossRef] [PubMed]
17. Beydon, N.; Davis, S.D.; Lombardi, E.; Allen, J.L.; Arets, H.G.; Aurora, P.; Bisgaard, H.; Davis, G.M.; Ducharme, F.M.; Eigen, H.; et al. An official American Thoracic Society/European Respiratory Society statement: Pulmonary function testing in preschool children. *Am. J. Respir. Crit. Care Med.* **2007**, *175*, 1304–1345. [CrossRef] [PubMed]
18. Konstantinou, G.N.; Xepapadaki, P.; Manousakis, E.; Makrinioti, H.; Kouloufakou-Gratsia, K.; Saxoni-Papageorgiou, P.; Papadopoulos, N.G. Assessment of airflow limitation, airway inflammation, and symptoms during virus-induced wheezing episodes in 4- to 6-year-old children. *J. Allergy Clin. Immunol.* **2013**, *131*, 87–93.e1-5. [CrossRef]
19. Oostveen, E.; MacLeod, D.; Lorino, H.; Farré, R.; Hantos, Z.; Desager, K.; Marchal, F. The forced oscillation technique in clinical practice: Methodology, recommendations and future developments. *Eur. Respir. J.* **2003**, *22*, 1026–1041. [CrossRef]
20. Dencker, M.; Malmberg, L.P.; Valind, S.; Thorsson, O.; Karlsson, M.K.; Pelkonen, A.; Pohjanpalo, A.; Haahtela, T.; Turpeinen, M.; Wollmer, P. Reference values for respiratory system impedance by using impulse oscillometry in children aged 2–11 years. *Clin. Physiol. Funct. Imaging* **2006**, *26*, 247–250. [CrossRef]

21. Nowowiejska, B.; Tomalak, W.; Radliński, J.; Siergiejko, G.; Latawiec, W.; Kaczmarski, M. Transient reference values for impulse oscillometry for children aged 3–18 years. *Pediatric Pulmonol.* **2008**, *43*, 1193–1197. [CrossRef]
22. Lándsér, F.J.; Nagles, J.; Demedts, M.; Billiet, L.; van de Woestijne, K.P. A new method to determine frequency characteristics of the respiratory system. *J. Appl. Physiol.* **1976**, *41*, 101–106. [CrossRef] [PubMed]
23. Gochicoa-Rangel, L.; Torre-Bouscoulet, L.; Martínez-Briseño, D.; Rodríguez-Moreno, L.; Cantú-González, G.; Vargas, M.H. Values of impulse oscillometry in healthy Mexican children and adolescents. *Respir. Care* **2015**, *60*, 119–127. [CrossRef]
24. Knihtilä, H.; Kotaniemi-Syrjänen, A.; Pelkonen, A.S.; Kalliola, S.; Mäkelä, M.J.; Malmberg, L.P. Small airway oscillometry indices: Repeatability and bronchodilator responsiveness in young children. *Pediatric Pulmonol.* **2017**, *52*, 1260–1267. [CrossRef] [PubMed]
25. Clément, J.; Dumoulin, B.; Gubbelmans, R.; Hendriks, S.; van de Woestijne, K.P. Reference values of total respiratory resistance and reactance between 4 and 26 Hz in children and adolescents aged 4–20 years. *Bull. Eur. De Physiopathol. Respir.* **1987**, *23*, 441–448.
26. De Assumpcao, M.S.; da Silva Goncalves, E.; Oliveira, M.S.; Ribeiro, J.D.; Dalbo Contrera Toro, A.A.; de Azevedo Barros-Filho, A.; de Monteiro, M.; Santos Schivinski, C.I. Impulse Oscillometry System and Anthropometric Variables of Preschoolers, Children and Adolescents Systematic Review. *Curr. Pediatric Rev.* **2017**, *13*, 126–135. [CrossRef] [PubMed]
27. Xepapadaki, P.; Bachert, C.; Finotto, S.; Jartti, T.; Konstantinou, G.N.; Kiefer, A.; Kowalski, M.; Lewandowska-Polak, A.; Lukkarinen, H.; Roumpedaki, E.; et al. Contribution of repeated infections in asthma persistence from preschool to school age: Design and characteristics of the PreDicta cohort. *Pediatric Allergy Immunol. Off. Publ. Eur. Soc. Pediatric Allergy Immunol.* **2018**, *29*, 383–393. [CrossRef] [PubMed]
28. Lands, L.C.; Allen, J.; Cloutier, M.; Leigh, M.; McColley, S.; Murphy, T.; Wilfond, B. Pediatric Assembly of American Thoracic Society Subcommittee. ATS Consensus Statement: Research opportunities and challenges in pediatric pulmonology. *Am. J. Respir. Crit. Care Med.* **2005**, *172*, 776–780. [CrossRef] [PubMed]

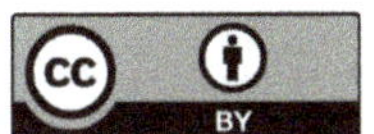

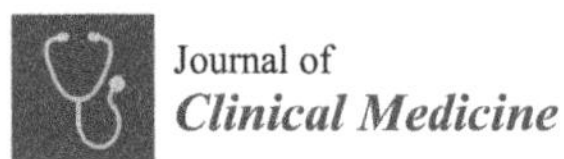
Journal of
Clinical Medicine

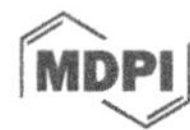

Article

Increased Ratio of Matrix Metalloproteinase-9 (MMP-9)/Tissue Inhibitor Metalloproteinase-1 from Alveolar Macrophages in Chronic Asthma with a Fast Decline in FEV_1 at 5-Year Follow-up

Fu-Tsai Chung [1,2,3,4], Hung-Yu Huang [1,3], Chun-Yu Lo [1,2], Yu-Chen Huang [1,2], Chang-Wei Lin [1,3], Chih-Chen He [1], Jung-Ru He [1,2], Te-Fang Sheng [1,2] and Chun-Hua Wang [1,2,*]

1 Department of Thoracic Medicine, Chang Gung Memorial Hospital, Taipei 105, Taiwan; vikingchung@yahoo.com.tw (F.-T.C.) compaction71@gmail.com (H.-Y.H.); mixova@yahoo.com (C.-Y.L.); yuchenhahaha@gmail.com (Y.-C.H.); naturewei@cgmh.org.tw (C.W.L.); heh0229@yahoo.com.tw (C.-C.H.); mitosenorico@gmail.com (J.-R.H.); rubysheng050@gmail.com (T.-F.S.)
2 College of Medicine, Chang Gung University, Taoyuan 333, Taiwan
3 Division of Pulmonary and Critical Care, Department of Internal Medicine, Saint Paul's Hospital, Taoyuan 330, Taiwan
4 Graduate Institute of Clinical Medical Sciences, College of Medicine, Chang Gung University, Taoyuan 333, Taiwan
* Correspondence: wchunhua@ms7.hinet.net; Tel.: +886-3-3281200 (ext. 8467)

Received: 9 August 2019; Accepted: 9 September 2019; Published: 12 September 2019

Abstract: Chronic asthma is associated with progressive airway remodeling, which may contribute to declining lung function. An increase in matrix metalloproteinases-9 (MMP-9)/tissue inhibitor metalloproteinase-1 (TIMP-1) may indicate airway inflammation and bronchial injury. Bronchial biopsy specimens and alveolar macrophages (AMs) were obtained from patients with asthma under regular treatment with inhaled corticosteroids or combination therapy and normal subjects ($n = 10$). Asthmatics included those with a slow forced expiratory volume in one second (FEV_1) decline (<30 mL/year, $n = 13$) and those with a fast FEV_1 decline (≥30 mL/year, $n = 8$) in 5-year follow-up. Immunostaining expression of MMP-9 and TIMP-1 was detected in airway tissues. MMP-9 and TIMP-1 was measured from AMs cultured for 24 h. After the 5-year treatment, the methacholine airway hyperresponsiveness of the slow FEV_1 decline group was decreased, but that of the fast FEV_1 decline group was increased (PC_{20}, provocative concentration causing a 20% decrease in FEV_1, 3.12 ± 1.10 to 1.14 ± 0.34 mg/dL, $p < 0.05$). AMs of asthma with a fast FEV_1 decline released a higher level of MMP-9 (8.52 ± 3.53 pg/mL, $p < 0.05$) than those of a slow FEV_1 decline (0.99 ± 0.20 pg/mL). The MMP-9/TIMP ratio in the fast FEV_1 decline group (0.089 ± 0.032) was higher than that of the slow FEV_1 decline group (0.007 ± 0.001, $p < 0.01$). The annual FEV_1 decline in 5 years was proportional to the level of MMP-9 (r = 57, $p < 0.01$) and MMP-9/TIMP-1 ratio (r = 0.58, $p < 0.01$). The airways of asthma with greater yearly decline in FEV_1 showed an increased thickness of submucosa and strong expression of MMP-9. An increase in MMP-9 and MMP-9/TIMP-1 in airways or AMs could be indicators of chronic airway inflammation and contribute to a greater decline in lung function of patients with chronic asthma.

Keywords: asthma; airway remodeling; matrix metalloproteinases-9; tissue inhibitor of metalloproteinase-1; alveolar macrophages

1. Introduction

Asthma is a chronic respiratory disease of airway inflammation that manifests as variable airflow limitation [1]. Patients with asthmatic airway inflammation develop tissue injury with subsequent structural changes, which is termed airway wall remodeling [2,3]. Elderly or longer duration of asthma is correlated to airway wall remodeling and contributes to a decline in lung function [4]. The features of airway remodeling include smooth muscle hypertrophy, goblet-cell hyperplasia, subepithelial fibrosis, inflammatory cell infiltration, as well as epithelial shedding [5].

Matrix metalloproteinases (MMPs) are a family of enzymes that can break down proteins of the extracellular matrix (ECM), thus contributing to pathological processes of inflammation, wound healing, and fibrosis [6]. The MMPs also play an important role in several lung or airway diseases, or even lung cancer [7–10]. Additionally, increased levels of MMP-9 in serum, sputum, or lavage fluid were observed in patients with asthma [11–13]. MMP-9-deficient animals could inhibit airway inflammation and the immunoreactivity of MMP-9 has also been reported to be correlated with asthma severity [14]. Nevertheless, a defensive function of MMP-9 in asthma was reported through a heightened inflammation in MMP9-deficient mice [15,16]. Taken together, MMP-9 may be an important factor involved in asthma, but the production of MMP-9 in chronic asthma with persistent airway obstruction is still undetermined.

The tissue inhibitors of matrix metalloproteinase (TIMPs) inhibit enzymatic activity of MMPs through binding to the MMPs [17,18]. The secretion of TIMP-1 is associated with MMP-9. TIMP-1 may possibly result in the thickening process of the basement membrane in asthma [19]. Therefore, MMP and TIMP imbalance may cause clinical differences in chronic airway diseases [20,21]. The ratio of MMP-9/TIMP-1 in the sputum of asthmatic patients has been shown to decrease after recovery from an acute exacerbation of asthma, which may imply that MMP9/TIMP has a negative correlation [22]. Through increasing the thickness of the airway wall by collagen deposition, a decreased ratio of MMP-9/TIMP-1 in chronic asthma may result in airway obstruction [4]. Vignola et al. [21] reported that the ratio of sputum MMP-9/TIMP-1 has a positive correlation with the forced expiratory volume in one second (FEV_1) of asthmatic patients. Additionally, a previous report [23] showed that a low serum MMP-9/TIMP-1 ratio was found in asthmatic patients who show little FEV_1 improvement with the treatment of corticosteroids. Despite some reports [22,23], which revealed the possibly negative correlation of MMP9, TIMP, and lung function in asthmatic patients, the relation among these parameters remains controversial. Some reports also presented no correlation between MMP9, TIMP, and lung functions [24], or positive correlations among MMP9, TIMP, and lung functions [25,26].

Our aim was to evaluate whether the ratio of MMP-9/TIMP-1 released from cultured alveolar macrophages was higher in chronic asthmatic patients who had a fast, yearly decline in FEV_1. We also investigate whether the ratio of MMP-9/TIMP-1 was correlated to the magnitude of yearly FEV_1 decline.

2. Materials and Methods

2.1. Patient Population

Non-smoking asthmatic patients, aged 18 to 65 years, were recruited from outpatient clinics of the Chang Gung Memorial Hospital. Asthma was defined according to the American Thoracic Society criteria [27]. All asthmatic subjects had a >12% improvement in forced expiratory volume in one second (FEV_1) with inhaled albuterol (400 μg) and bronchial hyperreactivity to methacholine (provocative concentration (PC) causing a 20% decrease in FEV_1, $PC_{20} < 8$ mg/L). These patients received anti-asthma medications, which included inhaled and/or oral corticosteroids, inhaled long-acting β_2-agonist, or a combination of these, and had been followed up at our clinics for more than 5 years. All of the patients with asthma had used inhaled corticosteroids all the time. All patients had been stable for at least 3 months and were taking their usual medications before entry into the study. Inhaled β_2-agonists were withheld for 12 hours before methacholine testing.

The asthmatic subjects were divided into 2 groups: 13 asthmatic subjects (7 women and 6 men, aged 49.2 ± 3.4 years) with a slow FEV_1 decline (< 30 mL/year) in the 5-year follow-up, and 8 asthmatic subjects (3 women and 5 men, aged 49.4 ± 3.7 years) with a fast FEV_1 (≥ 30 mL/year) in the 5-year follow-up, as previously described [28]. During the following years, one of the asthmatics with a slow FEV_1 decline and 4 asthmatics with a fast FEV_1 decline experienced difficulty in controlling their asthma symptoms despite taking the maximum recommended dose of inhaled corticosteroids and inhaled long-acting β_2-agonist. These patients needed additional therapy with long-term oral corticosteroids or a long-acting muscarinic antagonist. The calculation of annual FEV_1 decline (mL/year) was determined by subtracting FEV_1 at the first year by the second measurement 5 years later, then dividing this by 5 [28].

Ten normal non-smoking subjects (6 women and 4 men, aged 47.3 ± 2.8 years), who had normal pulmonary function and no evidence of bronchial hyperresponsiveness, allergic rhinitis, or asthma, were recruited. Their total IgE levels and eosinophil counts were normal and their serum-specific IgE was negative.

2.2. Study Protocol

All patients who satisfied the enrollment criteria performed routine pulmonary function tests and methacholine provocation testing after abstaining from short-acting oral or metered-dose inhaler bronchodilator use for 6 h, and long-acting β_2 agonist for 24–48 hours. Asthmatic subjects underwent the procedure of fiberoptic bronchoscopy with bronchial biopsy and bronchoalveolar lavage. Informed consent was obtained from all patients before entry into the study. The study was approved by the Chang Gung Memorial Hospital Ethics Committee (IRB number: 90-13).

2.3. Fiberoptic Bronchoscopy

All study patients received fiberoptic bronchoscopy under sedation. The procedure of bronchoscopy under sedation and administering of local anesthesia was performed in the study institution. Sedation with intravenous midazolam (5–10 mg), and local anesthesia with 2% xylocaine solution was performed during bronchoscopy. Oxygen saturation, blood pressure, and electrocardiography (ECG) were monitored during bronchoscopy. The bronchoscope was advanced through the nose and larynx, and then into the tracheal and bronchial lumen; bronchial biopsies were taken from the 4th or 5th subsegmental bronchus. The specimens were fixed by 4% paraformaldehyde for immunocytochemistry.

2.4. Preparation of BAL Cells

Bronchoalveolar lavage (BAL) was completed in subjects using 300 mL of 0.9% saline solution [29]. Sterile saline solution was instilled into the right fourth or fifth subsegmental bronchus. The lavage fluid was retrieved by gentle aspiration, collected, and filtered through two layers of sterile gauze. BAL fluid was kept on ice throughout processing. The collected BAL fluid was centrifuged at 600× *g* for 20 min at 4 °C. The cell pellet was obtained after centrifugation followed by consecutive washes and finally resuspended at 10^6 cells per mL in RPMI-1640 (GIBCO, Grand Island, New York, NY, USA) containing 5% heat-inactivated fetal calf serum (FCS, Flow Laboratories, Paisley, Scotland, UK). Trypan blue exclusion was used to determine cell viability. Differential cell counts were determined by counting 500 cells on cytocentrifuge preparations using a modified Wright–Giemsa stain. BAL fluids were stored at −70 °C until analysis. The purified alveolar macrophages were placed in 6-well plates at 10^6 cells/mL for 24 h at 37 °C and 5% CO_2. The culture supernatant was collected and frozen at −70 °C until use.

2.5. Immunocytochemistry

Immunoreactivity for tissues was performed with the use of the avidin–biotin peroxidase complex method. Tissue sections (5 μm) from asthmatic subjects were incubated overnight at 4 °C with a variety of primary antibodies, including anti-human MMP-9 (Oncogen Science Inc, Cambridge, MA, USA) and TIMP-1 antibodies (Fuji Pharmaceutical Co, Toyama, Japan) [30]. Mouse immunoglobulin G1 (Dako, Kyoto, Japan) was used for negative controls. After washing in PBS/Tween 20 twice, the slides were counterstained by hematoxylin. Positive immunostaining was visualized as brown granules contained in the cytoplasm. The scores corresponding to MMP-9 and TIMP-1 immunostaining expression were evaluated by a semi-quantitative assessment using the intensity and percentage of positively stained cells, such as epithelial cells, inflammatory cells, and mucus gland or smooth muscle. The intensity of MMP-9 and TIMP-1 staining was scored as follows: 1, weak; 2, moderate; and 3, strong (Figures 1 and 2). The percentage scores were determined by the following definition: 1, ≤25%; 2, 26–50%; 3, 51–75%; and 4, >75%. These scores were multiplied by the intensity and the percentage score. The range was between 1 and 12.

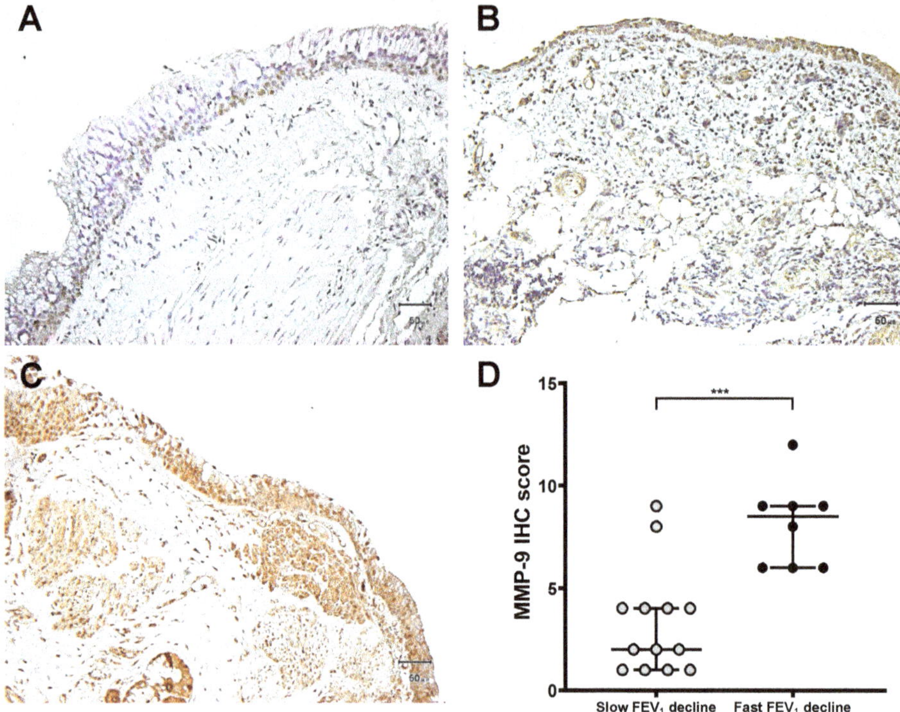

Figure 1. Immunohistochemical expression levels of MMP-9. An avidin–biotin complex immunohistochemical study for MMP-9 labeling was performed in airway tissues obtained from asthmatic patients with a slow FEV_1 decline (A) and a fast FEV_1 decline (B and C). Positive staining was defined as brown–yellow particles or tan–brown particles in the cytoplasm (magnification, 200×). (**A**) Airway tissue with weak staining (score 1); (**B**) airway tissue with moderate staining (score 6); (**C**) airway tissue with strong staining (score 12); (**D**) the immunohistochemistry score of MMP-9 was determined through a semi-quantitative assessment by calculating the intensity and percentage of positive cells. The central horizontal lines indicate the median, and the error bars (upper and lower horizontal lines) are the 75th percentile and 25th percentile, respectively, *** $p < 0.0001$. IHC, immunohistochemistry; MMP-9, matrix metalloproteinase-9.

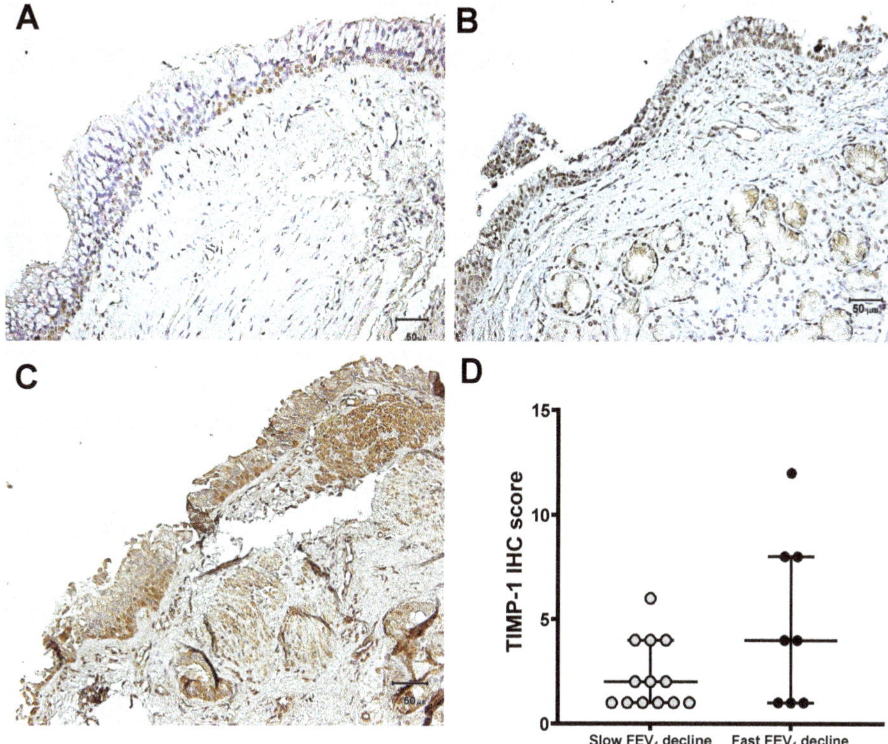

Figure 2. Immunohistochemical expression levels of TIMP-1. An avidin–biotin complex immunohistochemical study for TIMP-1 expression was performed in airway tissues derived from asthmatic patients with a slow FEV_1 decline (A and B) and a rapid FEV_1 decline (C). Positive staining was defined as brown–yellow particles or tan–brown particles in the cytoplasm (magnification, 200×). (**A**) airway tissue with weak staining (score 1); (**B**) airway tissue with moderate staining (score 6); (**C**) airway tissue with strong staining (score 12); (**D**) immunostaining of TIMP-1 was scored through a semi-quantitative assessment by calculating the intensity and percentage of positive cells. The central horizontal lines indicate the median, and the error bars (upper and lower horizontal lines) are the 75th percentile and 25th percentile, respectively. IHC, immunohistochemistry; TIMP-1, tissue inhibitor of matrix metalloproteinase-1.

2.6. Hematoxylin and Eosin Staining (H and E)

The thickness of the epithelium, basement membrane, and subepithelial layer was investigated by H and E staining for 20 min at room temperature. The results were visualized using an Olympus BX51 microscope (Olympus Corporation, Tokyo, Japan).

2.7. MMP-9 and TIMP-1 ELISA

Quantitative sandwich-type enzyme-linked immunoassay techniques (ELISA) were used to assay the secretory products in macrophage supernatants [26]. MMP-9 and TIMP-1 kits were used (Amersham Life Sciences, Arlington Heights, IL, USA) according to the manufacturer's instructions. The optical density was measured with a spectrophotometer set to 450 mM for all assays. Quantification was performed by interpolation from a standard curve.

2.8. Statistical Analysis

Data were presented as mean ± SEM. The data were analyzed using a Student's *t*-test for paired or unpaired data. For data with even or uneven or variation, a Mann–Whitney U test or Wilcoxon signed rank test was used for unpaired or paired data, respectively. ANOVA with post hoc analysis was used when comparing data from three groups; $p < 0.05$ was considered significant.

3. Results

3.1. Demographic Features of Patients

Table 1 summarizes pulmonary function tests on asthmatic patients and normal subjects. The FVC, FEV_1, and levels of PC_{20} in methacholine tests demonstrated no difference between the two groups of asthmatics. Initially, the PC_{20} was similar in both asthmatic groups. After 5 years, airway hyperresponsiveness of patients with a slow FEV_1 decline was significantly decreased (PC_{20} from 1.87 ± 0.52 to 3.52 ± 0.81 mg/dL, $n = 13$, $p < 0.05$), while that of asthmatics with a fast FEV_1 decline demonstrated an increased airway hyperresponsiveness (PC_{20} from 3.46 ± 1.02 to 1.14 ± 0.34 mg/dL, $n = 8$, $p < 0.05$) (Figure 3).

Table 1. Baseline characteristics of the normal subjects and asthmatics.

Clinical Features	Normal Subjects ($n = 10$)	Asthma ($n = 13$) Slow FEV_1 Decline	Asthma ($n = 8$) Fast FEV_1 Decline
Age, year	47.6 ± 2.8	49.2 ± 3.4	49.4 ± 3.7
Gender, F/M	5/5	5/8	4/4
FVC, L	3.4 ± 0.3	3.0 ± 0.3	3.3 ± 0.2
FVC, % pred.	95.2 ± 4.7	88.8 ± 5.7	94.0 ± 5.0
FEV_1, L	2.6 ± 0.3	2.1 ± 0.3	2.4 ± 0.2
FEV_1, % pred.	82.4 ± 4.5	72.2 ± 6.3	77.6 ± 4.8
FEV_1/FVC	83.3 ± 2.7	68.7 ± 3.6	73.8 ± 4.0
Annual FEV_1 decline, mL/year		−18.2 ± 9.7	135.8 ± 14.0 ***
PC_{20}, mg/dL	> 25	1.9 ± 0.5	3.5 ± 1.0

Values are mean ± SEM; F/M, female/male; FEV_1: forced expiratory volume in one second; FVC: forced vital capacity; % pred., percent of predicted value; L: liter; PC_{20}: value of methacholine provocative concentration causing a 20% decrease in FEV_1. *** $p < 0.0001$ compared with group A.

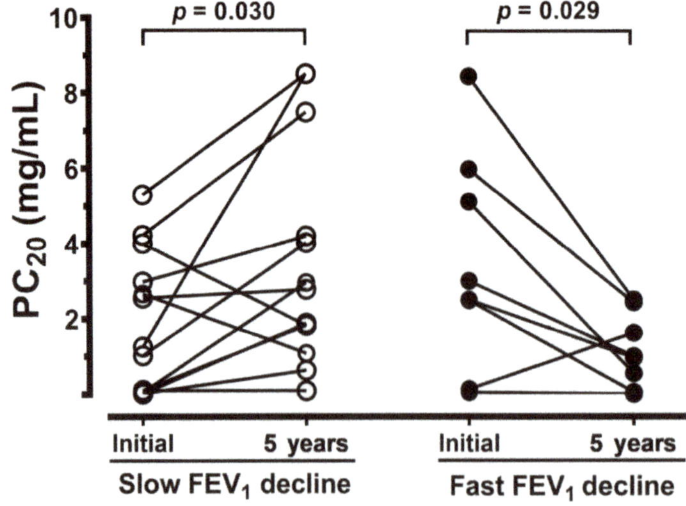

Figure 3. The individual concentration of methacholine provocation in asthmatic patients who had a slow FEV_1 decline (open circle, $n = 13$) or a fast FEV_1 decline (solid circle, $n = 8$) after receiving 5 years of inhaled anti-asthma medicine, compared with the initial values (initial). The significance is indicated.

3.2. Cellular Profile Analysis of Bronchoalveolar Lavage

The cellularity of lavage fluid was similar between the asthmatic groups but was significantly lower in normal subjects. Compared to normal subjects, there was an increase in the percentage of eosinophils and lymphocytes and a corresponding decrease in the proportion of alveolar macrophages in asthmatics with either a fast or a slow decline in FEV_1 (Table 2). The cellularity of different cell types in normal subjects and asthmatics is presented in Figure 4 and had the same result as the percentage of cell types. The asthmatic patients with a fast FEV_1 decline over 5 years had a marked rise in the proportion of neutrophils compared with those who exhibited a slow decline in FEV_1 or normal subjects (Table 2). In addition, the magnitude of the annual FEV_1 decline in asthmatics was highly correlated with the cellularity of neutrophils in BAL (r = 0.718, n = 21, p = 0.0002).

Table 2. Characteristics of bronchoalveolar lavage.

Cell Profile	Normal (n = 10)	Asthma (n = 13) Slow FEV_1 Decline	Asthma (n = 8) Fast FEV_1 Decline
Total cell count, $\times 10^6$ cells	11.9 ± 1.7	21.2 ± 6.6 **	34.2 ± 10.1 **
Recovered volume, %	62.9 ± 3.7	44.6 ± 5.0	47.5 ± 5.8
Cell viability, %	94.4 ± 1.4	94.1 ± 1.3	91.6 ± 2.5
AMs, %	97.5 ± 0.6	87.9 ± 2.3 **	84.3 ± 5.3 **
Lymphocytes, %	1.5 ± 0.5	8.2 ± 1.8 **	8.0 ± 3.6 **
Neutrophils, %	0.7 ± 0.2	1.4 ± 0.3	5.0 ± 1.5 **#
Eosinophils, %	0.2 ± 0.1	2.4 ± 1.1 *	2.6 ± 1.1 *

Abbreviation: AMs = alveolar macrophages; Values present as mean ± SEM; * $p < 0.05$, ** $p < 0.01$ compared with normal subjects. # $p < 0.05$ compared with normal subjects or asthma with a slow FEV_1 decline.

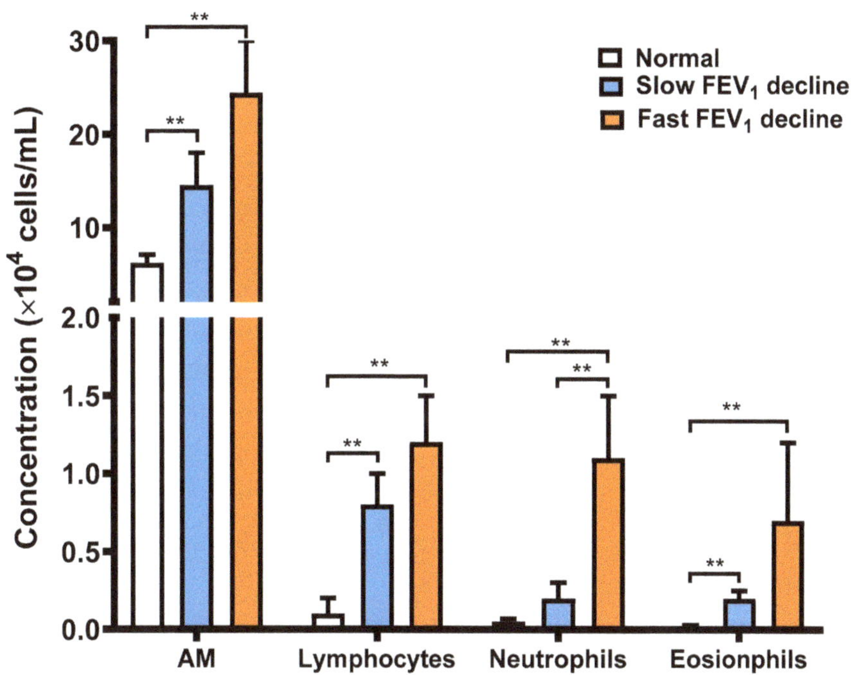

Figure 4. The concentration of different cell types in bronchoalveolar lavage fluid derived from normal subjects (Normal, n = 10), and asthmatic patients with a slow FEV_1 decline (Slow FEV_1 decline, n = 13) or a fast FEV_1 decline (Fast FEV_1 decline, n = 8); ** $p < 0.01$ is indicated.

3.3. Expression of MMP-9 and TIMP-1 in Bronchial Biopsies

MMP-9 was expressed in airway tissue obtained from asthmatics, especially in epithelial cells, inflammatory cells, or gland cells (Figure 1A–C). Furthermore, asthmatic patients with a rapid FEV_1 decline had a significantly higher immunohistochemistry (IHC) score of MMP-9 (median, 8.5; IQR, 6.5–9.0), when compared with asthmatic patients with a slow FEV_1 decline (median, 2.0; IQR, 1.0–4.0) ($p < 0.0001$, Figure 1D). The IHC score of TIMP-1 expression in the airway showed no significant difference between the two groups (Figure 2D). The thickness of the basement membrane (15.5 ± 2.2 µm, $n = 8$, $p = 0.0002$) and subepithelial layer (138.3 ± 12.2 µm, $n = 8$, $p < 0.0001$) in asthmatics with a fast FEV_1 decline was significantly increased (Table 3). However, the asthmatics with a slow FEV_1 decline had a thinner basement membrane and subepithelial layer.

Table 3. The thickness of airway structure in patients with asthma.

Airway Structure	Asthma (n = 13) Slow FEV_1 Decline	Asthma (n = 8) Fast FEV_1 Decline	p Value
Epithelium, µm	27.2 ± 6.3	23.8 ± 7.4	0.733
Basement membrane, µm	7.0 ± 0.6	15.5 ± 2.2	0.0002
Subepithelium, µm	37.8 ± 4.2	138.3 ± 12.2	<0.0001

Data expressed as mean ± SEM.

3.4. Generation of MMP-9 and TIMP-1 From Macrophages

Most importantly, alveolar macrophages (AMs) from chronic asthma with a fast FEV_1 decline spontaneously released a higher amount of MMP-9 (8.52 ± 3.53 ng/mL, $n = 8$, $p < 0.05$) than those of asthma with a slow FEV_1 decline (0.99 ± 0.20 ng/mL, $n = 13$) or normal subjects (0.47 ± 0.20 ng/mL, $n = 10$). The level of MMP-9 was significantly higher in asthma with a slow FEV_1 decline compared to normal subjects (Figure 5A). Compared with MMP-9, concentrations of the inhibitor, TIMP-1, were higher in supernatants from normal subjects and asthmatic groups (Figure 5B). A significantly higher level of TIMP-1 released from AMs into the culture medium in asthmatics with a slow FEV_1 decline over 5 years was observed when compared to that of asthmatics with a fast decline in FEV_1 or normal subjects (Figure 5B). When data are expressed as the molar ratio of enzyme to inhibitor, chronic asthmatics with a fast FEV_1 decline in 5 years had a significant increase in this ratio in AMs (Figure 6). The ratio of MMP-9/TIMP-1 showed no difference between the normal subjects and those suffering from chronic asthma with a slow FEV_1 decline at the 5-year follow-up (Figure 6).

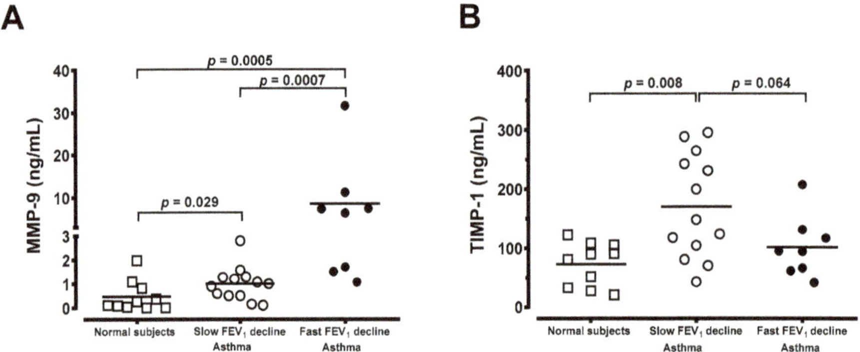

Figure 5. Individual concentration of (**A**) MMP-9 and (**B**) TIMP-1 spontaneously released from alveolar macrophages after 24 h culture in normal subjects (open square, $n = 10$), chronic asthma with a slow FEV_1 decline (open circle, $n = 13$), and chronic asthma with a fast FEV_1 decline in (solid circle, $n = 8$). The significance is indicated.

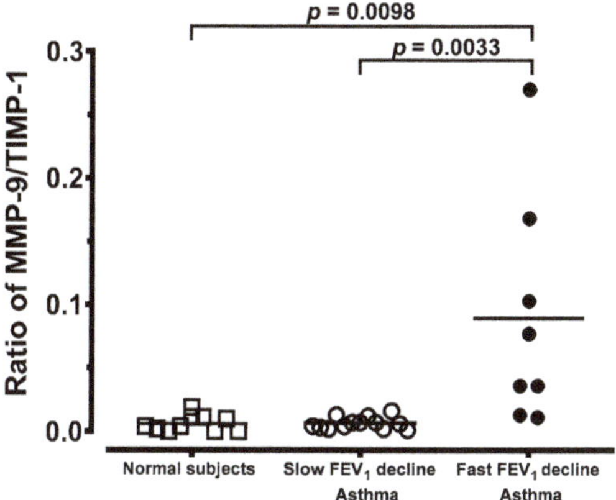

Figure 6. Ratio of MMP-9 to TIMP-1. Data are expressed as the individual value of MMP-9 to TIMP-1 ratio in normal subjects (open square, $n = 10$), chronic asthma with a slow FEV_1 decline (open circle, $n = 13$), and chronic asthma with a fast FEV_1 decline (solid circle, $n = 8$). The p values are presented.

The generation of MMP-9 released from AMs was positively associated with the annual decline in FEV_1 (r = 570, $n = 21$, $p < 0.01$) (Figure 7A). However, there was no correlation between the level of TIMP-1 and the annual decline in FEV_1 (Figure 6B). When the MMP-9/TIMP-1 ratios were plotted against the magnitude of FEV_1 change, the annual decline in FEV_1 was significantly proportional to the ratio of MMP-9/TIMP-1 (r = 0.584, $n = 21$, $p < 0.01$) (Figure 7C).

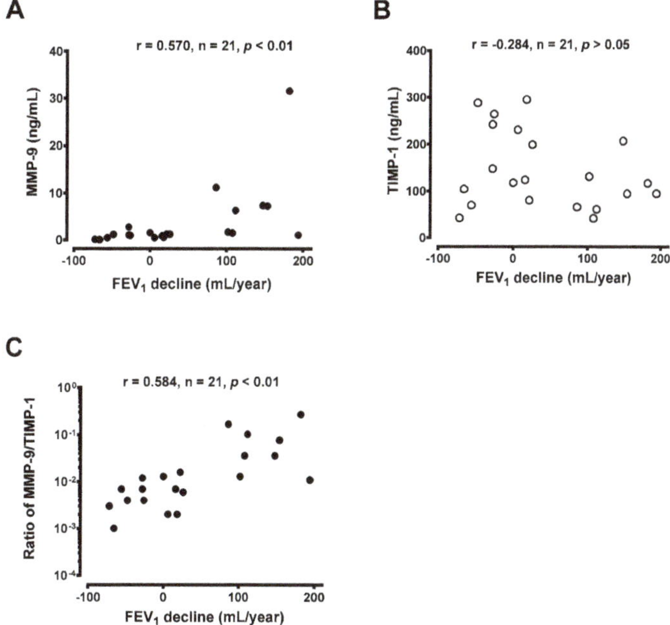

Figure 7. Correlation of the level of (**A**) MMP-9 and (**B**) TIMP-1 released from alveolar macrophages (AMs) cultured for 24 h with the magnitude of FEV_1 decline per year (mL/year) from patients with chronic asthma receiving inhaled corticosteroids. (**C**) Correlation of the MMP-9/TIMP-1 ratio in 24 h AM culture with the magnitude of FEV_1 decline per year over 5 years from patients with chronic asthma receiving inhaled corticosteroids.

4. Discussion

We demonstrated that the levels of MMP-9 expression in the epithelium, inflammatory cells, and submucosa as determined from immunostaining showed upregulation in asthmatic patients who regularly received inhaled corticosteroids and who had a rapid decline in pulmonary function at 5-year follow-up. The alveolar macrophages from these unstable asthmatics also spontaneously released higher amounts of MMP-9. Most importantly, the MMP-9 level and MMP-9/TIMP-1 ratio produced from AMs were significantly decreased in chronic asthma with a slow FEV_1 decline. The higher levels of TIMP-1 released from cultured AM were observed in clinically stable asthmatics. The magnitude of annual FEV_1 decline was proportional to the MMP-9 generation and the ratio of MMP-9/TIMP-1 released from alveolar macrophages, even though the patients had regularly received inhaled corticosteroids. An increased thickness of the basement membrane and subepithelial layer was observed in asthmatics with a fast FEV_1 decline. Taken together, MMPs (mainly MMP-9) and TIMP-1 may contribute to progressive loss of lung function and increased cellular matrix fibrosis of the airway wall in chronic asthmatics who demonstrated a poor response to anti-asthma treatments.

We reported that the generation of MMP-9 from alveolar macrophages and the ratio of MMP-9/TIMP-1 are strongly associated with the magnitude of FEV_1 decline in chronic asthma, which is in agreement with the data of Vignola et al. [21]. The same authors have stressed the potential importance of MMP-9 and TIMP-1 imbalance in asthma by showing that the basal airway caliber was related to the ratio of MMP-9 to TIMP-1. It was reported that concentrations of MMP-9 in airway neutrophils and BAL fluid revealed a significant correlation after allergen challenge [31]. We also observed that the BAL fluid of asthmatics with a rapid decline in FEV_1 exhibited a higher amount of neutrophils, while that of stable asthmatics did not show an increased amount of neutrophils. The cellularity of neutrophils in BAL was highly correlated to the annual FEV_1 decline in asthmatics. These observations raise the possibility that neutrophils may cause injury to the airway and result in further remodeling of chronic unstable asthma, as has been suggested by studies showing persistent bronchial neutrophilia in severe asthma and status asthmatics [32]. Our results strongly suggest that alveolar macrophages and neutrophils may be important sources of MMP-9 release, leading some asthmatic patients—who are poorly responsive to inhaled corticosteroid treatment—to develop progressive irreversible airway scarring and fibrosis. Accordingly, an excess of MMP-9 release in the airway was associated with impairment in the lung function of FEV_1.

It is thought that the imbalance between MMPs and TIMPs may play an important role in the process of the degradation and synthesis of the extracellular matrix of the airway. Hoshino et al. [33] reported that deposition of the basement membrane matrix components—including collagen III, collagen V, and tenascin—in asthma correlated to the upregulated expression of MMP-9 and, therefore, airway remodeling in asthma could cause airflow obstruction and airway hyperresponsiveness. As well as the consuming mechanisms of the extracellular matrix, MMP-9 may modulate cytokines and other proteases [34]. MMP-9 may degrade alpha1-antitrypsin and preserve neutrophil elastase activity [35], thus activating the function of fibroblasts [36]. In addition, the binding of MMP-9 to CD44 can result in the release of TGF-β1 and, therefore, regulate extracellular matrix remodeling via fibroblast activation [37]. MMP-9 may also potentiate angiogenesis by vascular endothelial growth factor activation [34,38] and increase the production of angiostatin [39]. Our results showed increased thickness in the submucosa and basement membrane, as well as higher expression of MMP-9 in chronic asthma with rapid pulmonary function decline. The asthmatics with a fast FEV_1 decline presented with higher airway hyperresponsiveness. Therefore, macrophages from these unstable asthmatics may release more MMP-9, leading to collagen deposition or neovascularization in the basement membrane of airways and contributing to airway hyperresponsiveness.

The TIMPs could bind to MMPs and inhibit their enzymatic activity. In our study, alveolar macrophages from chronic stable asthma patients responsive to inhaled corticosteroids released higher amounts of TIMP-1 than those of chronic unstable asthma patients who do not respond to inhaled corticosteroids or healthy subjects. Hoshino and colleagues [27] found that corticosteroid treatment can decrease the deposition of subepithelial collagen through downregulation of MMP-9 and upregulation of TIMP-1 in asthma. In addition, a higher level of TIMP in stable asthma potentially helps the airways to mitigate the degrading activities of MMPs [40]. Nevertheless, this process may restrict cell trafficking and tissue repair, and may cause increased deposition of the extracellular matrix through in vivo inhibition of MMP-9 or other MMPs. Russell et al. reported that the release and activity of MMP-9 and TIMP-1 by alveolar macrophages from patients with chronic obstructive pulmonary disease might be important in the development of COPD because these cells exhibit increased levels of MMP-9 elastolytic activity [41]. Meanwhile, Russell et al. also reported that dexamethasone prevented the increase in MMP-9 release, and increased TIMP-1 release. Similarly, alveolar macrophages released a higher amount of MMP-9 in chronic unstable asthma patients than those with stable asthma or normal subjects in our study (Figures 5 and 6). Asthmatic patients had higher cell counts of BAL, including total cell counts, macrophage, lymphocytes, neutrophils, and eosinophils than those observed in normal subjects in Table 2 and Figure 4. MMP-9 is known to be produced by several inflammatory or structural cells, including bronchial epithelial cells, eosinophils, mast cells, and alveolar macrophages, and these may have a greater contribution relative to neutrophils in chronic asthma. This means that persistent airway or lung inflammation of chronic unstable asthmatics may be less responsive to anti-asthma treatment, which may contribute to higher cellularity of inflammatory cells, thus leading to the increased amount of MMP-9.

Although our patients have received inhaled corticosteroids for more than 5 years, some of these patients still demonstrated a progressive decline in pulmonary function and persistent airway structure change. A report showed that a high dose of inhaled corticosteroids did not change the levels of MMP-1, MMP-9, and TIMP-1 in induced sputum [42], although other authors have described a significant decrease in MMP-9 in the bronchial biopsies of asthmatics treated with inhaled corticosteroids [27]. Our results revealed that inhaled corticosteroids do not modify the expression of MMP-9 and TIMP-1 in AMs in patients with chronic asthma exhibiting a rapid decline in FEV_1. Thus, inhaled corticosteroids cannot inhibit the airway remodeling of chronic asthma. Several reports have shown that neutrophil levels may increase in the airways in severe asthmatics or in patients with chronic asthma who exhibit a poor response to inhaled steroids [32,43]. Persistent generation of inflammatory products and their inhibitors in chronic asthma may cause airway injury and remodeling. The mechanisms should be further studied.

Previous reports revealed that MMP-9 increases in severe asthma [40,44], and that it may be the cause of airflow obstruction through the induction of airway structural changes [45]. The persistently high levels of MMP-9 indicate that the remodeling of airways may be initiated at the beginning of asthma development and may be expressed as severe asthma.

Extensive studies have revealed the role of MMPs in the pathogenesis of asthma, airway hyperresponsiveness (AHR), and asthma-associated airway remodeling [45,46]. MMP-9 was the first MMP to be investigated in depth for its role in the development of asthmatic pathology and was also the most highly expressed MMP in the BAL fluid and sputum of asthma patients [21,47]. Moreover, the high level of MMP-9 expression in bronchial biopsies from asthmatic patients [48] was associated with asthma severity [49] as well as the number of macrophages and neutrophils [50]. MMP-9 can degrade elastin and type IV collagen [51], an important component of the basement membrane and, thus, MMP-9 plays a role in the disruption of the basement membrane and contributes to increased ECM deposition, subepithelial fibrosis, and airway wall thickness [52]. Airway remodeling related to the thickness of the sub-basement membrane [45] has been linked to airway AHR and leads to the subsequent development of fixed airflow limitation and to a long-term decline in lung function in asthmatics [53]. Our recent study revealed that AMs produced excessive MMP-9 over TIMP-1, which was associated with increased AHR and was a predictor of the development of accelerated lung function decline [20]. Other MMPs, including MMP-1, -2, -3, or -12, are also studied as being involved in asthma [6]. MMP-1 is activated by mast cell tryptase, leading to a proproliferative extracellular matrix. The interactions of airway smooth muscle/mast cell contribute to asthma severity by transiently increasing MMP activation, thus inducing airway smooth muscle hyperplasia and AHR [54]. The potentially pro-remodeling roles for MMP-1 are involved in the promotion of airway smooth muscle proliferation. In stable mild-to-moderate asthma, MMP-2 in association with MMP-3 is released from bronchial fibroblasts and may have a negative effect on lung function and AHR [55]. However, studies on MMP-9 and MMP-2 double-knockout mice revealed that MMP-9, and not MMP-2, is the dominant airway MMP controlling inflammatory cell egression [56]. Although MMP-12 is suggested to be involved in asthma, this conclusion is based on studies in which mostly animal models are used [6]. In humans, the MMP-12-mediated pathological degradation of the ECM is associated with COPD patients [57]. Our study aimed to investigate whether the MMP released from AM was associated with AHR and increased expression in airways, thus contributing to subepithelial thickness and accelerated lung function decline. Therefore, our study focused on MMP-9. Nevertheless, a greater understanding of the involvement of MMPs in airway remodeling in asthma is indispensable and, thus, further studies are needed to examine the expression of other MMPs in airways and BAL fluid as well as their release from AMs.

Limitations

Alveolar macrophages are the predominant immune cells in the lung and are represented by the classically activated (or M1) and the alternatively activated (or M2) phenotypes according to their function [58]. Increased polarization and activation of M2 macrophages, which was induced by interleukin (IL)-4 and IL-13, are found in asthma and are suggested to be involved in asthma pathogenesis [59,60]. A previous study has shown that activation of M1 or M2 macrophages may upregulate a distinct group of MMPs and TIMP-3 [61]. A group of matrix metalloproteinases also influences M1/M2 polarization of macrophages [62]. However, our study did not investigate the association of MMP-9 with M1/M2 polarization in the asthma with accelerated lung function decline. Therefore, to understand the causal relationship of MMP-9 and M1/M2 macrophage activation in the development of airway remodeling in asthma, the macrophage polarization in BAL and airway tissue should be addressed in future studies.

5. Conclusions

We concluded that there was an increase in MMP-9 and MMP-9/TIMP-1 in airways and alveolar macrophages from chronic asthmatics with a rapid FEV_1 decline, despite having been regularly treated with inhaled corticosteroids. An increase in MMP-9 and MMP-9/TIMP-1 in airways or AMs could contribute to a greater decline in lung function in cases of chronic asthma and could therefore be used as an indicator of chronic airway inflammation.

Author Contributions: Conceptualization, F.-T.C., C.-Y.L., and C.-H.W.; Data curation, F.-T.C., C.-Y.L., C.-C.H., and J.-R.H.; Funding acquisition, C.-H.W.; Investigation, F.-T.C. and C.-H.W.; Methodology, C.-W.L., C.-C.H., J.-R.H., and T.-F.S.; Project administration, F.-T.C. and H.-Y.H.; Resources, C.-Y.L., C.-W.L., Y.-C.H., and C.-H.W.; Supervision, C.-H.W.; Validation, F.T.C. and C.-Y.L.; Writing—original draft, F.-T.C. and C.-H.W.; Review and editing, C.-H.W.

Funding: This research was funded by Chang Gung Memorial Hospital Research Project Grant (CMRPG3F1492, CMRPG3F1493, CMRPG3B1321, CMRPG3B1322, CMRPG3B1323, CMRPG3F1501, and CMRPG3F1502) and Taiwan National Science Research Project (NMRP) grant (NSC90-2314-B182A-036).

Conflicts of Interest: The authors declare no conflict of interest.

References

1. Sullivan, P.W.; Campbell, J.D.; Ghushchyan, V.H.; Globe, G. Outcomes before and after treatment escalation to Global Initiative for Asthma steps 4 and 5 in severe asthma. *Ann. Allergy Asthma Immunol.* **2015**, *114*, 462–469. [CrossRef] [PubMed]
2. Beasley, R.; Roche, W.; Holgate, S.T. Inflammatory processes in bronchial asthma. *Drugs* **1989**, *37* (Suppl. 1), 117–122. [CrossRef] [PubMed]

3. Prakash, Y.S.; Halayko, A.J.; Gosens, R.; Panettieri, R.A.; Camoretti-Mercado, B.; Penn, R.B. ATS Assembly on Respiratory Structure and Function. *Am. J. Respir. Crit. Care Med.* **2017**, *195*, e4–e19. [CrossRef] [PubMed]
4. Bai, T.R.; Cooper, J.; Koelmeyer, T.; Pare, P.D.; Weir, T.D. The effect of age and duration of disease on airway structure in fatal asthma. *Am. J. Respir. Crit. Care Med.* **2000**, *162*, 663–669. [CrossRef] [PubMed]
5. Holgate, S.T.; Lackie, P.; Wilson, S.; Roche, W.; Davies, D. Bronchial epithelium as a key regulator of airway allergen sensitization and remodeling in asthma. *Am. J. Respir. Crit. Care Med.* **2000**, *162*, S113–S117. [CrossRef]
6. Vandenbroucke, R.E.; Dejonckheer, E.; Libert, C. A therapeutic role for matrix metalloproteinase inhibitors in lung diseases? *Eur. Respir. J.* **2011**, *38*, 1200–1214. [CrossRef] [PubMed]
7. Chaudhuri, R.; McSharry, C.; Brady, J.; Donnelly, I.; Grierson, C.; McGuinness, S.; Jolly, L.; Weir, C.J.; Messow, C.M.; Spears, M.; et al. Sputum matrix metalloproteinase-12 in patients with chronic obstructive pulmonary disease and asthma: Relationship to disease severity. *J. Allergy Clin. Immunol.* **2012**, *129*, 655–663. [CrossRef]
8. Oka, S.; Furukawa, H.; Shimada, K.; Hayakawa, H.; Fukui, N.; Tsuchiya, N.; Tohma, S. Serum biomarker analysis of collagen disease patients with acute-onset diffuse interstitial lung disease. *BMC Immunol.* **2013**, *14*, 9. [CrossRef]
9. Hu, C.; Wang, J.; Xu, Y.; Li, X.; Chen, H.; Bunjhoo, H.; Xiong, W.; Xu, Y.; Zhao, J. Current evidence on the relationship between five polymorphisms in the matrix metalloproteinases (MMP) gene and lung cancer risk: A meta-analysis. *Gene* **2013**, *517*, 65–71. [CrossRef]
10. Craig, V.J.; Quintero, P.A.; Fyfe, S.E.; Patel, A.S.; Knolle, M.D.; Kobzik, L.; Owen, C.A. Profibrotic activities for matrix metalloproteinase-8 during bleomycin-mediated lung injury. *J. Immunol.* **2013**, *190*, 4283–4296. [CrossRef]
11. Ko, F.W.; Diba, C.; Roth, M.; Patel, A.S.; Knolle, M.D.; Kobzik, L.; Owen, C.A. A comparison of airway and serum matrix metalloproteinase-9 activity among normal subjects, asthmatic patients, and patients with asthmatic mucus hypersecretion. *Chest* **2005**, *127*, 1919–1927. [CrossRef] [PubMed]
12. Castano, R.; Miedinger, D.; Maghni, K.; Ghezzo, H.; Trudeau, C.; Castellanos, L.; Wattiez, M.; Vandenplas, O.; Malo, J.L. Matrix metalloproteinase-9 increases in the sputum from allergic occupational asthma patients after specific inhalation challenge. *Int. Arch. Allergy Immunol.* **2013**, *160*, 161–164. [CrossRef]
13. Hong, Z.; Lin, Y.M.; Qin, X.; Peng, J.L. Serum MMP-9 is elevated in children with asthma. *Mol. Med. Rep.* **2012**, *5*, 462–464. [CrossRef] [PubMed]
14. Bratcher, P.E.; Weathington, N.M.; Nick, H.J.; Jackson, P.L.; Snelgrove, R.J.; Gaggar, A. MMP-9 cleaves SP-D and abrogates its innate immune functions in vitro. *PLoS ONE* **2012**, *7*, e41881. [CrossRef] [PubMed]
15. Page, K.; Ledford, J.R.; Zhou, P.; Wills-Karp, M. A TLR2 agonist in German cockroach frass activates MMP-9 release and is protective against allergic inflammation in mice. *J. Immunol.* **2009**, *183*, 3400–3408. [CrossRef] [PubMed]
16. Barbaro, M.P.; Spanevello, A.; Palladino, G.P.; Salerno, F.G.; Lacedonia, D.; Carpagnano, G.E. Exhaled matrix metalloproteinase-9 (MMP-9) in different biological phenotypes of asthma. *Eur. J. Intern. Med.* **2014**, *25*, 92–96. [CrossRef] [PubMed]
17. Khokha, R.; Murthy, A.; Weiss, A. Metalloproteinases and their natural inhibitors in inflammation and immunity. *Nat. Rev. Immunol.* **2013**, *13*, 649–665. [CrossRef] [PubMed]
18. Fanjul-Fernández, M.; Folgueras, A.R.; Cabrera, S.; López-Otín, C. Matrix metalloproteinases: Evolution, gene regulation and functional analysis in mouse models. *Biochim. Biophys. Acta.* **2010**, *1803*, 3–19. [CrossRef] [PubMed]
19. Roche, W.R.; Beasley, R.; Williams, J.H.; Holgate, S.T. Subepithelial fibrosis in the bronchi of asthmatics. *Lancet* **1989**, *1*, 520–524. [CrossRef]
20. Lo, C.Y.; Huang, H.Y.; He, J.R.; Huang, T.T.; Heh, C.C.; Sheng, T.F.; Chung, K.F.; Kuo, H.P.; Wang, C.H. Increased matrix metalloproteinase-9 to tissue inhibitor of metalloproteinase-1 ratio in smokers with airway hyperresponsiveness and accelerated lung function decline. *Int. J. Chronic Obstr. Pulm. Dis.* **2018**, *13*, 1135–1144. [CrossRef]
21. Vignola, A.M.; Riccobono, L.; Mirabella, A.; Profita, M.; Chanez, P.; Bellia, V.; Mautino, G.; D'accardi, P.; Bousquet, J.; Bonsignore, G. Sputum metalloproteinase-9/tissue inhibitor of metalloproteinase-1 ratio correlates with airflow obstruction in asthma and chronic bronchitis. *Am. J. Respir. Crit. Care Med.* **1998**, *158*, 1945–1950. [CrossRef] [PubMed]

22. Tanaka, H.; Miyazaki, N.; Oashi, K.; Tanaka, S.; Ohmichi, M.; Abe, S. Sputum matrix metalloproteinase-9: Tissue inhibitor of metalloproteinase-1 ratio in acute asthma. *J. Allergy Clin. Immunol.* **2000**, *105*, 900–905. [CrossRef] [PubMed]
23. Bosse, M.; Chakir, J.; Rouabhia, M.; Boulet, L.P.; Audette, M.; Laviolette, M. Serum matrix metalloproteinase-9: Tissue inhibitor of metalloproteinase-1 ratio correlates with steroid responsiveness in moderate to severe asthma. *Am. J. Respir. Crit. Care Med.* **1999**, *159*, 596–602. [CrossRef] [PubMed]
24. Sagel, S.D.; Kapsner, R.K.; Osberg, I. Induced sputum matrix metalloproteinase-9 correlates with lung function and airway inflammation in children with cystic fibrosis. *Pediatric Pulmonol.* **2005**, *39*, 224–232. [CrossRef] [PubMed]
25. Matsumoto, H.; Niimi, A.; Takemura, M.; Ueda, T.; Minakuchi, M.; Tabuena, R.; Chin, K.; Mio, T.; Ito, Y.; Muro, S.; et al. Relationship of airway wall thickening to an imbalance between matrix metalloproteinase-9 and its inhibitor in asthma. *Thorax* **2005**, *60*, 277–281. [CrossRef] [PubMed]
26. Mercer, P.F.; Shute, J.K.; Bhowmik, A.; Donaldson, G.C.; Wedzicha, J.A.; Warner, J.A. MMP-9, TIMP-1 and inflammatory cells in sputum from COPD patients during exacerbation. *Respir. Res.* **2005**, *6*, 151. [CrossRef]
27. American Thoracic Society. Standards for the diagnosis and care of patients with chronic obstructive pulmonary disease (COPD) and asthma. This official statement of the American Thoracic Society was adopted by the ATS Board of Directors, November 1986. *Am. Rev. Respir. Dis.* **1987**, *136*, 225–244.
28. Broekema, M.; Volbeda, F.; Timens, W.; Dijkstra, A.; Lee, N.A.; Lee, J.J.; Lodewijk, M.E.; Postma, D.S.; Hylkema, M.N.; Ten Hacken, N.H. Airway eosinophilia in remission and progression of asthma: Accumulation with a fast decline of FEV(1). *Respir. Med.* **2010**, *104*, 1254–1262. [CrossRef]
29. Wang, C.H.; Liu, C.Y.; Lin, H.C.; Yu, C.T.; Chung, K.F.; Kuo, H.P. Increased exhaled nitric oxide in active pulmonary tuberculosis due to inducible NO synthase upregulation in alveolar macrophages. *Eur. Respir. J.* **1998**, *11*, 809–815. [CrossRef]
30. Hoshino, M.; Takahashi, M.; Takai, Y.; Sim, J. Inhaled corticosteroids decrease subepithelial collagen deposition by modulation of the balance between matrix metalloproteinase-9 and tissue inhibitor of metalloproteinase-1 expression in asthma. *J. Allergy Clin. Immunol.* **1999**, *104*, 356–363. [CrossRef]
31. Kelly, E.A.; Busse, W.W.; Jarjour, N.N. Increased matrix metalloproteinase-9 in the airway after allergen challenge. *Am. J. Respir. Crit. Care Med.* **2000**, *162*, 1157–1161. [CrossRef] [PubMed]
32. Ray, A.; Kolls, J.K. Neutrophilic inflammation in asthma and association with disease severity. *Trends Immunol.* **2017**, *38*, 942–954. [CrossRef] [PubMed]
33. Hoshino, M.; Nakamura, Y.; Sim, J.; Shimojo, J.; Isogai, S. Bronchial subepithelial fibrosis and expression of matrix metalloproteinase-9 in asthmatic airway inflammation. *J. Allergy Clin. Immunol.* **1998**, *102*, 783–788. [CrossRef]
34. Page-McCaw, A.; Ewald, A.J.; Werb, Z. Matrix metalloproteinases and the regulation of tissue remodelling. *Nat. Rev. Mol. Cell Biol.* **2007**, *8*, 221–233. [CrossRef] [PubMed]
35. Liu, Z.; Zhou, X.; Shapiro, S.D.; Shipley, J.M.; Twining, S.S.; Diaz, L.A.; Senior, R.M.; Werb, Z. The serpin alpha1-proteinase inhibitor is a critical substrate for gelatinase B/MMP-9 in vivo. *Cell* **2000**, *102*, 647–655. [CrossRef]
36. Zhu, Y.K.; Liu, X.D.; Skold, C.M.; Umino, T.; Wang, H.J.; Spurzem, J.R.; Kohyama, T.; Ertl, R.F.; Rennard, S.I. Synergistic neutrophil elastase-cytokine interaction degrades collagen in three-dimensional culture. *Am. J. Physiol. Lung Cell Mol. Physiol.* **2001**, *281*, L868–L878. [CrossRef] [PubMed]
37. Govindaraju, P.; Todd, L.; Shetye, S.; Monslow, J.; Pure, E. CD44-dependent inflammation, fibrogenesis, and collagenolysis regulates extracellular matrixremodeling and tensile strength during cutaneous wound healing. *Matrix Biol.* **2019**, *75–76*, 314–330. [CrossRef] [PubMed]
38. Lee, K.S.; Min, K.H.; Kim, S.R.; Park, S.J.; Park, H.S.; Jin, G.Y.; Lee, Y.C. Vascular endothelial growth factor modulates matrix metalloproteinase-9 expression in asthma. *Am. J. Respir. Crit. Care Med.* **2006**, *174*, 161–170. [CrossRef] [PubMed]
39. Basile, D.P.; Fredrich, K.; Weihrauch, D.; Hattan, N.; Chilian, W.M.; Patterson, B.C.; Sang, Q.A. Angiostatin and matrix metalloprotease expression following ischemic acute renal failure. *Am. J. Physiol. Ren. Physiol.* **2004**, *286*, F893–F902. [CrossRef]
40. Cataldo, D.D.; Gueders, M.; Munaut, C.; Rocks, N.; Bartsch, P.; Foidart, J.M.; Noël, A.; Louis, R. Matrix metalloproteinases and tissue inhibitors of matrix metalloproteinases mRNA transcripts in the bronchial secretions of asthmatics. *Lab. Investig.* **2004**, *84*, 418–424. [CrossRef]

41. Russell, R.E.; Culpitt, S.V.; DeMatos, C.; Donnelly, L.; Smith, M.; Wiggins, J.; Barnes, P.J. Release and activity of matrix metalloproteinase-9 and tissue inhibitor of metalloproteinase-1 by alveolar macrophages from patients with chronic obstructive pulmonary disease. *Am. J. Respir. Cell Mol. Biol.* **2002**, *26*, 602–609. [CrossRef] [PubMed]
42. Barnes, P.J. Corticosteroid resistance in airway disease. *Proc. Am. Thorac. Soc.* **2004**, *1*, 264–268. [CrossRef] [PubMed]
43. Wenzel, S.E. Asthma phenotypes: The evolution from clinical to molecular approaches. *Nat. Med.* **2012**, *18*, 716–725. [CrossRef] [PubMed]
44. The ENFUMOSA cross-sectional European multicentre study of the clinical phenotype of chronic severe asthma. European Network for Understanding Mechanisms of Severe Asthma. *Eur. Respir. J.* **2003**, *22*, 470–477.
45. Bergeron, C.; Tulic, M.K.; Hamid, Q. Airway remodelling in asthma: From bench side to clinical practice. *Can. Respir. J.* **2010**, *17*, e85–e93. [CrossRef]
46. Grzela, K.; Litwiniuk, M.; Zagorska, W.; Grzela, T. Airway remodeling in chronic obstructive pulmonary disease and asthma: The role of matrix metalloproteinase-9. *Arch. Immunol. Ther. Exp.* **2016**, *64*, 47–55. [CrossRef]
47. Mautino, G.; Oliver, N.; Chanez, P.; Bousquet, J.; Capony, F. Increased release of matrix metalloproteinase-9 in bronchoalveolar lavage fluid and by alveolar macrophages of asthmatics. *Am. J. Respir. Cell Mol. Biol.* **1997**, *17*, 583–591. [CrossRef]
48. Han, Z.; Zhong, N. Expression of matrix metalloproteinases MMP-9 within the airways in asthma. *Respir. Med.* **2003**, *97*, 563–567. [CrossRef]
49. Wenzel, S.E.; Balzar, S.; Cundall, M.; Chu, H.W. Subepithelial basement membrane immunoreactivity for matrix metalloproteinase 9: Association with asthma severity, neutrophilic inflammation, and wound repair. *J. Allergy Clin. Immunol.* **2003**, *111*, 1345–1352. [CrossRef]
50. Ventura, I.; Vega, A.; Chacón, P.; Chamorro, C.; Aroca, R.; Gómez, E.; Bellido, V.; Puente, Y.; Blanca, M.; Monteseirín, J. Neutrophils from allergic asthmatic patients produce and release metalloproteinase-9 upon direct exposure to allergens. *Allergy* **2014**, *69*, 898–905. [CrossRef]
51. Kostamo, K.; Tervahartiala, T.; Sorsa, T.; Richardson, M.; Toskala, E. Metalloproteinase function in chronic rhinosinusitis with nasal polyposis. *Laryngoscope* **2007**, *117*, 638–643. [CrossRef] [PubMed]
52. Vignola, A.M.; Kips, J.; Bousquet, J. Tissue remodeling as a feature of persistent asthma. *J. Allergy Clin. Immunol.* **2000**, *105*, 1041–1053. [CrossRef] [PubMed]
53. Ward, C.; Pais, M.; Bish, R.; Reid, D.; Feltis, B.; Johns, D.; Walters, E.H. Airway inflammation, basement membrane thickening and bronchial hyperresponsiveness in asthma. *Thorax* **2002**, *57*, 309–316. [CrossRef] [PubMed]
54. Naveed, S.U.; Clements, D.; Jackson, D.J.; Philp, C.; Billington, C.K.; Soomro, I.; Reynolds, C.; Harrison, T.W.; Johnston, S.L.; Shaw, D.E.; et al. Matrix metalloproteinase-1 activation contributes to airway smooth muscle growth and asthma severity. *Am. J. Respir. Crit. Care Med.* **2017**, *195*, 1000–1009. [CrossRef]
55. Todorova, L.; Bjermer, L.; Miller-Larsson, A.; Westergren-Thorsson, G. Relationship between matrix production by bronchial fibroblasts and lung function and AHR in asthma. *Respir. Med.* **2010**, *104*, 1799–1808. [CrossRef] [PubMed]
56. Corry, D.B.; Kiss, A.; Song, L.Z.; Song, L.; Xu, J.; Lee, S.H.; Werb, Z.; Kheradmand, F. Overlapping and independent contributions of MMP2 and MMP9 to lung allergic inflammatory cell egression through decreased CC chemokines. *FASEB J.* **2004**, *18*, 995–997. [CrossRef]
57. Churg, A.; Zhou, S.; Wright, J.L. Series "matrix metalloproteinases in lung health and disease": Matrix metalloproteinases in COPD. *Eur. Respir. J.* **2012**, *39*, 197–209. [CrossRef]
58. Gordon, S. Alternative activation of macrophages. *Nat. Rev. Immunol.* **2003**, *3*, 23–35. [CrossRef]
59. Melgert, B.N.; ten Hacken, N.H.; Rutgers, B.; Timens, W.; Postma, D.S.; Hylkema, M.N. More alternative activation of macrophages in lungs of asthmatic patients. *J. Allergy Clin. Immunol.* **2011**, *127*, 831–833. [CrossRef]
60. Girodet, P.O.; Nguyen, D.; Mancini, J.D.; Hundal, M.; Zhou, X.; Israel, E.; Cernadas, M. Alternative macrophage activation is increased in asthma. *Am. J. Respir. Cell Mol. Biol.* **2016**, *55*, 467–475. [CrossRef]

61. Huang, W.C.; Sala-Newby, G.B.; Susana, A.; Johnson, J.L.; Newby, A.C. Classical macrophage activation up-regulates several matrix metalloproteinases through mitogen activated protein kinases and nuclear factor-κB. *PLoS ONE* **2012**, *7*, e42507. [CrossRef]
62. Craig, V.J.; Zhang, L.; Hagood, J.S.; Owen, C.A. Matrix metalloproteinases as therapeutic targets for idiopathic pulmonary fibrosis. *Am. J. Respir. Cell Mol. Biol.* **2015**, *53*, 585–600. [CrossRef]

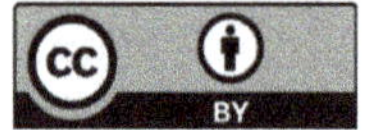

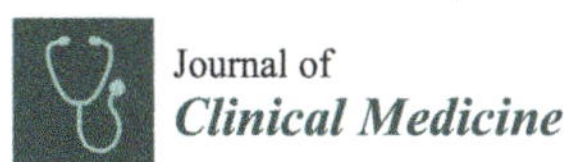

Journal of
Clinical Medicine

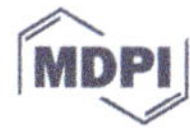

Review

Lung Microbiome in Asthma: Current Perspectives

Konstantinos Loverdos [1], Georgios Bellos [2], Louiza Kokolatou [2], Ioannis Vasileiadis [1], Evangelos Giamarellos [3], Matteo Pecchiari [4], Nikolaos Koulouris [1], Antonia Koutsoukou [1] and Nikoletta Rovina [1,*]

1 ICU, 1st Department of Pulmonary Medicine, "Sotiria" Hospital; Athens School of Medicine, National and Kapodistrian University of Athens, 11527 Athens, Greece; kloverdos@yahoo.com (K.L.); ioannisvmed@yahoo.gr (I.V.); koulnik@med.uoa.gr (N.K.); koutsoukou@yahoo.gr (A.K.)

2 Koropi Academic Health Care Center, Koropi, 19400 Attica, Greece; geobellos1010@yahoo.gr (G.B.); louikok@gmail.com (L.K.)

3 4th Department of Internal Medicine, Attikon University Hospital, 12462 Athens, Greece; egiamarel@med.uoa.gr

4 Dipartimento di Fisiopatologia e dei Trapianti, Università degli Studi di Milano, 20122 Milan, Italy; matteo.pecchiari@unimi.it

* Correspondence: nikrovina@med.uoa.gr; Tel.: +30-210-7763650

Received: 29 October 2019; Accepted: 12 November 2019; Published: 14 November 2019

Abstract: A growing body of evidence implicates the human microbiome as a potentially influential player actively engaged in shaping the pathogenetic processes underlying the endotypes and phenotypes of chronic respiratory diseases, particularly of the airways. In this article, we specifically review current evidence on the characteristics of lung microbiome, and specifically the bacteriome, the modes of interaction between lung microbiota and host immune system, the role of the "lung–gut axis", and the functional effects thereof on asthma pathogenesis. We also attempt to explore the possibilities of therapeutic manipulation of the microbiome, aiming at the establishment of asthma prevention strategies and the optimization of asthma treatment.

Keywords: microbiome; pathogenesis; inflammation; immune responses; asthma

---

1. Introduction

Asthma is the most common chronic respiratory disease, affecting more than 300 million people of all ages worldwide and killing about 250,000 of them each year [1], posing a substantial socioeconomic burden, especially in low- and middle-income countries. Asthma is a multifactorial and heterogeneous disease, comprising several different disease "phenotypes" and "endotypes" [2–4]. The current approach acknowledging that different phenotypes may share a common endotype and vice versa and, more important, that the disease phenotype may change over time has boosted our understanding on asthma pathogenesis and facilitated the development of novel targeted biological therapies, especially where they are most needed—that is severe corticosteroid-insensitive asthma [5]. However, while highly effective biologics are now available, and several more are in the pipeline for severe uncontrolled asthmatics with the Th2-high endotype [6], an almost-empty therapeutic arsenal is the case for those with the Th2-low endotype. Moreover, given the fact that Th2 inflammatory markers are absent in up to 50% of asthmatic patients (although an even higher corresponding percentage of 76% was reported in a very recent randomized controlled trial of patients with mild persistent asthma) [7,8], it is clear that further research is urgently needed to shed light on the biological pathways leading to non-eosinophilic asthma and, thus, promote the discovery of new treatment strategies for this large group of patients.

A growing body of evidence implicates the human microbiome as a potentially influential player that is actively engaged in shaping the pathogenetic processes underlying the aforementioned and other unresolved issues both in asthma [9,10] and in the other chronic respiratory diseases, particularly of the airways [11–13]. In contrast to earlier beliefs, a well-developed metabolically active microbial community, termed lung microbiota, resides in the lower respiratory tract of healthy humans. The entire habitat, including the microorganisms (bacteria, archaea, lower and higher eukaryotes, and viruses), their genomes (i.e., genes), and the surrounding environmental conditions are defined as the lung microbiome [14]. The latter is involved in a constant cross-talk with the host, and the same applies for the other bacterial communities residing in and on the human body, as well, with the most prominent being the gut microbiota, forming the "gut–lung axis" [15]. The diverse mechanisms mediating this cross-talk are now being gradually recognized. Under normal conditions; the interaction between the microbiota and the host confers mutual benefits for both ("symbiosis"). However, we are becoming increasingly cognizant of the fact that lung microbiota composition and diversity are affected in disease (including asthma) and that these changes can be translated in altered host immune responses, influencing asthma susceptibility, phenotype, exacerbation pattern, and treatment responsiveness ("dysbiosis" instead of "symbiosis").

In this article, we review current evidence on the characteristics of lung microbiome, the modes of interaction between lung microbiota and host immune system, the role of the "lung–gut axis" and the functional effects thereof on asthma pathogenesis. We also attempt to explore the possibilities of therapeutic manipulation of the microbiome, aiming at the establishment of asthma prevention strategies and the optimization of asthma treatment.

2. Microbiome

2.1. Historical Perspectives

The perception of the existence of bacteria inhabiting certain parts of the human body without causing disease is not new. For decades, diverse microbial genera were isolated after in vitro cultivation of biological samples collected from healthy individuals. However, the sensitivity of these traditional culture-dependent microbiological methods was severely limited. For instance, in an early study, it was estimated that only 24% of the entire microbiota present in an adult male fecal sample could be recovered by cultivation [16]. Using a variety of media and incubation methods, the corresponding sensitivity of in vitro cultivation for bacterial species identification in bronchoalveolar lavage samples of healthy individuals was substantially higher (61%), but it was still limited [17]. However, the exact role and teleology of this "normal (micro) flora" remained largely unknown, although it was postulated that changes in its composition could be detrimental, as in the case of antibiotic-induced *Clostridium difficile* overgrowth in the large intestine of patients with pseudomembranous colitis [18]. The advent of novel molecular techniques for microbiological profiling, with the most important being the implementation of polymerase chain reaction (PCR) amplification and sequencing of the highly specific and ubiquitous among bacteria 16S-rRNA gene, led to a tremendous progress in our understanding of the extent, diversity, composition, and location of the sum of microbial communities living inside or on the human organism (now termed microbiota instead of normal flora) [19]. Large-scale research collaborations, such as the two phases of the Human Microbiome Program (HMP), funded by the US National Institutes of Health (NIH), and the Metagenomics of the Human Intestinal Tract (MetaHIT) project, funded by the European Community, established enormous reference databases of human microbiota genomes and metagenomes, after analyzing dozens of thousands of samples derived from 48 primary sites (mostly feces) in hundreds of healthy individuals and patients with specific conditions or disorders [20–24]. Based on these advances, it is now estimated that human microbiome consists of approximately 3.8×10^{13} bacteria, probably marginally outnumbering human cells (3×10^{13} for the standard age and somatotype) [25,26]. As expected, the microbial community residing in the gut is the most abundant, comprising slightly more than 1000 bacterial species [24,27]. These commensal bacteria harbor about 3.3 million genes, surpassing in number the genes contained in the host genome by approximately 150 times [24]. It soon became evident that this incredibly rich microbial ecosystem could not be uninvolved in the biological processes underlying health and disease. Further evolution in molecular biology, namely the emergence of "-omics" technologies (genomics, transcriptomics, proteomics, and metabolomics), have now enabled the investigation of the functional effects of human microbiome by detecting and studying the functional genes encoded by the microbial community and their products (proteins, metabolites etc.) [19].

Amplicon-based sequencing of marker genes, such as 16S rRNA, is a powerful tool for assessing and comparing the structure of microbial communities at a high phylogenetic resolution. Because 16S rRNA sequencing is more cost-effective than whole-metagenome shotgun sequencing, marker gene analysis is frequently used for broad studies that involve a large number of different samples. With the expanded use of 16S rRNA sequencing for resident microbiota recognition on different human surfaces, organs such as the lungs, the stomach, and the uterus, previously considered sterile based on culture-dependent studies, were shown to host a substantial microbial burden under normal conditions. These findings gave birth to the notion of lung microbiome and primed tenacious research endeavors for its characterization.

2.2. The Lung Microbiome in Health

2.2.1. The Early Life Shaping

Although not specifically studied in humans, the development of the lung microbiome probably adheres to that of the rest of the human body microbial ecosystem. The exact starting time point for the bacterial colonization of the human body cannot be accurately determined. Until recently, amniotic fluid, which fills fetal lungs prenatally, was considered sterile. This historical belief was challenged by the discovery of bacterial DNA in amniotic fluid and placental samples [28], which may be suggestive of a prenatal initiation of lung microbial colonization and development, although the actual existence of an amniotic fluid microbiome remains controversial [29] and its potential significance vastly unknown. Detectable microbial communities in multiple body sites have been identified in newborns as early as <5 min after delivery, and their synthesis initially resembles the maternal vagina or skin microbiota composition, depending on the mode of delivery (vaginal or caesarian section) [30]. This premature microbiome has been shown to change in composition and diversity and mature functionally during the first two to three years of life, after which it gradually stabilizes to a pattern closely matching that of adults [31–33]. This early life microbiota instability, probably in parallel with the concurrent immune system immaturity, is believed to render microbiome particularly susceptible to the influence of diverse environmental factors, including diet (e.g., breastfeeding), day care, crowding, and antibiotic use [34,35], which ultimately shape the structure of the adult human microbiome and, presumably, confer predisposition or resistance to disease ("window of opportunity" theory) [36] (see Figure 1). A similar trajectory of diversity and composition changes with increasing age has recently been described in the lung microbiota of mice [37].

2.2.2. The Immigration/Elimination Balance

The synthesis of any bacterial (or other living organism) community at any given time is dictated by the interaction between three factors: (1) immigration, (2) elimination, and (3) local reproduction of community members (see Figure 2).

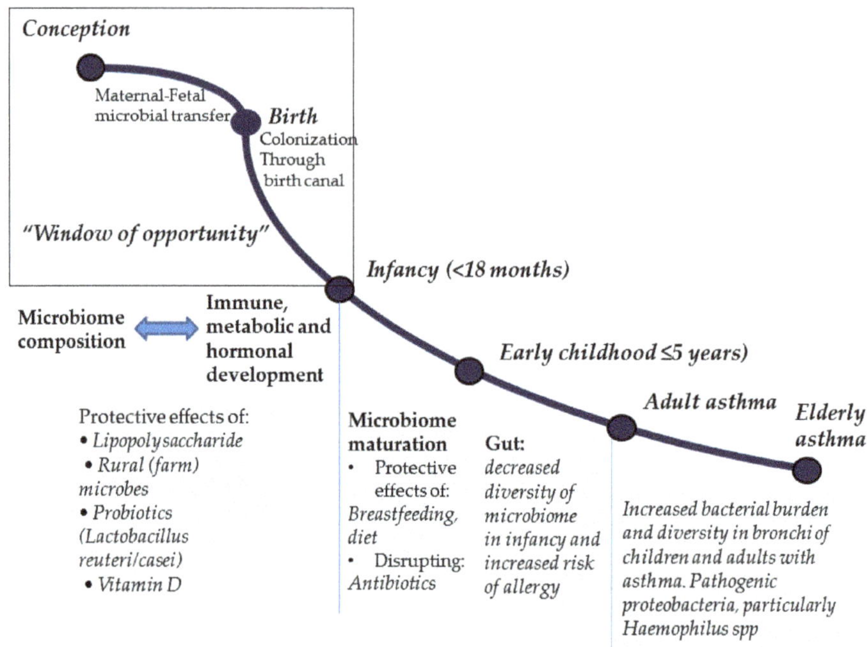

Figure 1. The natural history of microbiome development.

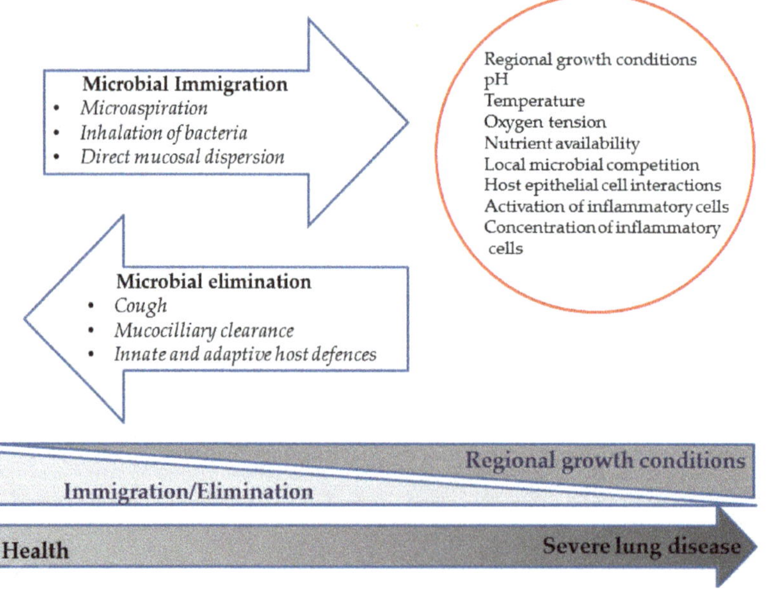

Figure 2. Factors determining the immigration/elimination balance.

With regard to lung microbiome, immigration mostly originates from subclinical micro-aspiration from the upper respiratory tract (URT), although other sources, including the inspired air (which carries approximately 10^5–10^6 bacteria/m^3) [38], and the upper gastrointestinal tract via aspiration of gastric contents [39], may also make minor contributions. The elimination of lung microbial community members can be assumed to be mediated by the complete armory of lung defense mechanisms, including cough reflex, mucociliary clearance, and innate and adaptive immunity [40], and, thus, to depend on its effectiveness. In health, the balance between dispersal of microbes from the URT and eradication of lung microbial community members via local defense mechanisms is considered the major determinant of lung microbiome characteristics, whereas local bacterial reproduction most probably plays a rather minor role. The URT as the major source of lung microbiome is strongly supported by data showing a close resemblance between upper and lower respiratory tract (LRT) microbiome composition in healthy individuals [41–43]. Further corroboration of these results comes from the study of Venkataraman et al., demonstrating that lung microbiome composition in healthy individuals could be best attributed to neutral dispersal of microbes from the oropharynx rather than active local bacterial selection in the lungs [16]. Even more so, in a study investigating the possibility of spatially determined intrapulmonary discrepancies in the characteristics of lung microbiome, Dickson et al. showed that microbial richness and Firmicutes phylum abundance in the right upper lobe was more similar to those of the supraglottic region compared with the other lung lobes sampled, in which microbiome is practically identical [44]. Given the closer vicinity of the right upper lobe to the URT, these findings suggest that not only is the LRT microbiome directly related to that of the URT, but also this association is probably inversely proportional to the distance from the oropharynx (i.e., the more proximal to the oropharynx, the closer the microbiome resemblance). Conversely, if intrapulmonary bacterial growth was a major determinant of lung microbiome synthesis, significant intra-subject variations in the microbiome characteristics of different lobes should have been expected, given the well-established between-lobes disparities in local growth conditions (e.g., oxygen tension, pH, temperature) [45]. This was not the case in the study of Dickson et al, in which all parts of the lung located distally from the URT, irrespective of exact lobe, had practically identical microbiome [44].

2.2.3. Composition and Structural Features

In contrast with the microbial communities residing in other parts of the human body, our knowledge on normal lung microbiome features, in terms of its development, composition (particularly at the genus and species levels), functional effects, and their determinants remains largely incomplete. To some extent, this reflects sampling difficulties, resulting in most relevant studies suffering from small-size limitations and lack of longitudinal data [13].

Lung microbiota is a relatively small bacterial community. Based on the findings of studies applying 16S rRNA sequencing in endobronchial brushing (EB) samples from healthy and diseased individuals, it is estimated that there are on average 10^3–10^5 bacterial genomes (or 16S copies) per cm^2 of bronchial tissue sampled, although with significant inter-subject variability [41,46]. Comparatively, colon microbiota, which is the most abundant microbial ecosystem in the human body, comprises up to 10^{11} CFU/gr of luminal content [47]. In a study evaluating the associations between the diverse microbial communities of the aero-digestive tract, bacterial density in bronchoalveolar lavage (BAL) fluid was found to be 100- to 1000-fold and 10- to 100-fold lower than in oral washes and gastric aspirates, respectively, of the same healthy subjects [43]. Sequencing of these 16S rRNA genes and comparison with established microbial genomic databases have led to the identification of 38 bacteria phyla, with 303 [48], or even more [49], genera residing in the human lung. However, these are far from equally represented with the top six phyla and the top 25 genera accounting for 86% and 65%, respectively, of all sequences identified [48]. Specifically, *Bacteroidetes* and *Firmicutes* are the most abundant phyla in the lung microbiota of healthy humans, followed by *Proteobacteria* and, to a lesser extent, *Actinobacteria* and *Fusobacteria* [41,43,46,48,50]. At the genus level, *Prevotella*, *Veillonella*, and *Streptococcus* are generally considered the most dominant taxa [41,42,46,51], although there is substantial variation in the relevant abundance of lung commensal microbes between studies and *Neisseria*, *Haemophilus*, *Fusobacterium*, or other genera (e.g., *Actinomyces*, *Porphyromonas*, and *Lactobacillus*) are occasionally found in comparable counts [42,46–49,52]. Although these discrepancies are probably, at least in part, due to the small sizes of the relevant studies, the presence of considerable inter-subject variability in lung microbiota composition has been documented in healthy individuals [44,52], so that, to date, it is not possible to define a typical ("normal") lung microbiome.

2.3. Potential Effects of Sampling Methods on the Assessment of Lung Microbiome Structure

The study of lung microbiota parameters requires bronchoscopy for BAL or EB samples acquisition. Induced sputum analysis may be a less invasive alternative, although differences in bacterial composition of sputum samples compared with those retrieved by bronchoscopic techniques, as a result of contamination by the rich oral/oropharyngeal microbiota, have been well documented [49]. Moreover, there is a certain degree of uncertainty surrounding putative effects of the specific bronchoscopic technique used for sampling on the characteristics of the derived microbiota. Denner et al. reported significant discrepancies in the extent, diversity, and relative affluence of the retrieved microbial communities between BAL and EB bronchoscopic sampling, the latter being associated with a denser and more diverse microbiome [48]. An earlier study comparing the microbial communities sampled by multiple respiratory tract sites of healthy individuals, demonstrated that the bacterial population of the left lower lobar bronchus retrieved by EB was generally larger than the populations of the right middle lobe segmental bronchi, which were sampled by consecutive BALs, although no differences were found in the corresponding bacterial communities' composition [41]. Other researchers have ruled out bronchoscopic-technique-specific effects on the lung microbiota synthesis after applying both BAL and EB in contralateral lobes of healthy volunteers [44]. Although the reported discrepancies could be merely the result of differences in the nature of the samples (and in the modes of their acquisition), along with small study sizes, they might also represent a shift in the microbiota characteristics of the small peripheral airways and the lung parenchyma (sampled by BAL) compared with the more proximal bronchi (sampled by EB). Until further research addresses these issues and establishes a standardized technique for lung microbiota derivation, sampling methods should be taken into account when designing or evaluating the results of human lung microbiome studies.

2.4. Spatial Discrepancies in the Structure of Lung Microbiome

Some degree of spatially dependent intra-subject variability in lung microbiota features has been demonstrated, although this is substantially more limited than the aforementioned between-subjects variability [44]. Specifically, it has been shown that the right upper lobe microbial community richness, composition, and variation are all significantly different from those of more distal parts of the lungs (left upper lobe, right middle lobe, and lingula) of the same healthy individuals and more closely resemble the upper respiratory tract microbiota [44]. Finally, it should be mentioned that, in contrast with the gut microbiome which has been shown to present significant geographical variation possibly associated with the regional lifestyle [32], there are no data suggesting a similar trend in lung microbiome. Despite the lack of direct comparisons between populations from different parts of the world, no dissimilarities have been found in the lung microbiome of HMP initiative participants from eight different US cities [42] and, to date, the relatively few studies conducted in non-Western populations do not seem to yield different results from the majority of lung microbiome studies, which have generally been confined to the Western world [53,54].

Cross-Talk between Lung Microbiota and the Host

The host immune system is primarily responsible for the conduct of most of the host–microbiome interplay, and there is now a growing body of evidence establishing the presence of an active and multiform cross-talk between the lung microbiome and the host immune system [11]. Invading pathogens activate the inflammasomes (multi-meric protein complexes) both directly and indirectly [55], to produce inflammasome associated pro-cytokines (IL-18, IL-1β), after the recognition of the pathogens by a family of receptors through pathogen-associated molecular patterns (PAMPs) [56]. Structural components of the bacterial cells and LPS (a ubiquitous structural component of Gram-negative bacteria outer membrane) are ligands for the pattern recognition receptors (PRRs) expressed by the host antigen-presenting cells. Upon stimulation, PRRs (with Toll-like receptors (TLRs)-2 and -4 being the principle representatives) may trigger diverse cellular processes regulating immune responses in the lung. Importantly, these responses appear to be bacterial species- or genus-specific, underscoring the potentially significant effects of lung microbiome composition alterations on the host immune regulation (see Figure 3).

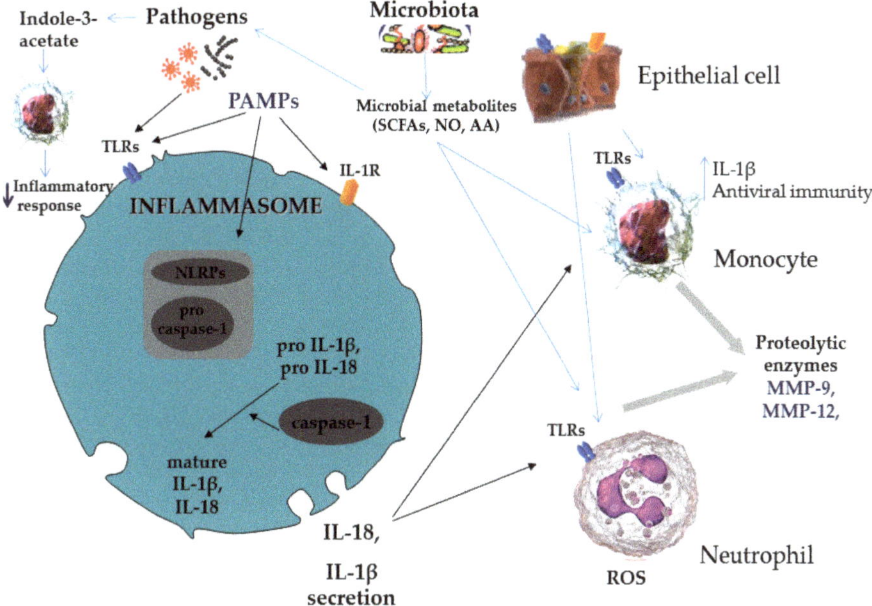

Figure 3. Respiratory microbiota produce metabolites (SCFAs, NO, or nitrite, aromatic amino acids), which influence host immune activity. Inflammasome-associated pro-cytokines can be produced and activated by a family of receptors which detect the presence of pathogens through PAMPs. SCFA: short chain fatty acids; NO: nitric oxide; AAs: aromatic amino acids; TLR: Toll-like receptors; ROS: reactive oxygen species; PAMP: pathogen associated molecular patterns; MMP: matrix metalloproteinase; MDC: macrophage-derived chemokine; MIP1α: macrophage inflammatory protein 1α.

Interspecies differences in LPS structure are thought to account for the corresponding variations in TLR subtype specificity and lung inflammatory capacity [57,58]. The Bacteroides *Prevotella*, one of the most abundant genera in the healthy lung microbiome, appears to exhibit a TLR2-dependent low inflammatory potential, whereas the Proteobacteria *Haemophilus influenzae* and *Moraxella catarrhalis*, linked with lung microbiome alterations in asthma and COPD, induce severe TLR2 independent (and probably TLR4-dependent) lung inflammation and injury in mice [57]. Other potentially pathogenic Proteobacteria residing in the lung, such as *Pseudomonas aeruginosa*, *Stenotrophomonas maltophilia*, and *Burkholderia* spp, possess flagella, the major structural component of which flagellin is recognized by host TLR5, leading to the induction of pro-inflammatory mediators' secretion [59]. Bacterial DNA may also stimulate host immune responses. This effect is mediated by the abundant in bacterial DNA sequences unmethylated CpG dinucleotides, which bind to the host TLR9, inducing an inflammatory response of the T-helper-1 (Th1) type [60]. Furthermore, all four major phyla of the lung microbiome (Bacteroidetes, Firmicutes, Proteobacteria, and Actinobacteria) have been shown to stimulate NOD2 receptors in vitro, and this effect is mediated by the bacterial cell wall component peptidoglycan [61].

Beyond structural microbial components, resident microbes-derived metabolites are also believed to be actively involved in the interplay between lung microbiome and the host immune system. Short-chain fatty acids (SCFAs) and amino acids metabolism products are the most extensively studied metabolites generated by human microbiota. SCFAs, such as butyrate, propionate, and acetate, are the main end-product of dietary fiber fermentation undertaken by the gastrointestinal tract microbiota. However, there are also data implying SCFAs production from lung microbiota, since active expression of bacterial genes associated with SCFAs metabolism has been described in bronchial brushings [62]. SCFAs have been implicated in numerous mechanisms promoting maintenance of homeostasis in health, including preservation of gut barrier integrity, control of appetite and energy intake, protection against autoimmunity and tumorigenesis in colon, and regulation of blood–brain barrier permeability, among others [63,64]. Importantly, they have also been shown to possess immunomodulatory properties [64,65]. The latter are mediated by G protein coupled receptors, particularly GPR41, GPR43, and GPR109a, which are all expressed on the surface of most types of inflammatory cells (macrophages/monocytes, dendritic cells, and neutrophils), as well as by direct inhibition of histone deacetylases (HDACs) [63–65], i.e., enzymes actively participating in post-translational modifications of the histones-DNA interaction inside the chromatin structure that regulates cell transcriptional activity and gene expression [66]. The principal immunomodulating effect of SCFAs appears to be the induction of differentiation and proliferation of extra-thymic regulatory T cells (Tregs) [67–69], a lymphocyte subset with established anti-inflammatory and anti-allergic effects [70,71]. Apart from the SCFAs, indole-3-acetate, a metabolite of the amino acid tryptophan produced by gut microbiota, was recently shown to attenuate LPS-induced pro-inflammatory cytokine and chemokine secretion in alveolar macrophages derived from smokers, and this observed anti-inflammatory action of indole-3-acetate was hypothesized to potentially mediate the effect of azithromycin on lowering exacerbation rates in COPD patients [72]. Indole-3-acetate and the other tryptophan metabolites are activators of the aryl hydrocarbon receptor [73], another well-known modulator of inflammation and immunity, with a proposed role in Treg generation [74].

We previously focused on microbiota-derived mediators engaged in shaping diverse aspects of host immune response. It must be realized that the opposite is most probably also valid. This means that numerous signaling molecules originating from host cells can be sensed by resident microbes and are capable of modifying the composition and diversity of lung microbiome. Indeed, there are data from several in vitro studies demonstrating potential influences of catecholamines and cytokines on the growth and virulence of various bacterial strains, perhaps with a species- or genus-specific manner [75–79]. This host-to-microbiome signaling pathway may be implicated in respiratory disease pathogenesis by contributing to lung microbiome alterations favoring the dominance of specific potentially pathogenic species. In this context, it has been shown that increased intra-alveolar levels of the catecholamines epinephrine and norepinephrine in BAL samples from lung-transplant recipients are significantly associated with both indices of acute infection and reduced lung microbiome diversity, characterized by the predominance of a single bacterial species, notably *Pseudomonas aeruginosa* [80].

2.5. Microbiome and Asthma Susceptibility

The "Gut–Lung Axis" and the Hygiene Hypothesis

Accumulated evidence arising from both human and animal studies suggests that the development of allergic diseases, including asthma, may, in fact, be dependent on the bacterial communities residing in the gut. Gut microbiota actively interact with the host immune system via bacterial structural components and secreted metabolites, and these interactions possess the ability to modulate immune responses both locally in the gastrointestinal tract and systemically, influencing various distal sites, including the lungs. The term "gut–lung axis" has been coined to account for these effects of gut microbiota on lung immunity, both in health and in disease [81] (see Figure 4).

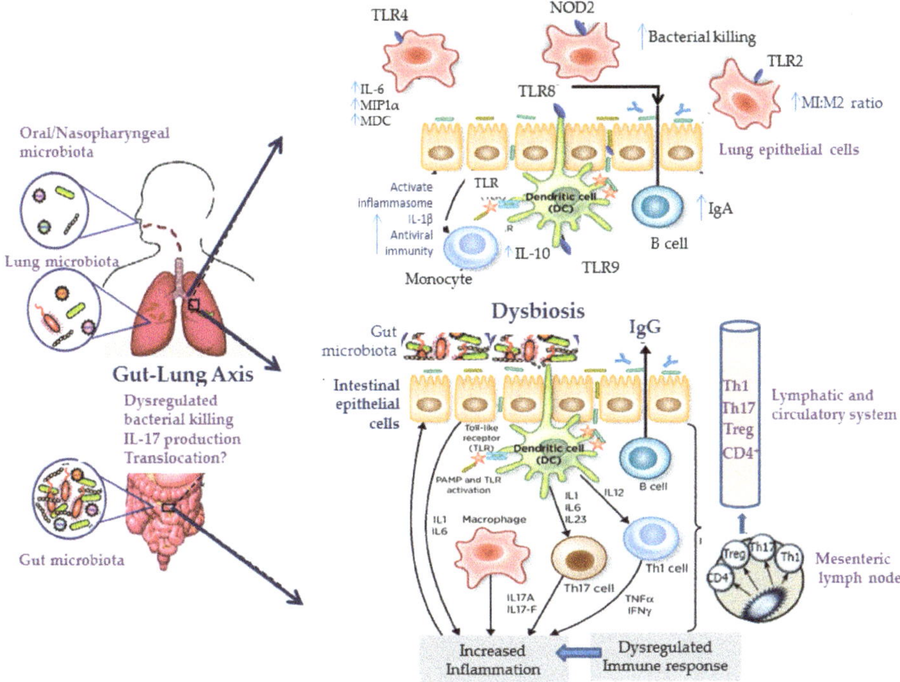

Figure 4. The "lung–gut" axis interactions with host immunity. TLR: Toll-like receptors; Treg: T regulatory cell; MDC: macrophage-derived chemokine; MIP1α: macrophage inflammatory protein 1α.

The presumable involvement of resident microbiota in allergic asthma development is primarily supported by data showing an exaggerated Th2 immunity-driven airway inflammation in germ-free (GF) mice sensitized with ovalbumin compared with specific pathogen-free (SPF) counterparts, which can be abrogated when GF mice are recolonized by the commensal flora of the SPF animals prior to sensitization [82]. Likewise, gut microbiota disruption as a result of antibiotics administration promotes allergic airway disease in experimental murine asthma [83,84]. Importantly, antibiotic-induced long-term alterations in gut microbiota diversity and composition have also been observed in humans [85–87] and both early life and maternal antibiotic use have been associated with an increased risk for recurrent wheeze and asthma development in childhood [88,89]. Aside from antibiotic exposure, formula feeding [90,91] and Caesarian-section delivery [92,93] have been correlated both with differences in infant gut microbiota composition and with a heightened childhood asthma susceptibility compared with breastfeeding and vaginal delivery. Other exposures operating in early life, when the microbiome and the host immune system are both in the process of maturation, might also be relevant (see Figures 1 and 5). For instance, living with dogs or cats as pets during the first year of life has been linked to a decreased prevalence of atopy at age six to seven [94], and dust from households with dogs has been shown to enrich cecal microbiota, together with downregulating Th2-mediated airway inflammation in a murine model of allergic sensitization [95]. Fujimura et al. [95] elegantly showed that exposure to pets may be associated with distinct gut microbiota composition characteristics conferring protection against airway allergen challenge [95]. Specifically, the cecal microbiome of mice exposed to dust derived from households with dogs was significantly enriched in Firmicutes compared with mice exposed to dust from residencies without pets, with *Lactobacillus johnsonii* being the most dominant taxon.

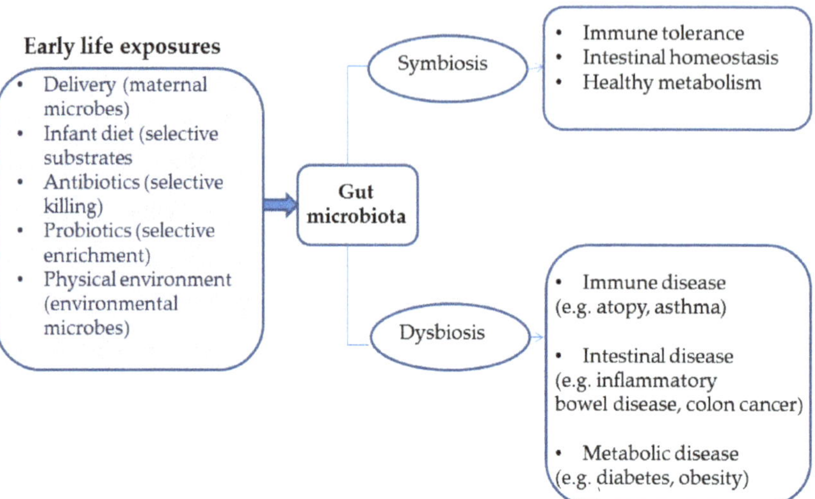

Figure 5. Early life exposures that may affect the symbiosis/dysbiosis balance and predispose to asthma.

The relative microbial diversity of the environment and the level of exposure during the first years of life have also been highlighted as important factors influencing subsequent allergy and asthma susceptibility. Several studies from around the world have consistently demonstrated that children growing up in rural settings with high-level exposure to bacterially enriched farming environments presented significantly lower rates of atopic asthma compared with their non-farm peers [96]. In a landmark study published in 2016, 60 schoolchildren from two reproductively isolated US agricultural communities, the Amish and the Hutterites, sharing strong similarities in terms of genetic background and lifestyle, but with diametrically opposite farming practices, were examined [97]. The children of the Amish, who practice a traditional type of farming, presented a significantly lower rate of allergic sensitization compared to those of Hutterites, who use highly industrialized farming infrastructure, and no asthma cases were identified among Amish, in contrast to the six asthmatic Hutterite children.

Short-chain fatty acids (SCFAs) have been proposed as pivotal mediators of the gut–lung interplay. Knockout mice lacking the *gpr43* receptor gene have been shown to present an exaggerated allergic airway inflammatory response upon ovalbumin challenge [98]. In a landmark study, Trompette et al. demonstrated that the dietary fiber content may influence the extent of allergic inflammatory changes in the lungs via SCFAs-mediated defects in DC activation, leading to an impaired Th2 cell differentiation [99]. Interestingly, they showed that high-fiber diet attenuated Th2-driven lung inflammation, as assessed by total and differential cell count in BAL fluid, Th2 cytokines mRNA levels in lung tissue, serum total IgE, metacholine challenge, and lung histological analysis. On the contrary, low-fiber diet aggravated allergic inflammation in the lungs. Furthermore, the administration of SCFAs to mice through drinking water led to an acceleration of Th2 inflammation resolution in propionate-supplemented wild-type mice compared with un-supplemented controls, which was abrogated in a separate group of GPR41-dedicient mice. These results indicate that circulating SCFAs (propionate in particular) produced by gut resident bacteria in direct proportion to the dietary fiber content may reduce susceptibility to allergic airway disease through the activation of the GRP41 receptor.

2.6. The Lung Microbiome in Asthma

During the last decade, an ever-growing number of studies have attempted to shed light on the features of lung microbiome in patients with asthma [46,48,50,62,100–108]; however, the small sample sizes, the lack of uniformity and standardization in the selection and processing of respiratory samples used for microbiome characterization in asthma, the scarcity of data on potential longitudinal changes in lung microbiome composition during the course of the disease and in association with treatment implementation, and finally, the absence of a clearly described 'normal' lung microbiome with which comparisons can be safely made pose limitations to the complete delineation and interpretation of lung microbiome in asthmatic patients. Despite these caveats, studies investigating the lung microbiome in asthma have been relatively successful in capturing microbiome alterations in a large part of the spectrum of disease severity and phenotypes, thus providing an initial premature understanding of a potential association between features of lung microbiome and specific disease characteristics.

Alterations of Lung Microbiome Structure in Asthma

The most constant finding of lung microbiome studies in asthma is probably an observed increase in the relative abundance of the Proteobacteria phylum in asthmatic lungs [9,46,62,106–109]. At the genus level, this change is seemingly driven by a corresponding increase in the prevalence of *Haemophilus* and/or *Neisseria* [46,62,103,105–107], although other potentially pathogenic genera belonging to the Proteobacteria phylum, such as *Moraxella*, *Pseudomonas*, and members of the *Enterobacteriaceae* family, might also be involved [48,103,106,108]. It appears, though, that this Proteobacteria expansion is rather specific to non-severe asthma, as studies directly comparing non-severe with severe asthmatics have demonstrated distinct patterns of lung microbiome composition in these two groups, with Proteobacteria dominating in the lung microbiome of non-severe asthmatics, while other phyla, possibly Actinobacteria [108] or Firmicutes (mainly *Streptococci*) [106], are more prevalent in severe asthma. However, an increased relative abundance of certain Proteobacteria, such as the *Pseudomonadaceae* and *Enterobacteriaceae* (most notably *Klebsiella* spp), has also been reported in severe asthma patients [104,108].

Other taxa, e.g., the common respiratory commensals *Prevotella* and *Veillonella*, have generally been shown to be less common in the lung microbiome of patients with both severe and non-severe asthma [46,48,50,106], although these findings are not universal [62]. Overall, asthma-associated alterations in lung microbiome composition are significantly less firmly determined at the genus level compared with the phylum level, possibly reflecting, at least in part, the corresponding variations described in the lung microbiome composition of healthy individuals.

The relationship between asthma and lung microbial community diversity is even more controversial. Earlier studies in patients with mild asthma have reported an increased bacterial burden and diversity in induced sputa and EBs compared with healthy individuals [101,102]. In line with these observations, Durack et al. found a marginally increased phylogenetic diversity in EB samples retrieved from 42 asthmatic patients compared with 21 healthy controls [62]. Likewise, Sverrild et al. showed bacterial diversity augmentation in BAL fluid specimens from 23 patients with non-eosinophilic asthma [107]. On the contrary, other studies having included patients with more severe or corticosteroids refractory disease failed to replicate these findings and occasionally came up with opposite results [50,105,106,108].

2.7. The Potential Role of Lung Microbiome in Shaping Asthma Phenotypes and Endotypes

Several clinical, physiological, and inflammatory characteristics involved in the definition of asthma phenotypes (and, to a lesser extent, endotypes) [3] have been linked with features of lung microbiome (see Figure 6).

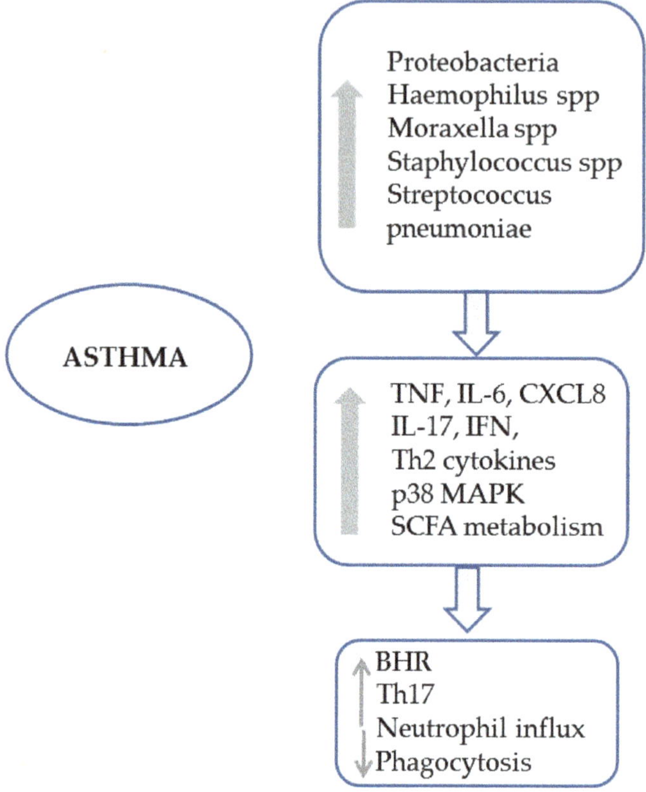

Figure 6. Implication of lung microbiome in asthma. TNF: Tumor necrosis factor; IL: Interleukin; IFN: Interferon; MAPK: Mitogen-activated protein kinase; SCFA: short chain fatty acid; BHR: bronchial hyperresponsiveness.

2.7.1. Inflammatory Profile

Eosinophilic Inflammation

Lung microbiota diversity and composition have been investigated in patients with both severe and non-severe eosinophilic asthma and compared with the corresponding features in non-eosinophilic asthma. In a cohort of mild corticosteroid (CS)-naïve asthma, Sverrild et al. reported increased α-diversity (a measure of bacterial taxa richness and evenness) and decreased β-diversity (an index of heterogeneity between bacterial communities) in the BAL microbiome of eosinophil-high asthmatic patients compared with eosinophil-low ones [107]. At the same time, various genera were significantly enriched (e.g., *Aeribacillus, Halomonas,* and *Sphingomonas*) or depleted (e.g., *Neisseria, Bacteroides,* and *Actinomyces*) in eosinophil-high as opposed to eosinophil-low asthma. On the contrary, in another cohort encompassing patients with both severe and non-severe asthma, the *Actinomycataceae* family members were significantly more abundant in eosinophilic compared with non-eosinophilic, asthma and their relative abundance was positively associated with the eosinophil count in sputa [108]. *Tropheryma whipplei* has also been identified as a prevalent member of the lung bacterial community in severe asthmatic patients of the eosinophilic inflammatory phenotype [105].

Instead of directly comparing lung microbiome composition in patients with eosinophilic and non-eosinophilic asthma, other groups have focused on the investigation of potential associations between features of microbiome and markers of eosinophilic airway inflammation. Eosinophil infiltration of bronchial tissue and eosinophil count in BAL fluid have been associated with lower total bacterial loads and diversity in EB samples from patients with mostly severe asthma [48,104]. Particularly, *Rickettsia* and certain Actinobacteria have been positively correlated with lung eosinophilia, whereas taxa negatively correlated mostly belong to Proteobacteria (including *Moraxellaceae*) and Firmicutes [48,104]. The bronchial epithelial cell expression of specific genes known to be involved in the Th2-mediated immune response (*CLCA1, SERPINB2* and *POSTN*) has also been examined in relation to lung microbiome composition [62,104]. These three gene expressions correlated negatively with total bacterial burden and relative abundance of certain taxa, including the previously mentioned *Moraxellaceae* [62,104].

Despite significant variability and, to some extent, rather contradictory results between studies, these data strongly support the existence of distinct features of lung microbiota burden, diversity, and composition in patients with the eosinophilic asthma subtype. Overall, it appears that both the eosinophilic inflammatory phenotype and the underlying Th2-high endotype correspond to lung microbial communities with comparatively low bacterial load, substantial diversity but limited heterogeneity, and possibly increased representation of Actinobacteria (perhaps most notably of the *Actinomyces* genus) and decreased representation of certain Proteobacteria (potentially including *Moraxella* sp) [110].

Neutrophilic Inflammation

Neutrophilic asthma, along with the paucigranulocytic inflammatory phenotype, belongs to the non-Th2 (or Th2-low) asthma endotype and Th1 and/or Th17 immune processes have been implicated in its pathogenesis [109,111], although therapeutic targeting of neither Th1- nor Th17-related cytokines, namely anti-TNFa [112] and anti-IL17A receptor agents [113], have proved effective. On the other hand, certain bacterial pathogens are established triggers of Th17-driven immune responses [114], and there are some data showing reduction of neutrophilic inflammatory markers (primarily IL-8) and quality-of-life improvement following treatment with clarithromycin in patients with severe refractory non-eosinophilic asthma [115]. These observations have drawn attention to the investigation of potential associations between lung microbiome and neutrophilic asthma in particular. In the most recent and largest to-date study of lung microbiome in asthma, Taylor et al. classified 167 patients with moderate-to-severe asthma in eosinophilic, neutrophilic, paucigranulocytic, and mixed granulocytic inflammatory phenotypes based on induced sputum differential cell count percentages and searched for interphenotype dissimilarities in sputum bacterial diversity and composition [110]. Although limited by the uneven distribution of participants across the different phenotypes (only 14 had neutrophilic asthma), the study provided evidence for a significantly decreased bacterial diversity, along with increased heterogeneity in patients with neutrophilic compared with both eosinophilic and paucigranulocytic asthma. This was accompanied by a strong inverse correlation between phylogenetic diversity and neutrophil percentage in sputum. *Haemophilus* and *Moraxella* genera were found enriched in neutrophilic asthma samples and significantly correlated with asthma inflammatory profile, with the opposite being the case for *Streptococcus*. In line with these results, Simpson et al. also demonstrated a decreased bacterial diversity in induced sputa collected from patients with severe neutrophilic compared with non-neutrophilic asthma in an earlier study [105]. Again, Proteobacteria, particularly *Haemophilus influenzae*, was the phylum dominating in the neutrophilic airway microbiota, with a relative depletion of Actinobacteria and Firmicutes. Similarly, others have shown positive correlations between *Moraxella catarrhalis*, *Haemophilus* sp, and *Streptococcus* sp total abundance and sputum neutrophils percentage and IL-8 concentration in severe asthma [103].

Although observational, and thus not establishing causality, these studies may support a case for lung microbiota dysbiosis in the pathogenesis of neutrophilic asthma. It appears that the LRT of asthmatic patients with predominantly neutrophilic airway inflammation harbors a relatively uniform microbiome, in which Proteobacteria, most prominently the potentially pathogenic *Haemophilus* and *Moraxella* genera, have outgrown the taxa normally over-distributed in the lung microbiota (e.g.,

Firmicutes). These gradually expanding new colonizers of the asthmatic airways may, in fact, constitute the triggering factor for the aberrant Th17 immune response, along with other inflammatory pathways activation, observed in neutrophilic asthma. Indeed, non-typeable *Haemophilus influenzae* intranasally administered at a sublethal dose has been shown to produce a robust Th17 response in the lungs of experimental mice [116] and, even more relevantly, infection with non-typeable *Haemophilus influenzae* may lead to reduced eosinophilic inflammation and increased neutrophilic infiltration of the airways in an IL-17-dependent manner in a murine model of allergic asthma [117]. Although the cause of Proteobacteria overgrowth in the LRT of certain asthmatics remains elusive and may be multifactorial (e.g., selective bacterial growth favored by structural changes and/or inflammatory mediators in the airways as a result of the underlying disease process), it must be noted that, as previously discussed, inhaled corticosteroid (ICS) treatment itself may promote Proteobacteria enrichment in the lung microbiota and, thus, contribute to the development of neutrophilic asthma [2]. Apparently, if this hypothetical association between respiratory dysbiosis and neutrophilic asthma pathogenesis stands true, strategies aiming at the manipulation of lung microbiome, possibly through Proteobacteria suppression and normal diversity restoration, may open up new avenues for the treatment of this, until now, untargeted asthma phenotype. Macrolides may be part of such strategies.

2.7.2. Corticosteroid Responsiveness

Several data support the correlation between lung microbiota burden and diversity and corticosteroid responsiveness. Goleva et al, in a study on CS sensitive and CS resistant asthmatics, demonstrated that, although bacterial composition both at the phylum and at the genus level was quite similar between the two groups overall, unique patterns of bacterial expansions were observed in the majority of patients with both CS-resistant and CS-sensitive asthma [50]. In CS-resistant asthmatics, the genera *Neisseria, Haemophilus,* and *Tropheryma* were abundant, while the genera *Pasteurella* and *Fusobacterium* were predominant in CS-sensitive asthma. Of note, CS-resistant patients had significantly higher levels of interleukin (IL)-8 mRNA in their BAL cells, implying that distinct lung microbiota profiles may be responsible for CS resistance in the neutrophilic asthma phenotype. To further validate their findings, the authors subsequently incubated alveolar macrophages isolated from BAL samples of asthmatic patients, with either *Haemophilus parainfluenzae* (a genus solely expanded in CS resistant patients) or *Prevotella melaninogenica*, and found a significantly reduced CS responsiveness in vitro following treatment with dexamethasone in cells cultured with *H. parainfluenzae,* but not *P. melaninogenica*. Durack et al. assessed bacterial composition in ten ICS responders and an equal number of ICS non-responders, both with mild ICS-naive asthma [62]. They reported significantly different microbiota profiles in the two groups, with responder's lung microbiome synthesis sharing more resemblance with that of healthy controls. In particular, the *Microbacteriaceae* and *Pasteurellaceae* (including *Haemophilus*) families were found enriched in ICS non-responders and expansions of the *Streptococcaceae, Fusobacteriaceae,* and *Sphingomonodaceae* families were shown in responders. Interestingly, in the same study, lack of CS responsiveness was associated functionally with increased expression of bacterial genes involved in biodegradation pathways, which may explain resistance to CS treatment.

Finally, Huang et al. demonstrated a significant positive correlation between lung microbiota diversity and *FKBP5* gene expression, a marker of steroid response [104]. In terms of bacterial composition, increased *FKBP5* gene expression was associated mainly with Actinobacteria and Proteobacteria phyla enrichment. These results suggesting an association between lung-microbial community diversity and CS responsiveness in severe asthma are further supported by more recent data showing a significant inverse correlation linking phylogenetic diversity in induced sputum specimens collected from patients with moderate-to-severe asthma and ICS dose with the use of both univariate and multivariate regression analyses [110].

2.7.3. Effect of Treatment

Data regarding the effect of asthma treatment on lung microbiome are scarce in literature. In their study, after initial bronchoscopic sampling (EBs) for lung microbiome assessment at enrollment, Durack et al. randomized (2:1 ratio) 42 patients with mild well-controlled asthma, who had not received ICS previously, to receive a six-week course of a medium dose of ICS (250mcg fluticasone propionate twice daily) or placebo and repeated EBs post-treatment [62]. Despite limitations related to sample quantity insufficiency, the authors did not discern changes in bacterial burden and diversity after ICS treatment. However, they did find fluticasone-induced alterations in the relative abundance of certain taxa, namely an expansion of the *Microbacteriaceae* family and the *Moraxella* and *Neisseria* genera and a depletion of *Fusobacterium*, in those who responded to ICS treatment.

In another study, patients with both mild and more severe asthma were stratified according to the use of corticosteroids (inhaled and oral) [48]. Both those on ICS only and those on combined ICS and OCS treatment regimens exhibited significant alterations in EBs bacterial composition at the phylum, as well as the genus, level compared with corticosteroid-naïve asthma patients. These alterations comprised Proteobacteria enrichment and Bacteroidetes (specifically *Prevotella*) and Fusobacteria depletion in all corticosteroid groups, with decreased *Veillonella* and increased *Pseudomonas* abundance in those on ICS only and OCS, respectively. Although limited and centered exclusively on corticosteroids, these data clearly imply that asthma treatment may modify important compositional characteristics of the lung microbiome, including selection of potentially pathogenic species, with as yet unknown potential consequences.

Interestingly, most recent studies have attempted to provide insights into the possible functional properties of lung microbiome in asthma. Durack et al. employed an algorithmic prediction model (PICRUSt) to infer lung bacterial metagenomic characteristics based on 16S-rRNA sequencing in patients with mild asthma and showed potentially increased expression of genes involved in pathways mediating the metabolism of amino acids and carbohydrates, particularly SCFAs, in these patients compared with healthy controls [62]. On the contrary, a relative reduction was predicted in the activation of LPS synthesis-specific processes. Using the same analytical method in severe asthmatic patients, Huang et al. managed to associate distinct metabolic (e.g., carbohydrate digestion, indole alkaloid biosynthesis) and immune (e.g., NOD-like and RIG-I-like receptor signaling) pathways with taxa (positively or negatively) correlated with specific phenotypical features of asthma, including body-mass index (BMI), asthma control assessed by Asthma Control Questionnaire (ACQ), corticosteroid responsiveness, and Th17-driven inflammation [104]. The authors concluded that concrete members of the asthmatic lung microbiota may be actively engaged in the pathogenetic mechanisms leading to the acquisition of different disease characteristics between asthmatics (i.e., phenotypes). Furthermore, Sverrild et al., again with the use of PICRUSt, showed different predicted functional profiles of lung microbiota associated with mild eosinophilic compared with non-eosinophilic asthma [107]. Clearly, further research taking advantage of the novel technologies in metagenomic analysis of lung microbiota is urgently needed to better describe the potential mechanistic role of lung microbiome alterations in asthma pathogenesis and disease phenotype/endotype determination.

2.7.4. Bronchial Hyperresponsiveness (BHR)

BHR to direct or indirect stimuli, in addition to airway inflammation, has long been considered inherent to asthma. However, neither its presence nor its severity is uniform or stable in all asthmatic individuals, and, thus, BHR may potentially constitute a contributing factor in asthma phenotyping [118]. BHR (indicated by metacholine PC20 concentrations) has been shown to correlate significantly with lung microbiota diversity in asthma, with greater bacterial diversity associated with lower metacholine PC20 concentrations [101]. In the same study, Proteobacteria comprised the majority of resident taxa correlated with greater BHR. Likewise, lung microbiota diversity was greater in those patients with asthma that exhibited the larger reductions in BHR following a course with clarithromycin [101].

2.7.5. Lung Function

The potential impact of lung microbiome composition on lung function in patients with asthma has mainly been addressed by the study of Denner et al. [48]. The authors stratified their cohort of asthmatic patients (from across the range of disease severity) according to FEV_1 and noticed a significantly decreased relative abundance of various bacterial phyla (Firmicutes, Bacteroidetes, and Actinobacteria) and genera (*Prevotella, Veillonella,* and *Gemella*) in the BAL fluid of those with the lowest FEV_1 values ($FEV_1 < 60\%$). In contrast, *Lactobacillus* was found to be enriched in patients with the most severely impaired lung function. Similar positive correlations between the abundance of the *Bacteroidaceae* family or lung microbiota phylogenetic diversity and FEV_1 have also been reported elsewhere [108,110]. Others have reached different conclusions with respect to taxa-specific associations with lung function in severe asthma, showing significantly reduced FEV_1 levels in those patients with *M. catarrhalis, Haemophilus* sp, or *Streptococcus* sp predominance in induced sputa microbiota compared with others who had different taxa dominating the bacterial communities of their sputa [103].

2.7.6. Obesity

Obesity has repeatedly been identified in cluster analyses of asthmatic populations as a key clinical feature discriminating a distinct subset of patients (mostly female) with adult onset, non-Th2 mediated, highly symptomatic and difficult-to-treat asthma from other asthma phenotypes [119–121]. Although the exact pathogenetic mechanisms linking obesity with asthma remain unknown, studies in obese asthmatics have shown improvements in BHR, asthma control, lung function, and inflammatory indices following bariatric surgery [122,123] or diet-induced [124,125] weight loss.

In a cohort of patients with severe asthma, high BMI was significantly associated with a distinctive lung microbiota composition, mainly consisting of Bacteroidetes (including *Prevotella* species) and Firmicutes (e.g., *Clostridium* species) [104]. As expected, these obese asthmatic individuals presented less bronchial eosinophilic infiltration in EB specimens (non-eosinophilic asthma). It is noteworthy that bacterial taxa associated with obesity in this study exhibited distinct predicted functions, including activation of pathways involved in host immune response, such as NOD-like receptor signaling. These data suggest a potential role for lung microbiome in shaping the obesity-related asthma phenotype.

2.7.7. Smoking Asthma

Although no significant difference has been reported in BAL bacterial communities composition between healthy smokers and non-smokers [42], an analysis of induced sputum microbiota profiles in patients with severe asthma demonstrated increased total bacterial diversity and relative abundance of Fusobacteria in ex-smokers compared with never smokers, while smoking intensity (assessed by pack–years of smoking) was directly associated with the prevalence of Actinobacteria [105]. These findings raise the possibility that smoking may be involved in shaping lung microbiome alterations observed in asthma.

2.8. Lung Microbiome and Asthma Exacerbations

The most common precipitating factor triggering asthma exacerbations is viral respiratory tract infections, particularly from rhinoviruses [126]. On the contrary, bacterial lung infections have not been shown to trigger asthma exacerbations but for in a minority of cases, with the possible exception of the self-limiting atypical bacterial infections caused by *Mycoplasma pneumoniae* and *Chlamydophila pneumoniae* for both of which a relative prevalence of 18% has been serologically detected during asthma attacks in adults and children, respectively [127]. On the other hand, considerably high rates of the potentially pathogenic Proteobacteria *Haemophilus influenzae* (the most prevalent), *Streptococcus pneumoniae,* and *Moraxella catarrhalis* have been detected by both culture-based and molecular techniques from upper- and lower-respiratory-tract samples of asthmatic children during exacerbation periods [128,129]. Moreover, a cluster analysis based on sputum cellular and mediator profiles in adult asthmatic patients during exacerbations has linked the predominance of different bacterial phyla in lung microbiota with specific clinical features and inflammatory markers [130] (see Figure 7).

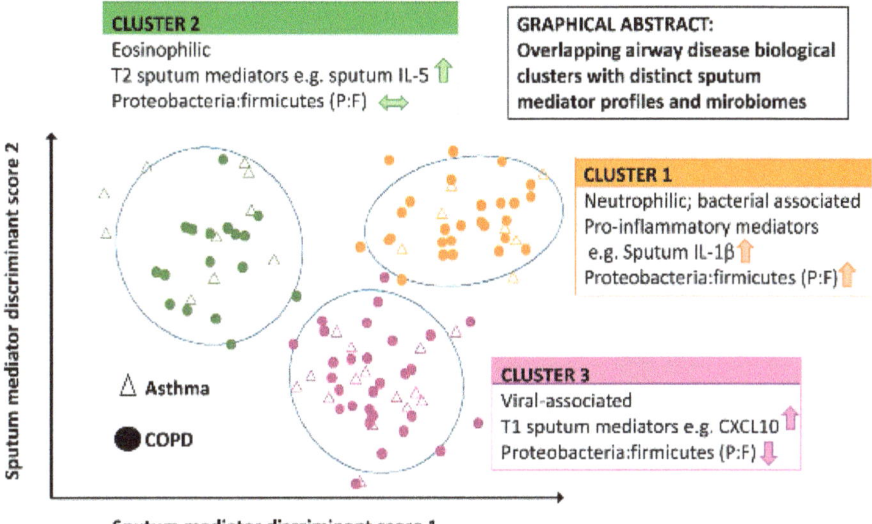

Figure 7. Exacerbation biologic clusters in asthmatic and COPD patients using the subjects' discriminant scores. Adapted from ref. [130], Creative Commons Attribution License (CC BY).

In order to provide an explanation for the above observations, a model of respiratory dysbiosis involving an altered lung microbiome and a dysregulated host immune response has been proposed to delineate the occurrence of asthma (and other chronic respiratory diseases) exacerbations [131]. According to this model, an acute stimulus, most commonly a viral infection, induces an immune-mediated inflammatory response, leading to a modification of local conditions in the airways, which may promote alteration of lung microbiota composition by favoring the predominance of specific previously underrepresented species and/or by predisposing to invasion by new potentially pathogenic strains. In turn, this deranged microbial growth may result in a further amplification of local airway inflammation, presumably via bacterial metabolite production and activation of signaling pathways mediated by the interaction between PAMPs and PRRs. Ultimately, a self-perpetuating vicious cycle arises, leading to the overwhelming inflammatory response that underlies asthma exacerbations.

Indeed, there is considerable evidence suggesting that viral infections can increase susceptibility to bacterial growth and invasion. Viral infections may impair mucociliary clearance through diverse mechanisms, including increased mucous production, ciliary dyskinesia, and cilia depletion [132,133]. Moreover, rhinoviral and possibly other viral infections have been reported to facilitate bacterial transmigration by increasing airway epithelial barrier permeability in vitro, and this effect has been attributed to the loss of occludins, a major component of tight junctions connecting adjacent epithelial cells [134,135]. Respiratory viruses alter the nasopharyngeal microbiome and may be associated with a distinct microbial signature. In the study by Rosas-Salazar et al. [136], which mostly included children <6 months of age, nasopharyngeal microbiome of infants during HRV and RSV acute respiratory tract infections (ARIs) was largely dominated by Moraxella, Streptococcus, Corynebacterium, Haemophilus, and Dolosigranulum. In addition, there was a higher abundance of Staphylococcus and a trend toward a higher abundance of Haemophilus in RSV-positive infants, and in the overall bacterial composition between infants with HRV and RSV ARIs. Furthermore, Santee et al. [137] showed that previous history of acute sinusitis influences the composition of the nasopharyngeal microbiota, characterized by a depletion in relative abundance of specific taxa. Diminished diversity was associated with more frequent upper-respiratory infections. These, among many other published data, highlight the possibility that virus-specific compositional shifts in the nasopharyngeal microbiome contribute to worse outcomes after early-life ARIs.

Various viruses, including human rhinovirus (HRV), respiratory syncytial virus (RSV), and influenza virus, can augment the expression of adhesion molecules, such as ICAM-1, CEACAM-1, CEACAM-6, and PAFR, on the surface of epithelial cells, thus promoting invasion by certain bacterial species, including *H influenza, S pneumoniae,* and *M catarrhalis* [138–140]. Apart from the upregulation of host receptors, some viral structures appear to directly promote bacterial binding to host tissues [141,142].

Furthermore, viral infections may interfere with host immune system integrity and function and, consequently, increase susceptibility to bacterial colonization and infection. For instance, HRV infection has been shown to attenuate the inflammatory response to *H. influenzae* and delay bacterial elimination by decreasing TLR2 responsiveness to bacterial insult [143]. An almost complete disappearance of alveolar macrophages has been observed after influenza infection in a murine model [144] and HRV and RSV have been found to compromise phagocytosis and diminish pro-inflammatory cytokine release from alveolar macrophages in response to bacterial products [145,146]. Dendritic cell (DC) as well as CD4 and CD8 T-cell numbers and/or function may also be impaired after influenza or other viral infections with detrimental effects on host defense against bacteria [147]. Finally, viral respiratory infections induce changes in the lung microenvironment, such as increased temperature, nutrient availability, and cytokine and catecholamine levels, all of which are potential enhancers of bacterial virulence and immunogenicity [78,79,148]. The above mechanisms may act synergistically to elicit potentially significant alterations in the composition and diversity of lung microbiota, thus resulting through the dynamic microbiome–host immune system interplay, in the amplified and deregulated inflammatory response characterizing asthma exacerbations and even predispose to recurrent exacerbations.

Conversely, there are data, albeit rather limited, suggesting that bacteria can influence susceptibility to viral infections. In this context, several experimental studies have provided evidence for a protective role of a healthy intact microbiome against influenza. Ichinohe et al. showed that mice with impaired microbiome as a result of pretreatment with antibiotics presented attenuated CD4 and CD8 T-cell responses and reduced antibody production following respiratory influenza virus infection [149]. Likewise, increased mortality has been reported in SPF mice intranasally infected with a lethal dose of influenza virus compared with non-SPF mice, and this finding could be replicated by priming mice with *Staphylococcus aureus,* used as a surrogate of upper-respiratory-tract commensal flora, before influenza virus inoculation [150]. TLR2 signaling and an M2 alveolar macrophage phenotype were essential for the relative insensitivity against influenza-induced lethal lung injury observed in this S aureus-primed murine model. Other studies focusing on the nasopharyngeal microbiota in children with RSV bronchiolitis have highlighted the potentially deleterious effects of a deranged Proteobacteria (*H influenzae, M catarrhalis*)-dominated microbiome on the risk of viral infection [151,152]. RSV infection occurrence and severity and pro-inflammatory cytokine concentrations were all found to be positively correlated with nasopharyngeal colonization with the potentially pathogenic *H. influenzae, M. catarrhalis,* and *Streptococcus species.* Similarly, *S. pneumoniae* colonization was associated with increased rates of seroconversion to human metapneumovirus in infants in an older study [153]. This viral infection predisposition conferred by the coexistence of potentially pathogenic bacteria could be the result of upregulation of viral entry receptors and/or impaired antiviral immune response induced by these bacteria. Such examples are the upregulation of the major HRV entry receptor ICAM-1 by *H. influenza* in airway epithelial cells [154] or the reduction of TLR3 expression and IFN secretion in bronchial epithelial cells infected with *M catarrhalis* [155].

Collectively, these data strengthen the hypothesis that lung microbiome alterations observed in asthma patients are actively involved in the pathogenesis of disease exacerbations and may represent a potential therapeutic target in asthma exacerbations management.

2.9. Therapeutic Implications of Microbiome Manipulation

Based on the above, the proposed role of human microbiome in shaping both asthma susceptibility and phenotypes renders exogenous manipulation of microbiome a potentially attractive therapeutic strategy for both asthma prevention and treatment. Interventions in microbiome composition have previously been recommended as putatively effective approaches in three areas of asthma management: (1) prevention of asthma development during early life by favoring factors that promote immune tolerance to allergens and minimizing those that predispose to the emergence of atopy; (2) management of Th2-low asthma phenotypes/endotype, particularly neutrophilic asthma with frequent exacerbations; and (3) reverse of CS resistance or prevention of its emergence [156]. As yet, potential interventions applied for these purposes comprise lifestyle measures, vaccinations, and pharmacological treatment, including (1) probiotics, (2) prebiotics, and (3) antibiotics. It must be emphasized that, until now, only scarce data are available for the exact impact of these interventions on human microbiome composition and function, and even less is known about their presumed ability to ameliorate clinically meaningful outcomes in asthmatic patients. Furthermore, the effects of medications currently used in asthma treatment, including CS and bronchodilators, on microbiome remain mostly undetermined, and microbiome manipulations could ideally enhance beneficial actions and/or minimize side effects possibly induced by these agents.

Theoretically, any environmental exposure capable of modifying the composition of human microbiome during the dynamic period of its acquisition and maturation starting in utero and extending to the first few years of life may influence the likelihood of subsequently developing allergic asthma. This means that there is a so-called 'window of opportunity' estimated to operate within the first 100 days of life, during which lifestyle interventions, as well as exogenously administered microbial agents, could promote the formation of a tolerogenic microbiome, thus limiting the risk of allergic asthma [157]. For instance, raw cow milk consumption and vitamin D and omega-3 fatty acids supplementation during pregnancy have all been shown to diminish the risk of asthma in the offspring, presumably by affecting the microbiome synthesis of the child [158]. Avoidance of unnecessary maternal antibiotic exposure is another potentially beneficial pre-birth measure linked with microbiome [89]. As previously mentioned, vaginal delivery, breastfeeding, reasonable antibiotic use, pet ownership, exposure to 'unhygienic' traditional farming environments, and high-fiber dietary content in infancy have, more or less consistently, been associated with favorable effects on human body microbiota composition and function (especially in the gut) and a reduced risk of allergic asthma development later in life. However, it must be stressed that available evidence is generally inconclusive and probably only a few of these associations can be considered definite. Moreover, implementation of some or even all of these measures may be practically unattainable for various reasons.

To overcome these limitations, more "interventional" approaches have been proposed. Probiotics are live microorganisms (bacteria or fungi) that may favorably affect the host health, whereas prebiotics are defined as non-digestible compounds that, after processing by intestinal microbiota, promote the expansion and/or activation of beneficial commensals. Symbiotics refer to preparations containing both probiotics and prebiotics [159]. A multitude of orally administered probiotics have been shown to attenuate allergic airway inflammation in mice [160–163]. As described above, high-fiber diets and SCFAs administration (which are essentially prebiotics) have also been found to mitigate inflammatory changes in experimental models of allergic airway disease [99,100]. The potential effect of these biologic agents with microbiome-modifying capacity on allergic asthma has further been studied in several randomized placebo-controlled trials (RCTs). Daily supplementation of asthmatic school children with the probiotic *Lactobacillus gasseri* A5 or a mixture of *Lactobacillus acidophilus, Bifidobacterium bifidum,* and *Lactobacillus delbrueckii* for two to three months have both been shown to improve asthma symptoms and lung function [164–168]. Similarly, a symbiotic preparation consisting of short-chain galacto-oligosaccharides, long-chain fructo-oligosaccharides, and the *Bifidobacterium breve* M-16V increased PEF and reduced serum IL-5 in an adult cohort of allergic asthma [168]. However, most [167–169], albeit not all [170], meta-analyses performed to date have failed to demonstrate a beneficial effect of preventive probiotic supplementation to mothers during pregnancy and/or infants during the first year of life on asthma risk. Further adequately powered and well-designed RCTs are warranted to clarify the role of probiotics/prebiotics on asthma prevention and treatment.

While the possible propitious effects of orally administered probiotics/prebiotics on asthma are thought to be derived by favorable alterations in the gut microbiota and the gut–lung axis, a more targeted approach involving direct interventions to lung microbiome via inhalational delivery of such agents remains relatively unexplored. In mice, intranasal administration of *Acinetobacter Iwoffii, Lactococcus lactis,* or *Staphylococcus sciuri*, all of which had previously been isolated from cowsheds in the context of farming asthma studies, have been shown to hinder eosinophilic airway inflammation induced by ovalbumin sensitization and challenge [2,171]. Similar findings have also been reported by another group for *Escherichia coli* administered via inhalation in the same murine model of allergic airway inflammation [172]. In all cases, allergy protection conferred by inhaled bacteria was associated with modifications in DC activation, leading to altered T-cell responses [172–174], in line with the previously presented observations on SCFAs administration. However, the effects of inhaled probiotic treatments on lung microbiota structure and function have not been addressed. In another experimental study assessing the potential influence of the administration route on the protective role of probiotics, *Lactobacillus paracasei* more efficiently suppressed eosinophilic inflammation when administered intranasally rather than via a feeding tube [175]. These results might suggest superior efficacy of microbiome-modifying therapeutic interventions, probiotics, and probably others (e.g., antibiotics) [176], when applied locally to the respiratory tract as compared to oral administration, which additionally may affect other organs. As yet, no human data are available for inhaled probiotic treatment in asthma.

The proposed role of human microbiome on shaping asthma phenotypes and exacerbation susceptibility, as analyzed above, may form the conceptual basis for the use of antibiotics as a means for therapeutic manipulation of the microbiome, aiming at the restoration of a symbiotic state between the host and the resident microbiota through the suppression of overgrown detrimental taxa and the foster of beneficial ones. This holds especially true for the Th2-low, CS-insensitive, exacerbation prone, severe neutrophilic asthma phenotype, the treatment options for which are particularly limited. As Proteobacteria-dominated changes in lung microbiome have quite consistently been identified in relation with this phenotype, with *Haemophilus influenzae* and *Moraxella catarrhalis* being the most prominent species involved, these taxa could probably be considered the primary targets of microbiome-modifying antibiotic treatment in neutrophilic asthma. The anticipated gradual advent of non-culture-based methods for lung microbiota identification in clinical practice may allow more personalized approaches in antibiotic targeting of dysbiotic lung bacteria in the future.

Both in asthma and in a growing list of other respiratory diseases, macrolides have become the subject of much attention due to the fact that they combine well-known antimicrobial activity along with multiform immunomodulatory properties, including attenuation of neutrophil chemotaxis, inhibition of biofilm formation, reduction of mucus hypersecretion, and even downregulation of viral entry receptors with amplification of viral infection-induced IFN production [177–179]. Overall, clinical trials of macrolides in asthma, most of which in patients with severe uncontrolled asthma, have yielded conflicting results. However, in a pre-specified subgroup analysis of the AZISAST multicenter randomized placebo-controlled trial, it was shown that a six-month course of azithromycin, given at a dose of 250 mg, three times a week, in patients with severe asthma and frequent exacerbation, significantly reduced a composite primary outcome comprising the rates of severe exacerbations and lower respiratory-tract infections requiring antibiotics in the non-eosinophilic asthma subgroup of patients [180]. More recently, the larger AMAZES randomized controlled trial (RCT) reported significantly decreased rates of exacerbations, along with improved asthma-related quality of life in patients with uncontrolled asthma despite therapy with medium-to-high doses of ICS plus LABA who received a higher dose of azithromycin (500 mg three times per week) for 12 months [181]. Interestingly, in this trial, azithromycin appeared equally effective in all studied subgroups, including both those of eosinophilic and non-eosinophilic asthma. Although these beneficial effects of azithromycin (and perhaps other macrolides) on asthma exacerbations could be attributed to the aforementioned immunomodulatory anti-inflammatory properties of macrolides, there are data showing alterations of microbiota composition following treatment with azithromycin. In a research letter published in 2014, Slater et al. described the longitudinal effects of six weeks of daily therapy with 250 mg azithromycin on lung microbiota characteristics, using bronchoscopic washings for sampling and DNA pyrosequencing analysis in five patients with moderate-to-severe asthma [182]. The study reported a reduction of lung microbiota diversity post-treatment, accompanied by an increased relative abundance of *Anaerococcus* and a decreased recognition of the potentially pathogenic genera of *Pseudomonas*, *Staphylococcus*, and *Haemophilus*. Furthermore, in a bacteriological sub-study of the AZISAST trial, azithromycin administration was associated with post-treatment changes in the microbiota composition of the oropharynx compared with both pretreatment status and control patients receiving placebo [183]. At the phylum level, Firmicutes increased and Fusobacteria decreased in oropharyngeal swabs derived from eight severe asthma patients after a six-month course of azithromycin. This finding corresponded to an increased abundance of *Streptococcus salivarius*, with a parallel reduction of *Leptotrichia wadei* at the species level. Of notice, in half of the washout samples collected one month following completion of azithromycin treatment, the microbiota composition was almost identical to the pretreatment oropharyngeal flora of the same patient, indicating a possibility for original microbiome recovery after cessation of antibiotics administration and a consequent requirement for long-term treatment.

Admittedly, there are considerable limitations in the long-term use of antibiotics as a therapeutic tool for favorable manipulations of the host microbiome. Apart from well-founded concerns with respect to potential adverse effects (sometimes irreversible or life threatening) and emergence of antimicrobial resistance arising from long-term antibiotic regimens, the lack of specificity in the elimination of resident bacteria does not allow currently available antimicrobial agents to eradicate exclusively dysbiotic members of the lung bacterial community while sparing beneficial commensals, and may, in fact, produce the opposite results. As previously noted, maternal and early life antibiotic usage has been associated with an increased risk of asthma development during childhood. The detrimental effects of antibiotic use (and not necessarily long-term) on gut microbiome are firmly established and involve the depletion of normal biodiversity and the overgrowth of potentially harmful bacterial strains, leading to dysbiosis. Occasionally, this can be expressed clinically in the form of antibiotic-associated diarrhea and pseudomembranous colitis. Such antibiotics-associated hazards (i.e., selection of potentially pathogenic microbiota) are also pertinent to the lung microbiome, and broad-spectrum antibiotic use may lead from a state of respiratory dysbiosis to another, each time dominated by different and probably more-resistant strains. Despite potentially abolishing systemic adverse effects, inhaled antibiotics are probably subject to these same limitations and cannot be considered as an ideal alternative to systemically administered agents.

Novel approaches to microbiome-modifying therapies have focused on the manipulation of metabolites known to be produced or processed by the (gut) microbiota and to act on the host [184,185]. Metabolite-targeting molecules are under development. Fecal transplantation has successfully been used as a means of gut microbiota manipulation in several intestinal disorders [186]. Its potential role in allergic and respiratory diseases remains unexplored.

The endeavor to therapeutically manipulate human microbiome is clearly still in its infancy, and, by all means, intensive innovative research applying to all stages of the treatment discovery and development pipeline is mandatory before any of these interventions could be incorporated into clinical practice guideline recommendations.

3. Conclusions

Studies conducted over the last two decades have dramatically changed our perspective on LRT microbiology, with the use of culture-independent molecular techniques. It is now universally accepted that the lung is far from a sterile organ. It has convincingly been shown that, in asthma, lung microbiome undergoes significant alterations in terms of diversity and composition, with certain species outgrowing others, functionally leading to a presumable state of respiratory dysbiosis. Many of these alterations have been associated with specific phenotypic features of asthma, including disease exacerbations, and aspects of this dysbiosis may represent the missing link in the pathogenesis of some expressions of the asthmatic disease, perhaps, in particular, the neutrophilic inflammatory phenotype. A considerably large body of evidence arising from both experimental and epidemiological studies is now available, suggesting that early life environmental exposures affecting the gut microbiome structure may be involved in shaping susceptibility for asthma development later in life by modifying microbiota-derived factors thought to be actively involved in the configuration of the gut–lung axis, such as the SCFAs. Given its proposed roles in influencing the risk for asthma development, as well as the phenotypic expression of an established disease, microbiome has emerged as a potential therapeutic target in asthma. As yet, interventions potentially modifying the microbiome have not clearly been shown to be efficacious in preventing and/or treating asthma, with few exceptions.

More accurate delineation of lung microbiota structural and functional characteristics, both in health and in asthma, remains an unmet need in the microbiome research. Larger longitudinal studies applying standardized sampling methods in well-characterized asthmatic cohorts are indispensable in this regard. Unquestionably, the impending widespread application of the novel "-omics" technologies can be expected to provide invaluable insights into the functional effects of lung microbiome and their presumable role in shaping asthma predisposition and phenotypes. Advancing our understanding on the mechanistic links between human microbiome and asthma will hopefully culminate in the discovery of novel therapeutic interventions targeting specific aspects of respiratory dysbiosis.

Author Contributions: Conceptualization, N.R.; literature search and data extraction, K.L., G.B., L.K., and N.R.; writing—original draft preparation, K.L., G.B., and L.K; writing, review, and editing, E.G., M.P., I.V., and N.R.; supervision, A.K., N.K., and N.R.

Acknowledgments: In this section you can acknowledge any support given which is not covered by the author contribution or funding sections. This may include administrative and technical support, or donations in kind (e.g., materials used for experiments).

Conflicts of Interest: The authors declare no conflicts of interest.

References

1. Croisant, S. Epidemiology of asthma: Prevalence and burden of disease. *Adv. Exp. Med. Biol.* **2014**, *795*, 17–29. [CrossRef] [PubMed]
2. Wenzel, S.E. Asthma phenotypes: The evolution from clinical to molecular approaches. *Nat. Med.* **2012**, *18*, 716–725. [CrossRef] [PubMed]
3. Desai, M.; Oppenheimer, J. Elucidating asthma phenotypes and endotypes: Progress towards personalized medicine. *Ann. Allergy Asthma Immunol.* **2016**, *116*, 394–401. [CrossRef] [PubMed]
4. Chung, K.F. Asthma phenotyping: A necessity for improved therapeutic precision and new targeted therapies. *J. Intern. Med.* **2016**, *279*, 192–204. [CrossRef] [PubMed]
5. Fahy, J.V. Type 2 inflammation in asthma–present in most, absent in many. *Nat. Rev. Immunol.* **2015**, *15*, 57–65. [CrossRef] [PubMed]
6. Diver, S.; Russell, R.J.; Brightling, C.E. New and emerging drug treatments for severe asthma. *Clin. Exp. Allergy* **2018**, *48*, 241–252. [CrossRef]
7. Robinson, D.; Humbert, M.; Buhl, R.; Cruz, A.A.; Inoue, H.; Korom, S.; Hanania, N.A.; Nair, P. Revisiting Type 2-high and Type 2-low airway inflammation in asthma: Current knowledge and therapeutic implications. *Clin. Exp. Allergy* **2017**, *47*, 161–175. [CrossRef]

8. Lazarus, S.C.; Krishnan, J.A.; King, T.S.; Lang, J.E.; Blake, K.V.; Covar, R.; Lugogo, N.; Wenzel, S.; Chinchilli, V.M.; Mauger, D.T.; et al. Mometasone or Tiotropium in Mild Asthma with a Low Sputum Eosinophil Level. *N. Engl. J. Med.* **2019**, *380*, 2009–2019. [CrossRef]
9. Chung, K.F. Potential Role of the Lung Microbiome in Shaping Asthma Phenotypes. *Ann. Am. Thorac. Soc.* **2017**, *14*, S326–S331. [CrossRef]
10. Ver Heul, A.; Planer, J.; Kau, A.L. The Human Microbiota and Asthma. *Clin. Rev. Allergy Immunol.* **2018**. [CrossRef]
11. Budden, K.F.; Shukla, S.D.; Rehman, S.F.; Bowerman, K.L.; Keely, S.; Hugenholtz, P.; Armstrong-James, D.P.H.; Adcock, I.M.; Chotirmall, S.H.; Chung, K.F.; et al. Functional effects of the microbiota in chronic respiratory disease. *Lancet Respir. Med.* **2019**. [CrossRef]
12. Caverly, L.J.; Huang, Y.J.; Sze, M.A. Past, Present, and Future Research on the Lung Microbiome in Inflammatory Airway Disease. *Chest* **2019**, *156*, 376–382. [CrossRef] [PubMed]
13. Faner, R.; Sibila, O.; Agusti, A.; Bernasconi, E.; Chalmers, J.D.; Huffnagle, G.B.; Manichanh, C.; Molyneaux, P.L.; Paredes, R.; Perez Brocal, V.; et al. The microbiome in respiratory medicine: Current challenges and future perspectives. *Eur. Respir. J.* **2017**, *49*. [CrossRef] [PubMed]
14. Marchesi, J.R.; Ravel, J. The vocabulary of microbiome research: A proposal. *Microbiome* **2015**, *3*, 31. [CrossRef] [PubMed]
15. Dang, A.T.; Marsland, B.J. Microbes, metabolites, and the gut-lung axis. *Mucosal Immunol.* **2019**, *12*, 843–850. [CrossRef] [PubMed]
16. Suau, A.; Bonnet, R.; Sutren, M.; Godon, J.J.; Gibson, G.R.; Collins, M.D.; Dore, J. Direct analysis of genes encoding 16S rRNA from complex communities reveals many novel molecular species within the human gut. *Appl. Environ. Microbiol.* **1999**, *65*, 4799–4807.
17. Venkataraman, A.; Bassis, C.M.; Beck, J.M.; Young, V.B.; Curtis, J.L.; Huffnagle, G.B.; Schmidt, T.M. Application of a neutral community model to assess structuring of the human lung microbiome. *mBio* **2015**, *6*. [CrossRef]
18. Cho, I.; Blaser, M.J. The human microbiome: At the interface of health and disease. *Nat. Rev. Genet.* **2012**, *13*, 260–270. [CrossRef]
19. Fujimura, K.E.; Lynch, S.V. Microbiota in allergy and asthma and the emerging relationship with the gut microbiome. *Cell Host Microbe* **2015**, *17*, 592–602. [CrossRef]
20. Turnbaugh, P.J.; Ley, R.E.; Hamady, M.; Fraser-Liggett, C.M.; Knight, R.; Gordon, J.I. The human microbiome project. *Nature* **2007**, *449*, 804–810. [CrossRef]
21. Human Microbiome Project Consortium. Structure, function and diversity of the healthy human microbiome. *Nature* **2012**, *486*, 207–214. [CrossRef] [PubMed]
22. Lloyd-Price, J.; Mahurkar, A.; Rahnavard, G.; Crabtree, J.; Orvis, J.; Hall, A.B.; Brady, A.; Creasy, H.H.; McCracken, C.; Giglio, M.G.; et al. Strains, functions and dynamics in the expanded Human Microbiome Project. *Nature* **2017**, *550*, 61–66. [CrossRef] [PubMed]
23. Integrative HMP (iHMP) Research Network Consortium. The Integrative Human Microbiome Project. *Nature* **2019**, *569*, 641–648. [CrossRef] [PubMed]
24. Qin, J.; Li, R.; Raes, J.; Arumugam, M.; Burgdorf, K.S.; Manichanh, C.; Nielsen, T.; Pons, N.; Levenez, F.; Yamada, T.; et al. A human gut microbial gene catalogue established by metagenomic sequencing. *Nature* **2010**, *464*, 59–65. [CrossRef] [PubMed]
25. Sender, R.; Fuchs, S.; Milo, R. Are We Really Vastly Outnumbered? Revisiting the Ratio of Bacterial to Host Cells in Humans. *Cell* **2016**, *164*, 337–340. [CrossRef] [PubMed]
26. Sender, R.; Fuchs, S.; Milo, R. Revised Estimates for the Number of Human and Bacteria Cells in the Body. *PLoS Biol.* **2016**, *14*, e1002533. [CrossRef]
27. Chotirmall, S.H.; Gellatly, S.L.; Budden, K.F.; Mac Aogain, M.; Shukla, S.D.; Wood, D.L.; Hugenholtz, P.; Pethe, K.; Hansbro, P.M. Microbiomes in respiratory health and disease: An Asia-Pacific perspective. *Respirology* **2017**, *22*, 240–250. [CrossRef]
28. Collado, M.C.; Rautava, S.; Aakko, J.; Isolauri, E.; Salminen, S. Human gut colonisation may be initiated in utero by distinct microbial communities in the placenta and amniotic fluid. *Sci. Rep.* **2016**, *6*, 23129. [CrossRef]
29. Lim, E.S.; Rodriguez, C.; Holtz, L.R. Amniotic fluid from healthy term pregnancies does not harbor a detectable microbial community. *Microbiome* **2018**, *6*, 87. [CrossRef]

30. Dominguez-Bello, M.G.; Costello, E.K.; Contreras, M.; Magris, M.; Hidalgo, G.; Fierer, N.; Knight, R. Delivery mode shapes the acquisition and structure of the initial microbiota across multiple body habitats in newborns. *Proc. Natl. Acad. Sci. USA* **2010**, *107*, 11971–11975. [CrossRef]

31. Koenig, J.E.; Spor, A.; Scalfone, N.; Fricker, A.D.; Stombaugh, J.; Knight, R.; Angenent, L.T.; Ley, R.E. Succession of microbial consortia in the developing infant gut microbiome. *Proc. Natl. Acad. Sci. USA* **2011**, *108*, 4578–4585. [CrossRef] [PubMed]

32. Yatsunenko, T.; Rey, F.E.; Manary, M.J.; Trehan, I.; Dominguez-Bello, M.G.; Contreras, M.; Magris, M.; Hidalgo, G.; Baldassano, R.N.; Anokhin, A.P.; et al. Human gut microbiome viewed across age and geography. *Nature* **2012**, *486*, 222–227. [CrossRef] [PubMed]

33. Biesbroek, G.; Tsivtsivadze, E.; Sanders, E.A.; Montijn, R.; Veenhoven, R.H.; Keijser, B.J.; Bogaert, D. Early respiratory microbiota composition determines bacterial succession patterns and respiratory health in children. *Am. J. Respir. Crit. Care Med.* **2014**, *190*, 1283–1292. [CrossRef] [PubMed]

34. Bosch, A.; de Steenhuijsen Piters, W.A.A.; van Houten, M.A.; Chu, M.; Biesbroek, G.; Kool, J.; Pernet, P.; de Groot, P.C.M.; Eijkemans, M.J.C.; Keijser, B.J.F.; et al. Maturation of the Infant Respiratory Microbiota, Environmental Drivers, and Health Consequences. A Prospective Cohort Study. *Am. J. Respir. Crit. Care Med.* **2017**, *196*, 1582–1590. [CrossRef]

35. Teo, S.M.; Mok, D.; Pham, K.; Kusel, M.; Serralha, M.; Troy, N.; Holt, B.J.; Hales, B.J.; Walker, M.L.; Hollams, E.; et al. The infant nasopharyngeal microbiome impacts severity of lower respiratory infection and risk of asthma development. *Cell Host Microbe* **2015**, *17*, 704–715. [CrossRef] [PubMed]

36. Gensollen, T.; Iyer, S.S.; Kasper, D.L.; Blumberg, R.S. How colonization by microbiota in early life shapes the immune system. *Science* **2016**, *352*, 539–544. [CrossRef] [PubMed]

37. Singh, N.; Vats, A.; Sharma, A.; Arora, A.; Kumar, A. The development of lower respiratory tract microbiome in mice. *Microbiome* **2017**, *5*, 61. [CrossRef]

38. Bowers, R.M.; McLetchie, S.; Knight, R.; Fierer, N. Spatial variability in airborne bacterial communities across land-use types and their relationship to the bacterial communities of potential source environments. *ISME J.* **2011**, *5*, 601–612. [CrossRef]

39. Qin, S.; Clausen, E.; Lucht, L.; Michael, H.; Beck, J.M.; Curtis, J.L.; Freeman, C.M.; Morris, A. Presence of Tropheryma whipplei in Different Body Sites in a Cohort of Healthy Subjects. *Am. J. Respir. Crit. Care Med.* **2016**, *194*, 243–245. [CrossRef]

40. Dickson, R.P.; Erb-Downward, J.R.; Huffnagle, G.B. Homeostasis and its disruption in the lung microbiome. *Am. J. Physiol. Lung Cell. Mol. Physiol.* **2015**, *309*, L1047–L1055. [CrossRef]

41. Charlson, E.S.; Bittinger, K.; Haas, A.R.; Fitzgerald, A.S.; Frank, I.; Yadav, A.; Bushman, F.D.; Collman, R.G. Topographical continuity of bacterial populations in the healthy human respiratory tract. *Am. J. Respir. Crit. Care Med.* **2011**, *184*, 957–963. [CrossRef] [PubMed]

42. Morris, A.; Beck, J.M.; Schloss, P.D.; Campbell, T.B.; Crothers, K.; Curtis, J.L.; Flores, S.C.; Fontenot, A.P.; Ghedin, E.; Huang, L.; et al. Comparison of the respiratory microbiome in healthy nonsmokers and smokers. *Am. J. Respir. Crit. Care Med.* **2013**, *187*, 1067–1075. [CrossRef] [PubMed]

43. Bassis, C.M.; Erb-Downward, J.R.; Dickson, R.P.; Freeman, C.M.; Schmidt, T.M.; Young, V.B.; Beck, J.M.; Curtis, J.L.; Huffnagle, G.B. Analysis of the upper respiratory tract microbiotas as the source of the lung and gastric microbiotas in healthy individuals. *mBio* **2015**, *6*, e00037. [CrossRef] [PubMed]

44. Dickson, R.P.; Erb-Downward, J.R.; Freeman, C.M.; McCloskey, L.; Beck, J.M.; Huffnagle, G.B.; Curtis, J.L. Spatial Variation in the Healthy Human Lung Microbiome and the Adapted Island Model of Lung Biogeography. *Ann. Am. Thorac. Soc.* **2015**, *12*, 821–830. [CrossRef]

45. Dickson, R.P.; Erb-Downward, J.R.; Huffnagle, G.B. Towards an ecology of the lung: New conceptual models of pulmonary microbiology and pneumonia pathogenesis. *Lancet. Respir. Med.* **2014**, *2*, 238–246. [CrossRef]

46. Hilty, M.; Burke, C.; Pedro, H.; Cardenas, P.; Bush, A.; Bossley, C.; Davies, J.; Ervine, A.; Poulter, L.; Pachter, L.; et al. Disordered microbial communities in asthmatic airways. *PLoS ONE* **2010**, *5*, e8578. [CrossRef]

47. Mathieu, E.; Escribano-Vazquez, U.; Descamps, D.; Cherbuy, C.; Langella, P.; Riffault, S.; Remot, A.; Thomas, M. Paradigms of Lung Microbiota Functions in Health and Disease, Particularly, in Asthma. *Front. Physiol.* **2018**, *9*, 1168. [CrossRef]

48. Denner, D.R.; Sangwan, N.; Becker, J.B.; Hogarth, D.K.; Oldham, J.; Castillo, J.; Sperling, A.I.; Solway, J.; Naureckas, E.T.; Gilbert, J.A.; et al. Corticosteroid therapy and airflow obstruction influence the bronchial microbiome, which is distinct from that of bronchoalveolar lavage in asthmatic airways. *J. Allergy Clin. Immunol.* **2016**, *137*, 1398–1405. [CrossRef]
49. Durack, J.; Huang, Y.J.; Nariya, S.; Christian, L.S.; Ansel, K.M.; Beigelman, A.; Castro, M.; Dyer, A.M.; Israel, E.; Kraft, M.; et al. Bacterial biogeography of adult airways in atopic asthma. *Microbiome* **2018**, *6*, 104. [CrossRef]
50. Goleva, E.; Jackson, L.P.; Harris, J.K.; Robertson, C.E.; Sutherland, E.R.; Hall, C.F.; Good, J.T., Jr.; Gelfand, E.W.; Martin, R.J.; Leung, D.Y. The effects of airway microbiome on corticosteroid responsiveness in asthma. *Am. J. Respir. Crit. Care Med.* **2013**, *188*, 1193–1201. [CrossRef]
51. Dickson, R.P.; Erb-Downward, J.R.; Martinez, F.J.; Huffnagle, G.B. The Microbiome and the Respiratory Tract. *Annu. Rev. Physiol.* **2016**, *78*, 481–504. [CrossRef] [PubMed]
52. Erb-Downward, J.R.; Thompson, D.L.; Han, M.K.; Freeman, C.M.; McCloskey, L.; Schmidt, L.A.; Young, V.B.; Toews, G.B.; Curtis, J.L.; Sundaram, B.; et al. Analysis of the lung microbiome in the "healthy" smoker and in COPD. *PLoS ONE* **2011**, *6*, e16384. [CrossRef] [PubMed]
53. Ren, L.; Zhang, R.; Rao, J.; Xiao, Y.; Zhang, Z.; Yang, B.; Cao, D.; Zhong, H.; Ning, P.; Shang, Y.; et al. Transcriptionally Active Lung Microbiome and Its Association with Bacterial Biomass and Host Inflammatory Status. *mSystems* **2018**, *3*. [CrossRef] [PubMed]
54. Liu, H.X.; Tao, L.L.; Zhang, J.; Zhu, Y.G.; Zheng, Y.; Liu, D.; Zhou, M.; Ke, H.; Shi, M.M.; Qu, J.M. Difference of lower airway microbiome in bilateral protected specimen brush between lung cancer patients with unilateral lobar masses and control subjects. *Int. J. Cancer* **2018**, *142*, 769–778. [CrossRef]
55. Zhou, R.; Yazdi, A.S.; Menu, P.; Tschopp, J. A role for mitochondria in NLRP3 inflammasome activation. *Nature* **2011**, *469*, 221–225. [CrossRef]
56. Ishii, K.J.; Koyama, S.; Nakagawa, A.; Coban, C.; Akira, S. Host innate immune receptors and beyond: Making sense of microbial infections. *Cell Host Microbe* **2008**, *3*, 352–363. [CrossRef]
57. Larsen, J.M. The immune response to Prevotella bacteria in chronic inflammatory disease. *Immunology* **2017**, *151*, 363–374. [CrossRef]
58. Huffnagle, G.B.; Dickson, R.P.; Lukacs, N.W. The respiratory tract microbiome and lung inflammation: A two-way street. *Mucosal Immunol.* **2017**, *10*, 299–306. [CrossRef]
59. Honko, A.N.; Mizel, S.B. Effects of flagellin on innate and adaptive immunity. *Immunol. Res.* **2005**, *33*, 83–101. [CrossRef]
60. Hemmi, H.; Takeuchi, O.; Kawai, T.; Kaisho, T.; Sato, S.; Sanjo, H.; Matsumoto, M.; Hoshino, K.; Wagner, H.; Takeda, K.; et al. A Toll-like receptor recognizes bacterial DNA. *Nature* **2000**, *408*, 740–745. [CrossRef]
61. Brown, R.L.; Sequeira, R.P.; Clarke, T.B. The microbiota protects against respiratory infection via GM-CSF signaling. *Nat. Commun.* **2017**, *8*, 1512. [CrossRef] [PubMed]
62. Durack, J.; Lynch, S.V.; Nariya, S.; Bhakta, N.R.; Beigelman, A.; Castro, M.; Dyer, A.M.; Israel, E.; Kraft, M.; Martin, R.J.; et al. Features of the bronchial bacterial microbiome associated with atopy, asthma, and responsiveness to inhaled corticosteroid treatment. *J. Allergy Clin. Immunol.* **2017**, *140*, 63–75. [CrossRef] [PubMed]
63. Chambers, E.S.; Preston, T.; Frost, G.; Morrison, D.J. Role of Gut Microbiota-Generated Short-Chain Fatty Acids in Metabolic and Cardiovascular Health. *Curr. Nutr. Rep.* **2018**, *7*, 198–206. [CrossRef] [PubMed]
64. Koh, A.; De Vadder, F.; Kovatcheva-Datchary, P.; Backhed, F. From Dietary Fiber to Host Physiology: Short-Chain Fatty Acids as Key Bacterial Metabolites. *Cell* **2016**, *165*, 1332–1345. [CrossRef] [PubMed]
65. Tan, J.; McKenzie, C.; Potamitis, M.; Thorburn, A.N.; Mackay, C.R.; Macia, L. The role of short-chain fatty acids in health and disease. *Adv. Immunol.* **2014**, *121*, 91–119. [CrossRef]
66. Castillo, J.; Lopez-Rodas, G.; Franco, L. Histone Post-Translational Modifications and Nucleosome Organisation in Transcriptional Regulation: Some Open Questions. *Adv. Exp. Med. Biol.* **2017**, *966*, 65–92. [CrossRef]
67. Furusawa, Y.; Obata, Y.; Fukuda, S.; Endo, T.A.; Nakato, G.; Takahashi, D.; Nakanishi, Y.; Uetake, C.; Kato, K.; Kato, T.; et al. Commensal microbe-derived butyrate induces the differentiation of colonic regulatory T cells. *Nature* **2013**, *504*, 446–450. [CrossRef]

68. Arpaia, N.; Campbell, C.; Fan, X.; Dikiy, S.; van der Veeken, J.; deRoos, P.; Liu, H.; Cross, J.R.; Pfeffer, K.; Coffer, P.J.; et al. Metabolites produced by commensal bacteria promote peripheral regulatory T-cell generation. *Nature* **2013**, *504*, 451–455. [CrossRef]
69. Smith, P.M.; Howitt, M.R.; Panikov, N.; Michaud, M.; Gallini, C.A.; Bohlooly, Y.M.; Glickman, J.N.; Garrett, W.S. The microbial metabolites, short-chain fatty acids, regulate colonic Treg cell homeostasis. *Science* **2013**, *341*, 569–573. [CrossRef]
70. Vignali, D.A.; Collison, L.W.; Workman, C.J. How regulatory T cells work. *Nat. Rev. Immunol.* **2008**, *8*, 523–532. [CrossRef]
71. Noval Rivas, M.; Chatila, T.A. Regulatory T cells in allergic diseases. *J. Allergy Clin. Immunol.* **2016**, *138*, 639–652. [CrossRef] [PubMed]
72. Segal, L.N.; Clemente, J.C.; Wu, B.G.; Wikoff, W.R.; Gao, Z.; Li, Y.; Ko, J.P.; Rom, W.N.; Blaser, M.J.; Weiden, M.D. Randomised, double-blind, placebo-controlled trial with azithromycin selects for anti-inflammatory microbial metabolites in the emphysematous lung. *Thorax* **2017**, *72*, 13–22. [CrossRef] [PubMed]
73. Cheng, Y.; Jin, U.H.; Allred, C.D.; Jayaraman, A.; Chapkin, R.S.; Safe, S. Aryl Hydrocarbon Receptor Activity of Tryptophan Metabolites in Young Adult Mouse Colonocytes. *Drug Metab. Dispos. Biol. Fate Chem.* **2015**, *43*, 1536–1543. [CrossRef] [PubMed]
74. Marshall, N.B.; Kerkvliet, N.I. Dioxin and immune regulation: Emerging role of aryl hydrocarbon receptor in the generation of regulatory T cells. *Ann. N. Y. Acad. Sci.* **2010**, *1183*, 25–37. [CrossRef] [PubMed]
75. Meduri, G.U.; Kanangat, S.; Stefan, J.; Tolley, E.; Schaberg, D. Cytokines IL-1beta, IL-6, and TNF-alpha enhance in vitro growth of bacteria. *Am. J. Respir. Crit. Care Med.* **1999**, *160*, 961–967. [CrossRef] [PubMed]
76. Lee, J.H.; Del Sorbo, L.; Khine, A.A.; de Azavedo, J.; Low, D.E.; Bell, D.; Uhlig, S.; Slutsky, A.S.; Zhang, H. Modulation of bacterial growth by tumor necrosis factor-alpha in vitro and in vivo. *Am. J. Respir. Crit. Care Med.* **2003**, *168*, 1462–1470. [CrossRef] [PubMed]
77. Belay, T.; Sonnenfeld, G. Differential effects of catecholamines on in vitro growth of pathogenic bacteria. *Life Sci.* **2002**, *71*, 447–456. [CrossRef]
78. Mahdavi, J.; Royer, P.J.; Sjolinder, H.S.; Azimi, S.; Self, T.; Stoof, J.; Wheldon, L.M.; Brannstrom, K.; Wilson, R.; Moreton, J.; et al. Pro-inflammatory cytokines can act as intracellular modulators of commensal bacterial virulence. *Open Biol.* **2013**, *3*, 130048. [CrossRef]
79. Marks, L.R.; Davidson, B.A.; Knight, P.R.; Hakansson, A.P. Interkingdom signaling induces Streptococcus pneumoniae biofilm dispersion and transition from asymptomatic colonization to disease. *mBio* **2013**, *4*. [CrossRef]
80. Dickson, R.P.; Erb-Downward, J.R.; Prescott, H.C.; Martinez, F.J.; Curtis, J.L.; Lama, V.N.; Huffnagle, G.B. Intraalveolar Catecholamines and the Human Lung Microbiome. *Am. J. Respir. Crit. Care Med.* **2015**, *192*, 257–259. [CrossRef]
81. Budden, K.F.; Gellatly, S.L.; Wood, D.L.; Cooper, M.A.; Morrison, M.; Hugenholtz, P.; Hansbro, P.M. Emerging pathogenic links between microbiota and the gut-lung axis. *Nat. Rev. Microbiol.* **2017**, *15*, 55–63. [CrossRef] [PubMed]
82. Herbst, T.; Sichelstiel, A.; Schar, C.; Yadava, K.; Burki, K.; Cahenzli, J.; McCoy, K.; Marsland, B.J.; Harris, N.L. Dysregulation of allergic airway inflammation in the absence of microbial colonization. *Am. J. Respir. Crit. Care Med.* **2011**, *184*, 198–205. [CrossRef] [PubMed]
83. Noverr, M.C.; Falkowski, N.R.; McDonald, R.A.; McKenzie, A.N.; Huffnagle, G.B. Development of allergic airway disease in mice following antibiotic therapy and fungal microbiota increase: Role of host genetics, antigen, and interleukin-13. *Infect. Immun.* **2005**, *73*, 30–38. [CrossRef] [PubMed]
84. Russell, S.L.; Gold, M.J.; Hartmann, M.; Willing, B.P.; Thorson, L.; Wlodarska, M.; Gill, N.; Blanchet, M.R.; Mohn, W.W.; McNagny, K.M.; et al. Early life antibiotic-driven changes in microbiota enhance susceptibility to allergic asthma. *EMBO Rep.* **2012**, *13*, 440–447. [CrossRef] [PubMed]
85. Dethlefsen, L.; Relman, D.A. Incomplete recovery and individualized responses of the human distal gut microbiota to repeated antibiotic perturbation. *Proc. Natl. Acad. Sci. USA* **2011**, *108*, 4554–4561. [CrossRef] [PubMed]
86. Zaura, E.; Brandt, B.W.; Teixeira de Mattos, M.J.; Buijs, M.J.; Caspers, M.P.; Rashid, M.U.; Weintraub, A.; Nord, C.E.; Savell, A.; Hu, Y.; et al. Same Exposure but Two Radically Different Responses to Antibiotics: Resilience of the Salivary Microbiome versus Long-Term Microbial Shifts in Feces. *mBio* **2015**, *6*, e01693-15. [CrossRef]

87. Abeles, S.R.; Jones, M.B.; Santiago-Rodriguez, T.M.; Ly, M.; Klitgord, N.; Yooseph, S.; Nelson, K.E.; Pride, D.T. Microbial diversity in individuals and their household contacts following typical antibiotic courses. *Microbiome* **2016**, *4*, 39. [CrossRef]
88. Dom, S.; Droste, J.H.; Sariachvili, M.A.; Hagendorens, M.M.; Oostveen, E.; Bridts, C.H.; Stevens, W.J.; Wieringa, M.H.; Weyler, J.J. Pre- and post-natal exposure to antibiotics and the development of eczema, recurrent wheezing and atopic sensitization in children up to the age of 4 years. *Clin. Exp. Allergy* **2010**, *40*, 1378–1387. [CrossRef]
89. Stensballe, L.G.; Simonsen, J.; Jensen, S.M.; Bonnelykke, K.; Bisgaard, H. Use of antibiotics during pregnancy increases the risk of asthma in early childhood. *J. Pediatr.* **2013**, *162*, 832–838 e833. [CrossRef]
90. Harmsen, H.J.; Wildeboer-Veloo, A.C.; Raangs, G.C.; Wagendorp, A.A.; Klijn, N.; Bindels, J.G.; Welling, G.W. Analysis of intestinal flora development in breast-fed and formula-fed infants by using molecular identification and detection methods. *J. Pediatric Gastroenterol. Nutr.* **2000**, *30*, 61–67. [CrossRef]
91. Scholtens, S.; Wijga, A.H.; Brunekreef, B.; Kerkhof, M.; Hoekstra, M.O.; Gerritsen, J.; Aalberse, R.; de Jongste, J.C.; Smit, H.A. Breast feeding, parental allergy and asthma in children followed for 8 years. The PIAMA birth cohort study. *Thorax* **2009**, *64*, 604–609. [CrossRef] [PubMed]
92. Francino, M.P. Birth Mode-Related Differences in Gut Microbiota Colonization and Immune System Development. *Ann. Nutr. Metab.* **2018**, *73*, 12–16. [CrossRef] [PubMed]
93. Kolokotroni, O.; Middleton, N.; Gavatha, M.; Lamnisos, D.; Priftis, K.N.; Yiallouros, P.K. Asthma and atopy in children born by caesarean section: Effect modification by family history of allergies—A population based cross-sectional study. *BMC Pediatr.* **2012**, *12*, 179. [CrossRef] [PubMed]
94. Ownby, D.R.; Johnson, C.C.; Peterson, E.L. Exposure to dogs and cats in the first year of life and risk of allergic sensitization at 6 to 7 years of age. *JAMA* **2002**, *288*, 963–972. [CrossRef] [PubMed]
95. Fujimura, K.E.; Demoor, T.; Rauch, M.; Faruqi, A.A.; Jang, S.; Johnson, C.C.; Boushey, H.A.; Zoratti, E.; Ownby, D.; Lukacs, N.W.; et al. House dust exposure mediates gut microbiome Lactobacillus enrichment and airway immune defense against allergens and virus infection. *Proc. Natl. Acad. Sci. USA* **2014**, *111*, 805–810. [CrossRef]
96. Von Mutius, E. The microbial environment and its influence on asthma prevention in early life. *J. Allergy Clin. Immunol.* **2016**, *137*, 680–689. [CrossRef] [PubMed]
97. Stein, M.M.; Hrusch, C.L.; Gozdz, J.; Igartua, C.; Pivniouk, V.; Murray, S.E.; Ledford, J.G.; Marques Dos Santos, M.; Anderson, R.L.; Metwali, N.; et al. Innate Immunity and Asthma Risk in Amish and Hutterite Farm Children. *N. Engl. J. Med.* **2016**, *375*, 411–421. [CrossRef]
98. Maslowski, K.M.; Vieira, A.T.; Ng, A.; Kranich, J.; Sierro, F.; Yu, D.; Schilter, H.C.; Rolph, M.S.; Mackay, F.; Artis, D.; et al. Regulation of inflammatory responses by gut microbiota and chemoattractant receptor GPR43. *Nature* **2009**, *461*, 1282–1286. [CrossRef]
99. Trompette, A.; Gollwitzer, E.S.; Yadava, K.; Sichelstiel, A.K.; Sprenger, N.; Ngom-Bru, C.; Blanchard, C.; Junt, T.; Nicod, L.P.; Harris, N.L.; et al. Gut microbiota metabolism of dietary fiber influences allergic airway disease and hematopoiesis. *Nat. Med.* **2014**, *20*, 159–166. [CrossRef]
100. Cait, A.; Hughes, M.R.; Antignano, F.; Cait, J.; Dimitriu, P.A.; Maas, K.R.; Reynolds, L.A.; Hacker, L.; Mohr, J.; Finlay, B.B.; et al. Microbiome-driven allergic lung inflammation is ameliorated by short-chain fatty acids. *Mucosal Immunol.* **2018**, *11*, 785–795. [CrossRef]
101. Huang, Y.J.; Nelson, C.E.; Brodie, E.L.; Desantis, T.Z.; Baek, M.S.; Liu, J.; Woyke, T.; Allgaier, M.; Bristow, J.; Wiener-Kronish, J.P.; et al. Airway microbiota and bronchial hyperresponsiveness in patients with suboptimally controlled asthma. *J. Allergy Clin. Immunol.* **2011**, *127*, 372–381. [CrossRef] [PubMed]
102. Marri, P.R.; Stern, D.A.; Wright, A.L.; Billheimer, D.; Martinez, F.D. Asthma-associated differences in microbial composition of induced sputum. *J. Allergy Clin. Immunol.* **2013**, *131*, 346–352. [CrossRef] [PubMed]
103. Green, B.J.; Wiriyachaiporn, S.; Grainge, C.; Rogers, G.B.; Kehagia, V.; Lau, L.; Carroll, M.P.; Bruce, K.D.; Howarth, P.H. Potentially pathogenic airway bacteria and neutrophilic inflammation in treatment resistant severe asthma. *PLoS ONE* **2014**, *9*, e100645. [CrossRef] [PubMed]
104. Huang, Y.J.; Nariya, S.; Harris, J.M.; Lynch, S.V.; Choy, D.F.; Arron, J.R.; Boushey, H. The airway microbiome in patients with severe asthma: Associations with disease features and severity. *J. Allergy Clin. Immunol.* **2015**, *136*, 874–884. [CrossRef] [PubMed]

105. Simpson, J.L.; Daly, J.; Baines, K.J.; Yang, I.A.; Upham, J.W.; Reynolds, P.N.; Hodge, S.; James, A.L.; Hugenholtz, P.; Willner, D.; et al. Airway dysbiosis: Haemophilus influenzae and Tropheryma in poorly controlled asthma. *Eur. Respir. J.* **2016**, *47*, 792–800. [CrossRef] [PubMed]
106. Zhang, Q.; Cox, M.; Liang, Z.; Brinkmann, F.; Cardenas, P.A.; Duff, R.; Bhavsar, P.; Cookson, W.; Moffatt, M.; Chung, K.F. Airway Microbiota in Severe Asthma and Relationship to Asthma Severity and Phenotypes. *PLoS ONE* **2016**, *11*, e0152724. [CrossRef] [PubMed]
107. Sverrild, A.; Kiilerich, P.; Brejnrod, A.; Pedersen, R.; Porsbjerg, C.; Bergqvist, A.; Erjefalt, J.S.; Kristiansen, K.; Backer, V. Eosinophilic airway inflammation in asthmatic patients is associated with an altered airway microbiome. *J. Allergy Clin. Immunol.* **2017**, *140*, 407–417 e411. [CrossRef]
108. Li, N.; Qiu, R.; Yang, Z.; Li, J.; Chung, K.F.; Zhong, N.; Zhang, Q. Sputum microbiota in severe asthma patients: Relationship to eosinophilic inflammation. *Respir. Med.* **2017**, *131*, 192–198. [CrossRef]
109. Thomson, N.C. Novel approaches to the management of noneosinophilic asthma. *Ther. Adv. Respir. Dis.* **2016**, *10*, 211–234. [CrossRef]
110. Taylor, S.L.; Leong, L.E.X.; Choo, J.M.; Wesselingh, S.; Yang, I.A.; Upham, J.W.; Reynolds, P.N.; Hodge, S.; James, A.L.; Jenkins, C.; et al. Inflammatory phenotypes in patients with severe asthma are associated with distinct airway microbiology. *J. Allergy Clin. Immunol.* **2018**, *141*, 94–103 e115. [CrossRef]
111. Carr, T.F.; Zeki, A.A.; Kraft, M. Eosinophilic and Noneosinophilic Asthma. *Am. J. Respir. Crit. Care Med.* **2018**, *197*, 22–37. [CrossRef] [PubMed]
112. Wenzel, S.E.; Barnes, P.J.; Bleecker, E.R.; Bousquet, J.; Busse, W.; Dahlen, S.E.; Holgate, S.T.; Meyers, D.A.; Rabe, K.F.; Antczak, A.; et al. A randomized, double-blind, placebo-controlled study of tumor necrosis factor-alpha blockade in severe persistent asthma. *Am. J. Respir. Crit. Care Med.* **2009**, *179*, 549–558. [CrossRef] [PubMed]
113. Busse, W.W.; Holgate, S.; Kerwin, E.; Chon, Y.; Feng, J.; Lin, J.; Lin, S.L. Randomized, double-blind, placebo-controlled study of brodalumab, a human anti-IL-17 receptor monoclonal antibody, in moderate to severe asthma. *Am. J. Respir. Crit. Care Med.* **2013**, *188*, 1294–1302. [CrossRef] [PubMed]
114. Bettelli, E.; Korn, T.; Oukka, M.; Kuchroo, V.K. Induction and effector functions of T(H)17 cells. *Nature* **2008**, *453*, 1051–1057. [CrossRef]
115. Simpson, J.L.; Powell, H.; Boyle, M.J.; Scott, R.J.; Gibson, P.G. Clarithromycin targets neutrophilic airway inflammation in refractory asthma. *Am. J. Respir. Crit. Care Med.* **2008**, *177*, 148–155. [CrossRef]
116. Li, W.; Zhang, X.; Yang, Y.; Yin, Q.; Wang, Y.; Li, Y.; Wang, C.; Wong, S.M.; Wang, Y.; Goldfine, H.; et al. Recognition of conserved antigens by Th17 cells provides broad protection against pulmonary Haemophilus influenzae infection. *Proc. Natl. Acad. Sci. USA* **2018**, *115*, E7149–E7157. [CrossRef]
117. Essilfie, A.T.; Simpson, J.L.; Horvat, J.C.; Preston, J.A.; Dunkley, M.L.; Foster, P.S.; Gibson, P.G.; Hansbro, P.M. Haemophilus influenzae infection drives IL-17-mediated neutrophilic allergic airways disease. *PLoS Pathog.* **2011**, *7*, e1002244. [CrossRef]
118. Chapman, D.G.; Irvin, C.G. Mechanisms of airway hyper-responsiveness in asthma: The past, present and yet to come. *Clin. Exp. Allergy* **2015**, *45*, 706–719. [CrossRef]
119. Haldar, P.; Pavord, I.D.; Shaw, D.E.; Berry, M.A.; Thomas, M.; Brightling, C.E.; Wardlaw, A.J.; Green, R.H. Cluster analysis and clinical asthma phenotypes. *Am. J. Respir. Crit. Care Med.* **2008**, *178*, 218–224. [CrossRef]
120. Moore, W.C.; Meyers, D.A.; Wenzel, S.E.; Teague, W.G.; Li, H.; Li, X.; D'Agostino, R., Jr.; Castro, M.; Curran-Everett, D.; Fitzpatrick, A.M.; et al. Identification of asthma phenotypes using cluster analysis in the Severe Asthma Research Program. *Am. J. Respir. Crit. Care Med.* **2010**, *181*, 315–323. [CrossRef]
121. Wu, W.; Bleecker, E.; Moore, W.; Busse, W.W.; Castro, M.; Chung, K.F.; Calhoun, W.J.; Erzurum, S.; Gaston, B.; Israel, E.; et al. Unsupervised phenotyping of Severe Asthma Research Program participants using expanded lung data. *J. Allergy Clin. Immunol.* **2014**, *133*, 1280–1288. [CrossRef] [PubMed]
122. Dixon, A.E.; Pratley, R.E.; Forgione, P.M.; Kaminsky, D.A.; Whittaker-Leclair, L.A.; Griffes, L.A.; Garudathri, J.; Raymond, D.; Poynter, M.E.; Bunn, J.Y.; et al. Effects of obesity and bariatric surgery on airway hyperresponsiveness, asthma control, and inflammation. *J. Allergy Clin. Immunol.* **2011**, *128*, 508–515. [CrossRef] [PubMed]
123. Van Huisstede, A.; Rudolphus, A.; Castro Cabezas, M.; Biter, L.U.; van de Geijn, G.J.; Taube, C.; Hiemstra, P.S.; Braunstahl, G.J. Effect of bariatric surgery on asthma control, lung function and bronchial and systemic inflammation in morbidly obese subjects with asthma. *Thorax* **2015**, *70*, 659–667. [CrossRef] [PubMed]

124. Dias-Junior, S.A.; Reis, M.; de Carvalho-Pinto, R.M.; Stelmach, R.; Halpern, A.; Cukier, A. Effects of weight loss on asthma control in obese patients with severe asthma. *Eur. Respir. J.* **2014**, *43*, 1368–1377. [CrossRef] [PubMed]
125. Scott, H.A.; Gibson, P.G.; Garg, M.L.; Pretto, J.J.; Morgan, P.J.; Callister, R.; Wood, L.G. Dietary restriction and exercise improve airway inflammation and clinical outcomes in overweight and obese asthma: A randomized trial. *Clin. Exp. Allergy* **2013**, *43*, 36–49. [CrossRef] [PubMed]
126. Singh, A.M.; Busse, W.W. Asthma exacerbations. 2: Aetiology. *Thorax* **2006**, *61*, 809–816. [CrossRef]
127. Sutherland, E.R.; Martin, R.J. Asthma and atypical bacterial infection. *Chest* **2007**, *132*, 1962–1966. [CrossRef]
128. De Schutter, I.; Dreesman, A.; Soetens, O.; De Waele, M.; Crokaert, F.; Verhaegen, J.; Pierard, D.; Malfroot, A. In young children, persistent wheezing is associated with bronchial bacterial infection: A retrospective analysis. *BMC Pediatr.* **2012**, *12*, 83. [CrossRef]
129. Kloepfer, K.M.; Lee, W.M.; Pappas, T.E.; Kang, T.J.; Vrtis, R.F.; Evans, M.D.; Gangnon, R.E.; Bochkov, Y.A.; Jackson, D.J.; Lemanske, R.F., Jr.; et al. Detection of pathogenic bacteria during rhinovirus infection is associated with increased respiratory symptoms and asthma exacerbations. *J. Allergy Clin. Immunol.* **2014**, *133*, 1301–1307. [CrossRef]
130. Ghebre, M.A.; Pang, P.H.; Diver, S.; Desai, D.; Bafadhel, M.; Haldar, K.; Kebadze, T.; Cohen, S.; Newbold, P.; Rapley, L.; et al. Biological exacerbation clusters demonstrate asthma and chronic obstructive pulmonary disease overlap with distinct mediator and microbiome profiles. *J. Allergy Clin. Immunol.* **2018**, *141*, 2027–2036 e2012. [CrossRef]
131. Dickson, R.P.; Martinez, F.J.; Huffnagle, G.B. The role of the microbiome in exacerbations of chronic lung diseases. *Lancet* **2014**, *384*, 691–702. [CrossRef]
132. Vareille, M.; Kieninger, E.; Edwards, M.R.; Regamey, N. The airway epithelium: Soldier in the fight against respiratory viruses. *Clin. Microbiol. Rev.* **2011**, *24*, 210–229. [CrossRef] [PubMed]
133. Smith, C.M.; Kulkarni, H.; Radhakrishnan, P.; Rutman, A.; Bankart, M.J.; Williams, G.; Hirst, R.A.; Easton, A.J.; Andrew, P.W.; O'Callaghan, C. Ciliary dyskinesia is an early feature of respiratory syncytial virus infection. *Eur. Respir. J.* **2014**, *43*, 485–496. [CrossRef] [PubMed]
134. Sajjan, U.; Wang, Q.; Zhao, Y.; Gruenert, D.C.; Hershenson, M.B. Rhinovirus disrupts the barrier function of polarized airway epithelial cells. *Am. J. Respir. Crit. Care Med.* **2008**, *178*, 1271–1281. [CrossRef]
135. Kilani, M.M.; Mohammed, K.A.; Nasreen, N.; Hardwick, J.A.; Kaplan, M.H.; Tepper, R.S.; Antony, V.B. Respiratory syncytial virus causes increased bronchial epithelial permeability. *Chest* **2004**, *126*, 186–191. [CrossRef]
136. Santee, C.A.; Nagalingam, N.A.; Faruqi, A.A.; DeMuri, G.P.; Gern, J.E.; Wald, E.R.; Lynch, S.V. Nasopharyngeal microbiota composition of children is related to the frequency of upper respiratory infection and acute sinusitis. *Microbiome* **2016**, *4*, 34. [CrossRef]
137. Rosas-Salazar, C.; Shilts, M.H.; Tovchigrechko, A.; Schobel, S.; Chappell, J.D.; Larkin, E.K.; Shankar, J.; Yooseph, S.; Nelson, K.E.; Halpin, R.A.; et al. Differences in the Nasopharyngeal Microbiome During Acute Respiratory Tract Infection with Human Rhinovirus and Respiratory Syncytial Virus in Infancy. *J. Infect. Dis.* **2016**, *214*, 1924–1928. [CrossRef]
138. Avadhanula, V.; Rodriguez, C.A.; Devincenzo, J.P.; Wang, Y.; Webby, R.J.; Ulett, G.C.; Adderson, E.E. Respiratory viruses augment the adhesion of bacterial pathogens to respiratory epithelium in a viral species- and cell type-dependent manner. *J. Virol.* **2006**, *80*, 1629–1636. [CrossRef]
139. Ishizuka, S.; Yamaya, M.; Suzuki, T.; Takahashi, H.; Ida, S.; Sasaki, T.; Inoue, D.; Sekizawa, K.; Nishimura, H.; Sasaki, H. Effects of rhinovirus infection on the adherence of Streptococcus pneumoniae to cultured human airway epithelial cells. *J. Infect. Dis.* **2003**, *188*, 1928–1939. [CrossRef]
140. Kc, R.; Shukla, S.D.; Walters, E.H.; O'Toole, R.F. Temporal upregulation of host surface receptors provides a window of opportunity for bacterial adhesion and disease. *Microbiology* **2017**, *163*, 421–430. [CrossRef]
141. Avadhanula, V.; Wang, Y.; Portner, A.; Adderson, E. Nontypeable Haemophilus influenzae and Streptococcus pneumoniae bind respiratory syncytial virus glycoprotein. *J. Med. Microbiol.* **2007**, *56*, 1133–1137. [CrossRef] [PubMed]
142. Hament, J.M.; Aerts, P.C.; Fleer, A.; van Dijk, H.; Harmsen, T.; Kimpen, J.L.; Wolfs, T.F. Direct binding of respiratory syncytial virus to pneumococci: A phenomenon that enhances both pneumococcal adherence to human epithelial cells and pneumococcal invasiveness in a murine model. *Pediatr. Res.* **2005**, *58*, 1198–1203. [CrossRef] [PubMed]

143. Unger, B.L.; Faris, A.N.; Ganesan, S.; Comstock, A.T.; Hershenson, M.B.; Sajjan, U.S. Rhinovirus attenuates non-typeable Hemophilus influenzae-stimulated IL-8 responses via TLR2-dependent degradation of IRAK-1. *PLoS Pathog.* **2012**, *8*, e1002969. [CrossRef] [PubMed]
144. Ghoneim, H.E.; Thomas, P.G.; McCullers, J.A. Depletion of alveolar macrophages during influenza infection facilitates bacterial superinfections. *J. Immunol.* **2013**, *191*, 1250–1259. [CrossRef]
145. Oliver, B.G.; Lim, S.; Wark, P.; Laza-Stanca, V.; King, N.; Black, J.L.; Burgess, J.K.; Roth, M.; Johnston, S.L. Rhinovirus exposure impairs immune responses to bacterial products in human alveolar macrophages. *Thorax* **2008**, *63*, 519–525. [CrossRef]
146. Arrevillaga, G.; Gaona, J.; Sanchez, C.; Rosales, V.; Gomez, B. Respiratory syncytial virus persistence in macrophages downregulates intercellular adhesion molecule-1 expression and reduces adhesion of non-typeable Haemophilus influenzae. *Intervirology* **2012**, *55*, 442–450. [CrossRef]
147. Bellinghausen, C.; Rohde, G.G.U.; Savelkoul, P.H.M.; Wouters, E.F.M.; Stassen, F.R.M. Viral-bacterial interactions in the respiratory tract. *J. Gen. Virol.* **2016**, *97*, 3089–3102. [CrossRef]
148. Wu, L.; Estrada, O.; Zaborina, O.; Bains, M.; Shen, L.; Kohler, J.E.; Patel, N.; Musch, M.W.; Chang, E.B.; Fu, Y.X.; et al. Recognition of host immune activation by Pseudomonas aeruginosa. *Science* **2005**, *309*, 774–777. [CrossRef]
149. Ichinohe, T.; Pang, I.K.; Kumamoto, Y.; Peaper, D.R.; Ho, J.H.; Murray, T.S.; Iwasaki, A. Microbiota regulates immune defense against respiratory tract influenza A virus infection. *Proc. Natl. Acad. Sci. USA* **2011**, *108*, 5354–5359. [CrossRef]
150. Wang, J.; Li, F.; Sun, R.; Gao, X.; Wei, H.; Li, L.J.; Tian, Z. Bacterial colonization dampens influenza-mediated acute lung injury via induction of M2 alveolar macrophages. *Nat. Commun.* **2013**, *4*, 2106. [CrossRef]
151. Suarez-Arrabal, M.C.; Mella, C.; Lopez, S.M.; Brown, N.V.; Hall, M.W.; Hammond, S.; Shiels, W.; Groner, J.; Marcon, M.; Ramilo, O.; et al. Nasopharyngeal bacterial burden and antibiotics: Influence on inflammatory markers and disease severity in infants with respiratory syncytial virus bronchiolitis. *J. Infect.* **2015**, *71*, 458–469. [CrossRef]
152. De Steenhuijsen Piters, W.A.; Heinonen, S.; Hasrat, R.; Bunsow, E.; Smith, B.; Suarez-Arrabal, M.C.; Chaussabel, D.; Cohen, D.M.; Sanders, E.A.; Ramilo, O.; et al. Nasopharyngeal Microbiota, Host Transcriptome, and Disease Severity in Children with Respiratory Syncytial Virus Infection. *Am. J. Respir. Crit. Care Med.* **2016**, *194*, 1104–1115. [CrossRef] [PubMed]
153. Verkaik, N.J.; Nguyen, D.T.; de Vogel, C.P.; Moll, H.A.; Verbrugh, H.A.; Jaddoe, V.W.; Hofman, A.; van Wamel, W.J.; van den Hoogen, B.G.; Buijs-Offerman, R.M.; et al. Streptococcus pneumoniae exposure is associated with human metapneumovirus seroconversion and increased susceptibility to in vitro HMPV infection. *Clin. Microbiol. Infect.* **2011**, *17*, 1840–1844. [CrossRef] [PubMed]
154. Gulraiz, F.; Bellinghausen, C.; Bruggeman, C.A.; Stassen, F.R. Haemophilus influenzae increases the susceptibility and inflammatory response of airway epithelial cells to viral infections. *FASEB J.* **2015**, *29*, 849–858. [CrossRef] [PubMed]
155. Heinrich, A.; Haarmann, H.; Zahradnik, S.; Frenzel, K.; Schreiber, F.; Klassert, T.E.; Heyl, K.A.; Endres, A.S.; Schmidtke, M.; Hofmann, J.; et al. Moraxella catarrhalis decreases antiviral innate immune responses by down-regulation of TLR3 via inhibition of p53 in human bronchial epithelial cells. *FASEB J.* **2016**, *30*, 2426–2434. [CrossRef]
156. Huang, Y.J. Asthma microbiome studies and the potential for new therapeutic strategies. *Curr. Allergy Asthma Rep.* **2013**, *13*, 453–461. [CrossRef]
157. Stiemsma, L.T.; Turvey, S.E. Asthma and the microbiome: Defining the critical window in early life. *Allergy Asthma Clin. Immunol.* **2017**, *13*, 3. [CrossRef]
158. Perdijk, O.; Marsland, B.J. The microbiome: Toward preventing allergies and asthma by nutritional intervention. *Curr. Opin. Immunol.* **2019**, *60*, 10–18. [CrossRef]
159. Patel, R.; DuPont, H.L. New approaches for bacteriotherapy: Prebiotics, new-generation probiotics, and synbiotics. *Clin. Infect. Dis.* **2015**, *60*, S108–S121. [CrossRef]
160. Karimi, K.; Inman, M.D.; Bienenstock, J.; Forsythe, P. Lactobacillus reuteri-induced regulatory T cells protect against an allergic airway response in mice. *Am. J. Respir. Crit. Care Med.* **2009**, *179*, 186–193. [CrossRef]

161. Sagar, S.; Morgan, M.E.; Chen, S.; Vos, A.P.; Garssen, J.; van Bergenhenegouwen, J.; Boon, L.; Georgiou, N.A.; Kraneveld, A.D.; Folkerts, G. Bifidobacterium breve and Lactobacillus rhamnosus treatment is as effective as budesonide at reducing inflammation in a murine model for chronic asthma. *Respir. Res.* **2014**, *15*, 46. [CrossRef] [PubMed]
162. Wang, X.; Hui, Y.; Zhao, L.; Hao, Y.; Guo, H.; Ren, F. Oral administration of Lactobacillus paracasei L9 attenuates $PM_{2.5}$-induced enhancement of airway hyperresponsiveness and allergic airway response in murine model of asthma. *PLoS ONE* **2017**, *12*, e0171721. [CrossRef] [PubMed]
163. Raftis, E.J.; Delday, M.I.; Cowie, P.; McCluskey, S.M.; Singh, M.D.; Ettorre, A.; Mulder, I.E. Bifidobacterium breve MRx0004 protects against airway inflammation in a severe asthma model by suppressing both neutrophil and eosinophil lung infiltration. *Sci. Rep.* **2018**, *8*, 12024. [CrossRef] [PubMed]
164. Chen, Y.S.; Jan, R.L.; Lin, Y.L.; Chen, H.H.; Wang, J.Y. Randomized placebo-controlled trial of lactobacillus on asthmatic children with allergic rhinitis. *Pediatric Pulmonol.* **2010**, *45*, 1111–1120. [CrossRef] [PubMed]
165. Gutkowski, P.M.; Madaliński, K.; Grek, M.; Dmenska, H.; Syczewska, M.; Michalkiewicz, J. Effect of orally administered probiotic strains Lactobacillus and Bifidobacterium in children with atopic asthma. *Cent. Eur. J. Immunol.* **2010**, *35*, 233–238.
166. Van de Pol, M.A.; Lutter, R.; Smids, B.S.; Weersink, E.J.; van der Zee, J.S. Symbiotics reduce allergen-induced T-helper 2 response and improve peak expiratory flow in allergic asthmatics. *Allergy* **2011**, *66*, 39–47. [CrossRef]
167. Azad, M.B.; Coneys, J.G.; Kozyrskyj, A.L.; Field, C.J.; Ramsey, C.D.; Becker, A.B.; Friesen, C.; Abou-Setta, A.M.; Zarychanski, R. Probiotic supplementation during pregnancy or infancy for the prevention of asthma and wheeze: Systematic review and meta-analysis. *BMJ* **2013**, *347*, f6471. [CrossRef]
168. Elazab, N.; Mendy, A.; Gasana, J.; Vieira, E.R.; Quizon, A.; Forno, E. Probiotic administration in early life, atopy, and asthma: A meta-analysis of clinical trials. *Pediatrics* **2013**, *132*, e666–e676. [CrossRef]
169. Wei, X.; Jiang, P.; Liu, J.; Sun, R.; Zhu, L. Association between probiotic supplementation and asthma incidence in infants: A meta-analysis of randomized controlled trials. *J. Asthma* **2019**, 1–12. [CrossRef]
170. Du, X.; Wang, L.; Wu, S.; Yuan, L.; Tang, S.; Xiang, Y.; Qu, X.; Liu, H.; Qin, X.; Liu, C. Efficacy of probiotic supplementary therapy for asthma, allergic rhinitis, and wheeze: A meta-analysis of randomized controlled trials. *Allergy Asthma Proc.* **2019**, *40*, 250–260. [CrossRef]
171. Debarry, J.; Garn, H.; Hanuszkiewicz, A.; Dickgreber, N.; Blumer, N.; von Mutius, E.; Bufe, A.; Gatermann, S.; Renz, H.; Holst, O.; et al. Acinetobacter lwoffii and Lactococcus lactis strains isolated from farm cowsheds possess strong allergy-protective properties. *J. Allergy Clin. Immunol.* **2007**, *119*, 1514–1521. [CrossRef] [PubMed]
172. Nembrini, C.; Sichelstiel, A.; Kisielow, J.; Kurrer, M.; Kopf, M.; Marsland, B.J. Bacterial-induced protection against allergic inflammation through a multicomponent immunoregulatory mechanism. *Thorax* **2011**, *66*, 755–763. [CrossRef] [PubMed]
173. Hagner, S.; Harb, H.; Zhao, M.; Stein, K.; Holst, O.; Ege, M.J.; Mayer, M.; Matthes, J.; Bauer, J.; von Mutius, E.; et al. Farm-derived Gram-positive bacterium Staphylococcus sciuri W620 prevents asthma phenotype in HDM- and OVA-exposed mice. *Allergy* **2013**, *68*, 322–329. [CrossRef] [PubMed]
174. Stein, K.; Brand, S.; Jenckel, A.; Sigmund, A.; Chen, Z.J.; Kirschning, C.J.; Kauth, M.; Heine, H. Endosomal recognition of Lactococcus lactis G121 and its RNA by dendritic cells is key to its allergy-protective effects. *J. Allergy Clin. Immunol.* **2017**, *139*, 667–678. [CrossRef] [PubMed]
175. Pellaton, C.; Nutten, S.; Thierry, A.C.; Boudousquie, C.; Barbier, N.; Blanchard, C.; Corthesy, B.; Mercenier, A.; Spertini, F. Intragastric and Intranasal Administration of Lactobacillus paracasei NCC2461 Modulates Allergic Airway Inflammation in Mice. *Int. J. Inflamm.* **2012**, *2012*, 686739. [CrossRef]
176. Barfod, K.K.; Vrankx, K.; Mirsepasi-Lauridsen, H.C.; Hansen, J.S.; Hougaard, K.S.; Larsen, S.T.; Ouwenhand, A.C.; Krogfelt, K.A. The Murine Lung Microbiome Changes During Lung Inflammation and Intranasal Vancomycin Treatment. *Open Microbiol. J.* **2015**, *9*, 167–179. [CrossRef]
177. Friedlander, A.L.; Albert, R.K. Chronic macrolide therapy in inflammatory airways diseases. *Chest* **2010**, *138*, 1202–1212. [CrossRef]
178. Spagnolo, P.; Fabbri, L.M.; Bush, A. Long-term macrolide treatment for chronic respiratory disease. *Eur. Respir. J.* **2013**, *42*, 239–251. [CrossRef]
179. Wong, E.H.; Porter, J.D.; Edwards, M.R.; Johnston, S.L. The role of macrolides in asthma: Current evidence and future directions. *Lancet Respir. Med.* **2014**, *2*, 657–670. [CrossRef]

180. Brusselle, G.G.; Vanderstichele, C.; Jordens, P.; Deman, R.; Slabbynck, H.; Ringoet, V.; Verleden, G.; Demedts, I.K.; Verhamme, K.; Delporte, A.; et al. Azithromycin for prevention of exacerbations in severe asthma (AZISAST): A multicentre randomised double-blind placebo-controlled trial. *Thorax* **2013**, *68*, 322–329. [CrossRef]
181. Gibson, P.G.; Yang, I.A.; Upham, J.W.; Reynolds, P.N.; Hodge, S.; James, A.L.; Jenkins, C.; Peters, M.J.; Marks, G.B.; Baraket, M.; et al. Effect of azithromycin on asthma exacerbations and quality of life in adults with persistent uncontrolled asthma (AMAZES): A randomised, double-blind, placebo-controlled trial. *Lancet* **2017**, *390*, 659–668. [CrossRef]
182. Slater, M.; Rivett, D.W.; Williams, L.; Martin, M.; Harrison, T.; Sayers, I.; Bruce, K.D.; Shaw, D. The impact of azithromycin therapy on the airway microbiota in asthma. *Thorax* **2014**, *69*, 673–674. [CrossRef] [PubMed]
183. Lopes Dos Santos Santiago, G.; Brusselle, G.; Dauwe, K.; Deschaght, P.; Verhofstede, C.; Vaneechoutte, D.; Deschepper, E.; Jordens, P.; Joos, G.; Vaneechoutte, M. Influence of chronic azithromycin treatment on the composition of the oropharyngeal microbial community in patients with severe asthma. *BMC Microbiol.* **2017**, *17*, 109. [CrossRef] [PubMed]
184. Suez, J.; Elinav, E. The path towards microbiome-based metabolite treatment. *Nat. Microbiol.* **2017**, *2*, 17075. [CrossRef]
185. Wong, A.C.; Levy, M. New Approaches to Microbiome-Based Therapies. *mSystems* **2019**, *4*. [CrossRef]
186. Ooijevaar, R.E.; Terveer, E.M.; Verspaget, H.W.; Kuijper, E.J.; Keller, J.J. Clinical Application and Potential of Fecal Microbiota Transplantation. *Annu. Rev. Med.* **2019**, *70*, 335–351. [CrossRef]

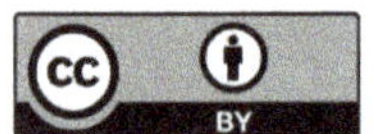

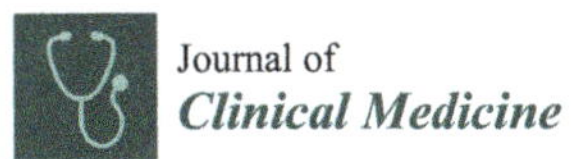
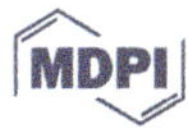

Review

Targeting NLRP3 Inflammasome Activation in Severe Asthma

Efthymia Theofani [1], Maria Semitekolou [1], Ioannis Morianos [1], Konstantinos Samitas [2] and Georgina Xanthou [1,*]

[1] Cellular Immunology Laboratory, Center for Basic Research, Biomedical Research Foundation of the Academy of Athens, 11527 Athens, Greece
[2] 7th Respiratory Clinic and Asthma Center, 'Sotiria' Athens Chest Hospital, 11527 Athens, Greece
* Correspondence: gxanthou@bioacademy.gr; Tel.: +30-210-6597-336

Received: 31 July 2019; Accepted: 26 September 2019; Published: 4 October 2019

Abstract: Severe asthma (SA) is a chronic lung disease characterized by recurring symptoms of reversible airflow obstruction, airway hyper-responsiveness (AHR), and inflammation that is resistant to currently employed treatments. The nucleotide-binding oligomerization domain-like Receptor Family Pyrin Domain Containing 3 (NLRP3) inflammasome is an intracellular sensor that detects microbial motifs and endogenous danger signals and represents a key component of innate immune responses in the airways. Assembly of the NLRP3 inflammasome leads to caspase 1-dependent release of the pro-inflammatory cytokines IL-1β and IL-18 as well as pyroptosis. Accumulating evidence proposes that NLRP3 activation is critically involved in asthma pathogenesis. In fact, although NLRP3 facilitates the clearance of pathogens in the airways, persistent NLRP3 activation by inhaled irritants and/or innocuous environmental allergens can lead to overt pulmonary inflammation and exacerbation of asthma manifestations. Notably, administration of NLRP3 inhibitors in asthma models restrains AHR and pulmonary inflammation. Here, we provide an overview of the pathophysiology of SA, present molecular mechanisms underlying aberrant inflammatory responses in the airways, summarize recent studies pertinent to the biology and functions of NLRP3, and discuss the role of NLRP3 in the pathogenesis of asthma. Finally, we contemplate the potential of targeting NLRP3 as a novel therapeutic approach for the management of SA.

Keywords: severe asthma; innate immunity; immune regulation; NLRP3; IL-1β; allergic airway inflammation

---

1. Introduction

Asthma represents a serious global health problem that affects 1%–18% of the population of all age groups. Its prevalence has increased in the last decades, especially among children [1]. Asthma is characterized by variable symptoms of wheezing, dyspnea, chest tightness, coughing, and reversible airflow obstruction, and is usually associated with airway hyperresponsiveness (AHR) to innocuous environmental allergens and chronic airway inflammation. Factors, such as allergen or irritant exposure, respiratory infections, exercise, climate changes, and stress, are responsible for the disparities and severity of asthma symptoms [1]. Asthma has been long considered as a heterogeneous chronic lung disease that encompasses multiple groups of patients characterized by varying features or phenotypes [2,3]. A small percentage of asthmatics exhibit severe disease exacerbations despite the fact that they are already under treatment with high doses of inhaled and/or systemic corticosteroids [2,3]. These patients suffer from severe asthma (SA) that is poorly controlled and, in some cases, life-threatening [4,5]. Although patients with SA comprise a small percentage of the total asthma population (5%–10%), they denote 50% of total healthcare costs, rendering SA a substantial health and socioeconomic burden [6,7]. SA is characterized by marked thickening and structural changes of the airway wall, excessive airway narrowing, and fixed airflow obstruction [6,7]. An in-depth understanding of the heterogeneity of SA and the immunological mechanisms underlying its pathophysiology is critical for the identification of novel biomarkers and molecular pathways that can be targeted in novel treatment modalities.

In the lung, innate immune responses provide the first line of defense against environmental signals, including pathogens, allergens, and other irritants, and act through downstream signaling by numerous extracellular and intracellular receptors, termed pattern recognition receptors (PRRs) [8–10]. NOD-like Receptor Family Pyrin Domain Containing 3 (NLRP3) is an intracellular PRR that detects microbial motifs, endogenous danger signals, and environmental irritants, and induces the formation and activation of the NLRP3 inflammasome. Although the NLRP3 inflammasome is essential for providing protective immunity, overactivation of inflammasome-mediated responses can cause excessive inflammation, tissue damage, and lead to chronic inflammatory diseases, including asthma [10,11]. In this review, we describe the immunological mechanisms underlying aberrant inflammatory responses in the airways and their link to SA pathogenesis. We also present the biology and functions of NLRP3 and discuss its role in the initiation and propagation of SA features. Finally, we present recent findings pertinent to targeting NLRP3 functions as a novel therapeutic approach for the control of inflammatory responses in the airways.

2. Severe Asthma Pathogenesis

2.1. Type 2 Asthma

To address SA complexity, the concept of asthma endotyping has emerged [12–14]. Depending on the type of immune cell responses implicated in disease pathogenesis, asthma endotypes are categorized as (a) type 2 asthma, characterized predominantly by T helper type 2 (Th2) cell-mediated inflammation and (b) nontype 2 asthma, associated with Th1 and/or Th17 cell inflammation [15–17].

Upon allergen exposure, dendritic cells (DCs) in the lung mucosa take up allergens, reach the mediastinal lymph nodes, and present allergen components to naive T cells in the context of major histocompatibility complex class II [18]. Allergens with proteolytic activity, such as those derived from house dust mites (HDM), pollen grains, fungi, and occupational sensitizers activate protease activated receptors expressed on DCs, disrupt epithelial tight junctions, and initiate inflammatory responses [18]. Moreover, certain allergens and airborne particulates contain microbial components which interact with PRRs, including Toll-like receptors (TLRs) and NOD-like receptors (NLRs), on DCs and airway epithelial cells, and serve as "danger signals" for the host immune response [18]. Upon interaction with allergen-loaded DCs, naive Th cells differentiate into Th1, Th2, Th9, or Th17 cells, depending on the type and dose of allergen and the local cytokine milieu [18]. Allergen-specific Th2 cells, generated in the presence of type 2 cytokines, migrate into the airways wherein upon allergen re-exposure, secrete cytokines and promote mucus secretion, subepithelial fibrosis, bronchial remodeling, and AHR [19]. The production of Th2 cytokines also leads to the recruitment of innate effector cells, including mast cells, basophils, and eosinophils, as well as to isotype switching of B cell-secreted IgG to allergen-specific IgE [19]. Additionally, Th9 cells, a recently identified Th cell subset characterized by high levels of IL-9, exacerbate allergic airway inflammation (AAI), predominantly through activation of mast cell functions [20,21]. More specifically, experimental studies have shown that IL-9 production by Th9 cells and by type 2 innate lymphoid cells (ILC2s) enhances the production of IL-2 by mast cells, leading to further expansion of ILC2s, which activate Th9 cells, in a positive feedback loop [22]. Of clinical relevance, increased numbers of Th9 cells were demonstrated in peripheral blood mononuclear cells (PBMCs) isolated from HDM or pollen allergic subjects and correlated with IgE levels [23]. Moreover, elevated IL-9-secreting T lymphocytes were observed in the bronchoalveolar lavage (BAL) of asthmatics [24].

Apart from DCs, the asthmatic airway epithelium represents a major source of cytokines termed "alarmins", such as, IL-25, IL-33, and thymic stromal lymphopoietin (TSLP), and chemokines, including

RANTES (Regulated on Activation, Normal T cell Expressed and Secrete or CCL5), TARC (Thymus- and Activation-Regulated Chemokine or CCL17), eotaxins (CCL11, CCL24 and CCL26), and MCP-3 (Monocyte Chemotactic Protein-3 or CCL7) that trigger Th2 cell polarization upon exposure to allergens, pollutants, viral, fungal, and bacterial components [18]. As mentioned above, recent studies have highlighted a key role for ILC2s in asthma immunopathogenesis [25]. ILC2s are activated in response to TSLP, IL-25, and IL-33 signaling [25], and produce IL-5, IL-13, and prostaglandin [26], further propagating Th2-cell mediated responses in the airways.

Type 2 asthma is characterized by any combination of the following processes: eosinophilia in the sputum or blood, atopy and a high level of fractional exhaled nitric oxide (FeNO) [16]. Several biomarkers of type 2 inflammation, such as FeNO, serum IgE, blood or sputum eosinophils, and serum periostin distinguish type 2-high and type 2-low asthma phenotypes and also predict the responsiveness to type 2 cytokine-targeted therapy [27]. Eosinophils play a crucial role in the initiation and propagation of inflammatory responses in asthma [16]. Asthmatic patients with increased numbers of eosinophils in the periphery suffer from more severe disease exacerbations and poorer disease control [16]. FeNO represents an indicator of IL-13-mediated and corticosteroid-responsive airway inflammation, as the presence of IL-13 activates inducible nitric oxide synthase (iNOS), leading to increased FeNO production in the airways [16]. Approximately 70% of patients with asthma have an allergic phenotype, characterized by allergen-specific IgE and elevated total IgE levels [16]. Periostin, an extracellular matrix protein, induced by IL-4 and IL-13 signaling, is secreted by bronchial epithelial cells and represents another important biomarker for severe eosinophilic type 2 asthma [28]. Periostin is involved in airway remodeling, sub-epithelial fibrosis, eosinophil recruitment, and mucus production. Notably, a high serum concentration of periostin denotes one of the most significant indicators of eosinophilic inflammation in asthma [29].

Clustering studies revealed that one of the major reasons SA patients remain unresponsive to corticosteroid treatment is that apart from Th2 inflammation, other mediators are also implicated in disease pathogenesis [12,30]. Indeed, enhanced Interferon gamma *IFNG* expression was detected in BAL cells, accompanied by increased secretion in SA patients compared to mild-to-moderate asthmatics (MMA) [31]. The same study also showed elevated percentages of $CD4^{+}IFN\text{-}\gamma^{+}$ T cells in the BAL [31]. In line with above, increased IFN-γ mRNA levels were observed in lung tissue and sputum of SA patients [32,33]. It must be asked what triggers these IFN-γ-mediated responses in the airways of SA patients? It is known that persistent viral (especially rhinoviruses) and bacterial (*Chlamydia pneumoniae, Streptococcus pneumoniae, Mycoplasma pneumoniae, Haemophilus influenzae, Moraxella catarrhalis* and *Staphylococcus aureus*) infections augment IFN-γ secretion in SA patients, highlighting a key role for respiratory tract infections in disease severity and asthma exacerbations [34].

2.2. Nontype 2 Asthma

The pathophysiology of nontype 2 asthma remains less well characterized. Nontype 2 asthma is denoted by the absence of type 2 biomarkers, such as eosinophils and IgE, and the predominance of Th17 cells and neutrophils in the airways [35]. In fact, growing evidence has highlighted a key role for IL-17 in the pathogenesis of nontype 2 asthma [35]. Tissue-infiltrating $CD4^{+}$ T cells isolated from bronchial biopsies of SA patients produce copious amounts of IL-17 and IL-22 upon ex vivo polyclonal stimulation [36,37]. Another study revealed that in vitro administration of recombinant human IL-17 enhanced the secretion of IL-8 by human bronchial epithelial cells (HBECs) and venous endothelial cells [38]. Moreover, conditioned medium from IL-17-treated HBECs increased neutrophil migration in vitro [38]. Increased IL-17 mRNA levels are also observed in the sputum of SA patients [39]. In addition, IL-17 levels in the peripheral blood (PB) of SA patients positively correlate with disease severity [40]. A very interesting recent study revealed that an IL-4Rα polymorphism associated with SA leads to the conversion of regulatory T cells (Tregs) to Th17 cells in vitro [41]. In brief, the authors isolated from the PB of asthmatics and healthy controls that were either wild type (WT) (IL4RQ576/Q576), heterozygous (IL4RQ576/R576), or homozygous (IL4RR576/R576) for the mutated allele, naive T cells, and differentiated them into Treg cells. Interestingly, naive $CD4^{+}$ T cells from asthmatics bearing the IL4RR576 mutation exhibited defective induction of Treg cells and were skewed towards a Th17-like phenotype, exemplified by increased secretion of IL-17 [41]. Still, targeting IL-17 has failed to improve disease symptoms in SA patients as opposed to anti-type 2 cytokine therapy, suggesting that other mechanisms compensate for its pathogenic effects or that targeting pathogenic Th17 cells specifically would be more appropriate [42,43].

To date, biomarkers of type 2-low or neutrophilic asthma have not been identified. Several studies have shown that there is no inverse correlation between sputum eosinophil and neutrophil numbers in SA patients and that eosinophils are present in excess, additionally to neutrophilic accumulation, in the airways [44]. Moreover, although measuring eosinophil numbers in the periphery correlates with the percentages of eosinophils in induced sputum, blood neutrophil parameters represent poor surrogates for the proportion of neutrophils in the sputum [45,46]. Recent studies showed that the levels of the chitinase-like protein YKL-40 in the blood of SA patients could potentially be used as a marker for nontype 2 neutrophilic asthma [47]. In fact, combining the measurement of YKL-40 with other clinical parameters of the disease may provide a more reliable strategy for defining nontype 2 asthma. Tumor necrosis factor (TNF)-α has been also shown to have a critical role in nontype 2 asthma through acting on smooth muscle cells or by modifying the release of the cysteinyl leukotrienes, LTC4 and LTD4 [48]. TNF-α is increased in the BAL and bronchial biopsies in SA patients compared to MMAs [49]. Importantly, the administration of inhaled recombinant TNF-α to normal subjects led to the development of AHR and airway neutrophilia [50,51]. Subsequent clinical trials utilizing antiTNF-α therapeutic administration contributed to the elucidation of the role of this cytokine in vivo [52]. Indeed, improvement in patient quality of life, lung function, and a reduction in AHR and exacerbation frequency was observed in patients treated with antiTNF-α [52]. Still, considering the significant heterogeneity observed in SA patients, benefit from antiTNF-α therapy is likely to occur only in a small group of patients.

Apart from type 2 and nontype 2, asthma can be categorized into four endotypes (eosinophilic, neutrophilic, mixed granulocytic, and paucigranulocytic) based on the type of airway infiltrating immune cells [53]. Among these endotypes, paucigranulocytic asthma (PGA) presents no evidence of increased eosinophils or neutrophils in induced sputum, and instead is characterized by low-grade airway inflammation associated with airway smooth muscle (ASM) dysfunction, persistent airflow limitation, and AHR [54,55]. Molecules involved in oxidative stress, matrix metalloproteinases, neutrophil elastase, and galectin-3, commonly used for the discrimination between eosinophilic and neutrophlic asthma, also remain unaltered in patients with PGA [56–59]. Moreover, patients with PGA display lower FeNO levels compared to those with eosinophilic asthma [60]. Notably, Wang and colleagues documented that PGA was the most common endotype observed in children with stable asthma [61]. Corticosteroids do not seem to exert beneficial effects in this cohort of asthmatics, irrespective of the dose used [62]. Considering that symptoms dominating in this cohort are mostly due to ASM phenotypic changes and/or neuronal dysfunction, therapies directed toward ASM responses, including mast cell-targeted therapies and/or bronchial thermoplasty, might benefit PGA patients [63]. Although the precise mechanisms of action remain incompletely understood, bronchial thermoplasty is considered to diminish ASM mass through the delivery of localized thermal energy [63]. In addition, factors associated with dysregulated ASM functions, as well as mediators involved in the thickening of the subepithelial basement membrane, could be used as disease biomarkers and guide the design of effective therapeutic approaches for PGA [56].

In sharp contrast to adult asthma, wherein the type of airway inflammation has been extensively investigated due to the use of invasive and semi-invasive techniques, such as bronchial biopsies, BAL, and induced sputum, the majority of analyses in childhood asthma have been performed only in severe forms of disease [64–67]. The most common endotype of childhood asthma is the eosinophilic, characterized by unrestrained symptoms, atopy, impaired lung function, enhanced AHR, increased numbers of exacerbations, and steroid responsiveness [68]. The percentages of eosinophils in induced sputum significantly vary over time in children with SA, and these variations are not associated with asthma therapy [69]. Importantly, persistent airway eosinophilia has been detected in a small cohort of children with SA, even after a high dose of systemic corticosteroids [70]. Regarding neutrophilic pediatric asthma, the functional role of airway neutrophils in asthma pathophysiology remains elusive. Infiltration of neutrophils in the airways in pediatric SA represents a feature of airway inflammation at all ages and is triggered by viral and/or bacterial infections, exacerbating asthma symptoms [71]. Increased numbers of intraepithelial neutrophils, along with enhanced epithelial and submucosal expression of IL-17R, have been observed in lung biopsies of a subgroup of children with therapy-resistant SA. These findings correlate with improved lung function suggesting a potential beneficial rather than adverse role for neutrophils in pediatric SA pathophysiology [72]. Other studies show that neutrophils coexist with eosinophils in the airways of a group of children with SA, highlighting the complexity of defining the distinct endotypes in children [73]. Overall, it becomes evident that a more detailed and careful assessment of all the inflammatory endotypes is essential for the characterization and management of severe pediatric asthma.

3. Targeted Therapies For Severe Asthma

In-depth investigation of the molecular and cellular mechanisms underlying SA pathophysiology has significantly contributed to the development of novel therapeutic strategies for disease management. Indeed, antibodies targeting factors involved in SA pathology are already being used as a first line medication. An excellent example is omalizumab, a monoclonal antibody directed against IgE that has become an established add-on therapy for patients with uncontrolled allergic asthma [74]. In addition, monoclonal antibodies against IL-5 (reslizumab, mepolizumab), IL-5R (benralizumab), and IL-4R (dupilumab) have been approved as add-on treatments for uncontrolled type 2 eosinophilic asthma [74]. Although these therapies have proven effective in certain asthma cohorts, some patients that suffer from severe allergic and/or eosinophilic asthma, as well as most patients with severe non type 2 asthma, experience weakly-regulated disease manifestations [74]. Notably, the reported adverse effects of these monoclonal antibody therapies should be also considered. For example, administration of omalizumab has been associated with an anaphylaxis rate of 0.09% that most frequently occurs within 2 hours after the first dose and 30 min after subsequent doses, necessitating the close monitoring of patients [75,76]. Moreover, a higher incidence of cardiovascular and cerebrovascular adverse effects (AEs) has been observed upon omalizumab administration [77]. Mepolizumab, the first anti-IL-5 monoclonal antibody approved for eosinophilc asthma, has been associated with headaches, injection site reactions, back pain, and fatigue [78]. The most common AEs of reslizumab, another FDA-approved anti-IL-5 antibody, are a 0.3% anaphylaxis rate, elevated serum creatinine kinase, and musculoskeletal and oropharyngeal pain [79]. Regarding benralizumab, an anti-IL-5R antibody that is currently undergoing phase 3 trials, there have been no documented AEs apart from nasopharyngitis and injection site reactions [80]. AEs in patients receiving dupilumab, a monoclonal antibody that targets the common receptor for IL-4 and IL-13, include nasopharyngitis, injection site reactions, and headaches [81]. Monoclonal antibodies targeting TSLP, IL-33 and its receptor ST2, the receptor for stem cell factors on mast cells, and a DNA enzyme directed at GATA3 are currently being evaluated for their efficacy in SA. It is worth mentioning that a number of antagonists directed against other potential targets, such as, IL-25, IL-6, TNF-like ligand 1A, CD6, and activated cell adhesion molecules are under consideration for future clinical trials [74]. Results from these clinical trials will be of great importance as they may introduce novel treatment modalities that will successfully replace the existing ones and lead to the efficient management of SA.

Taken together, it becomes evident that as the airway lumen is continually exposed to external and endogenous stimuli, its ability to distinguish between innocuous environmental allergens and pathogenic agents is crucial for the maintenance of immune tolerance and lung homeostasis. In fact, the complex interactions between innate and adaptive immune responses in the lung micromilieu represent a major determinant of the development of tolerance or allergic inflammation. Innate immune responses have considerable bearing on ensuing adaptive responses, and if left uncontrolled, can lead to detrimental pathological consequences. Hence, delineation of the precise mechanisms involved in the regulation of innate immune reponses in the airways is essential for the design of more efficient treatment modalities for SA patients.

4. Inflammasomes: A Key Component of Innate Immunity

The innate immune system acts as the first line of defense during exposure to environmental pathogens. In the lung, innate immune responses act through downstream signaling by numerous extracellular and intracellular receptors termed pattern recognition receptors (PRRs). PRRs recognize pathogen-associated molecular patterns (PAMPs), such as lipopolysaccharide (LPS), bacterial and viral RNA, danger-associated molecular patterns (DAMPs) in damaged and/or dying cells, including reactive oxygen species (ROS), ATP and mitochondrial DNA, and homeostasis-altering molecular processes (HAMPs) that detect alterations in cell homeostasis and elicit inflammatory responses in the host [8,9]. PRRs are expressed on macrophages, monocytes, DCs, and on tissue-resident cells, including airway epithelial cells, and upon ligand binding, induce the secretion of inflammatory cytokines and chemokines [82,83]. PRRs consist of the Toll-like receptors (TLRs), the RIG-I-like receptors (RLRs), the nucleotide-binding oligomerization domain-like receptors (NLRs), the Scavenger receptors, the C-type lectin receptors (CLRs), and the absent-in-melanoma (AIM)-like receptors (ALRs). Among PPRs, TLRs and NLRs represent the most well-known and studied receptors [83,84]. TLRs are located at the cell membrane and the intracellular compartment, while NLRs are located solely in the cytosol [84]. Signaling through these receptors enables the innate immune system to monitor and respond to infectious agents and other damage-inducing stimuli, eliciting protective immunity.

NLRs consist of a conserved nucleotide binding and oligomerization domain (NACHT), a carboxy-terminal ligand-binding region, composed of leucine-rich repeats (LRRs), involved in ligand binding or activator sensing, and an amino-terminal effector domain required for protein–protein interactions [85–87]. The human NLR gene family consists of 22 members, classified into four subfamilies depending on their N-terminal regions: NLRA, NLRB, NLRC, and NLRP. The NLRA region contains an acidic transactivation domain, the NLRB a baculoviral inhibitory repeat-like domain, NLRC contains a caspase activation and recruitment domain (CARD), and NLRP contains a pyrin domain (PYD) [85–87]. The detection of PAMPs, DAMPs, and HAMPs by NLRs leads to the formation of a large multimolecular signaling platform called the inflammasome. Inflammasomes respond to a constellation of endogenous and pathogenic signals and are critical inducers of host defense. Five major inflammasomes have been identified so far: NLRP1, NLRC4, RIG-I, AIM2, and NLRP3. These consist of an active NLRP receptor, the inflammasome adaptor protein, Apoptosis-associated Speck-like protein Containing CARD (ASC), and caspase-1 [88]. NLRP6, NLRP7, NLRP12, and IFI16, can also form inflammasomes, but their composition remains unclear. Apart from the physiological role of inflammasomes in providing protective immunity, inflammasomes also regulate cell proliferation and tissue repair processes [11]. Still, overactivation of inflammasome-mediated responses can cause excessive inflammation, tissue damage, and lead to chronic inflammatory diseases and metabolic disorders.

5. Nlrp3 Biology and Functions

NLRP3 is expressed in granulocytes, monocytes, DCs, T cells, and epithelial cells [89]. The NLPR3 inflammasome consists of the NLRP3 receptor, the adaptor protein ASC, also known as Pycard, and caspase-1 that acts as an effector protein [89]. The NLRP3 receptor is a tripartite protein that contains an amino-terminal PYD, a nucleotide-binding NACHT, and a carboxy-terminal LRR domain. ASC has two domains, an amino-terminal PYD and a carboxy-terminal CARD domain. NLRP3 activation leads to protein–protein interactions between the NLRP3 and ASC via PYD domains. This facilitates ASC polymerization to form long helical filaments that are condensed into an intracellular macromolecular aggregate, known as ASC speck [90]. Subsequently, the ASC CARD domain associates with the CARD domain of caspase-1, inducing caspase-1 self-cleavage and activation [91]. A serine–threonine kinase known as NIMA-related kinase 7 (NEK 7) binds to NLRP3 directly and oligomerizes with NLRP3 into a complex that is essential for ASC speck formation and caspase-1 activation [92]. Activated caspase-1 cleaves the inactive pro-IL-1β and pro-IL-18 forms into bioactive cytokines that activate downstream inflammatory pathways [93] (Figure 1). Recent studies have shown that ASC specks can be exocytosed and accumulated in the extracellular space, retaining their ability to produce IL-1β. Extracellular ASC specks can also be internalized by macrophages, further activating IL-1β production [94,95]. Moreover, ASC specks isolated from cells can induce the aggregation of other ASC specks located intracellularly, a feature shared with prionoid proteins. These findings suggest that extracellular ASC can propagate inflammatory responses even at distinct sites, promoting systemic inflammation. Of note, increased extracellular ASC specks were documented in bone marrow from patients with myelodysplastic syndrome [96]. Pertinent to lung diseases, increased extracellularly-assembled ASC specks were observed in the BAL of patients with chronic obstructive pulmonary disease and pneumonia compared to patients with pulmonary hypertension and healthy controls [94]. Considering the documented effects of extracellular ASC specks on the activation of distant cell populations, their presence in SA patients may have important implications, and warrants further investigation.

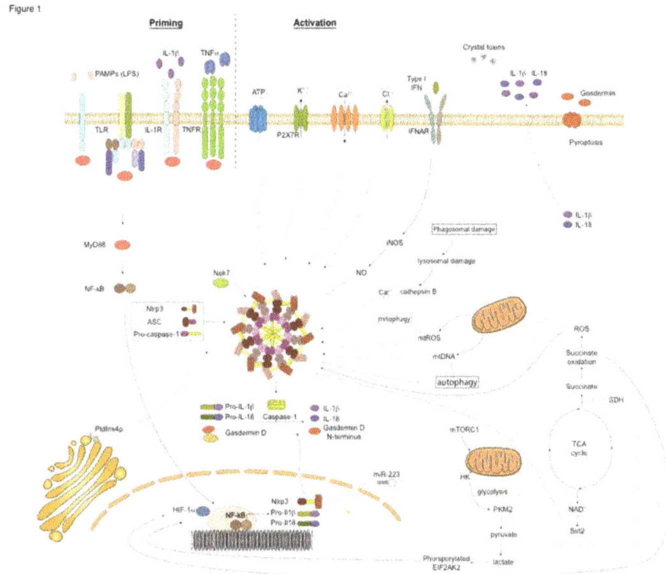

Figure 1. Mechanisms involved in activation and regulation of NLRP3 canonical pathway. NLRP3 inflammasome activation requires two signals. The "priming" signal is triggered by PAMP/DAMP recognition by PPRs (e.g. TLRs) and certain cytokines (e.g. TNF-α, IL-1β) and activates NF-κB in the cell nucleus. This leads to NLRP3, pro-IL1-β and pro-IL-18 gene transcription. The second signal induces the assembly of NLRP3, ASC, and caspase-1 to form an active NLRP3 inflammasome and ultimately leads to the release of mature IL-1β and IL-18. Gasdermin D is cleaved and becomes inserted into the cell membrane, forming pores and inducing pyroptosis. The mechanisms proposed for the second NLRP3 activating signals are shown and include: a) changes in cytosolic levels of ions, such as K^+, Cl^- and Ca^{+2}, b) lysosomal destabilization and the release of cathepsins, c) mitochondrial dysfunction-derived signals such as mtROS, mtDNA and d) metabolic changes. PtdIns4P on dTGN drive NLRP3 activation. Aerobic glycolysis pathways and the TCA cycle also activate NLRP3. Autophagy and mitophagy inhibit NLRP3 inflammasome activation. IFNs also inhibit NLRP3 activation through NO production. IL-1R, IL-1β receptor; TLR, Toll-like receptor; TNFR, tumor necrosis factor receptor; IFNAR, IFNα/β receptor; NEK7, NIMA- related kinase 7; NF- κB, nuclear factor- κB; P2X7, P2X purinoceptor 7; PtdIns4P, phosphatidylinositol-4-phosphate; PYD, pyrin domain; ROS, reactive oxygen species; HK1, hexokinase; mTORC1, rapamycin complex 1; SDH, succinate dehydrogenase; EIF2AK2, eukaryotic translation initiation factor 2-alpha kinase 2.

IL-1β secretion upon NLRP3 inflammasome activation initiates acute phase reactions, including the recruitment of inflammatory cells at the site of infection and expression of proinflammatory cytokines, such as, IL-6, TNF-α, and chemokines [97]. Briefly, active IL-1β binds to the extracellular domain of the IL-1 type 1 receptor (IL-1R) that recruits the second receptor chain, termed IL-1R accessory protein (IL-1RAcP) [98]. This leads to the activation of intracellular signaling molecules, such as the myeloid differentiation primary response 88 (MYD88), TNF receptor-associated factor 6 (TRAF6) and IL-1R-associated kinases (IRAK), which, in turn, activate the nuclear factor-κB (NF-κB) transcription factor, eliciting cytokine gene expression [99]. Active IL-1β exerts its functions through both autocrine and paracrine mechanisms, and therefore its regulation is under tight control to circumvent pathologic implications. IL-1β signaling is also involved in Th2 and Th17 cell differentiation and is implicated in the pathogenicity of allergic airway inflammation [100]. The biological role of IL-18 is different from that of IL-1β. IL-18 induces Th1 cell responses and the production of IFN-γ by $CD4^+$ and $CD8^+$ T cells, natural killer cells, and macrophages, and is essential for antiviral immunity. IL-18 also plays a role in Th2 cell differentiation and is involved in AHR in experimental models, as well as in asthmatic patients [101,102].

Apart from proinflammatory cytokine release, a key outcome of NLRP3 inflammasome activation is pyroptosis, a form of lytic cell death characterized by cell swelling, membrane rupture, and release of proinflammatory cellular contents [103,104]. The formation of plasma membrane pores during pyroptosis drives ion changes, inducing increased osmotic pressure, water influx, and cell swelling. Pyroptosis is triggered by caspase-1-driven cleavage of the pore-forming protein gasdermin D (GSDMD) that leads to the formation of the GSDM N-terminal fragment, that, in turn, introduces pore formation upon insertion into the plasma membrane, thus killing cells from within [103,104]. Pyroptosis is a highly inflammatory process that is accompanied by the release of IL-1β, IL-18, IL-1α, high mobility group box 1 protein, and lactate dehydrogenase to the extracellular milieu [103,105] (Figure 1). NLRP3 inflammasome activation occurs through three distinct molecular pathways: the canonical, the noncanonical, and the alternative pathways [11,86,89,92,105,106] (Table 1).

Table 1. Key characteristics of canonical, noncanonical and alternative NLRP3 activation.

Pathways of NLRP3 Inflammasome Activation	Canonical	Noncanonical	Alternative
NLRP3-ASC-Casp1 signaling	Yes	Yes	Yes
Caspase-1 cleavage, IL-1β maturation	Yes	Yes	Yes
Caspase-11, 4, 5 cleavage	No	Yes	No
Caspase-8 cleavage	No	No	Yes
Signal 2 requirement	Yes	No	No
Pyroptosome formation	Yes	Yes	No
Cell Death	Yes	Yes	No

6. Activation of the Canonical Nlrp3 Pathway

Activation of the NLRP3 inflammasome through the canonical pathway requires 2 steps: a priming signal and a second activating signal (Figure 1). The priming signal is crucial for the transcription of the inflammasome components, *NLRP3*, *CASP1*, and the *IL1B* and *IL18* genes. The priming signal is usually a PAMP, such as, LPS, lipoproteins, carbohydrates, and flagellin [107]. IL-1β and TNF-α signaling can also induce NLRP3 priming, known as sterile priming. Gene transcription upon priming is mediated predominantly through NF-κB activation and nuclear translocation [108,109]. Interestingly, recent studies have discovered a nontranscriptional priming process that relies on post-translational modifications (PTMs), such as ubiquitylation, phosphorylation, and sumoylation of NLRP3 components [110].

A wide variety of secondary stimuli activate the NLRP3 inflammasome, including bacteria, viruses, environmental nanoparticles such as alum and silica, and endogenous molecules, including ATP, monosodium urate (MSU), and cholesterol crystals. The main mechanisms through which these

PAMPs and DAMPs trigger NLRP3 inflammasome activation are associated with: a) changes in cytosolic levels of ions, such as, K^+, Ca^{+2}, and Cl^-, b) lysosomal destabilization, c) ROS production, and d) mitochondrial dysfunction [92,111]. The second activation signal leads to the assembly of the NLRP3 complex, the activation of caspase-1, and the release of the mature forms of IL-1β and IL-18 (Figure 1).

Decreased extracellular K^+ levels trigger NLRP3 activation, while high extracellular K^+ concentrations block NLRP3 signaling [112]. For example, extracellular ATP, upon binding to its receptor, the purine-dependent phenoxin-1 channel P2X7, induces K^+ efflux and initiates NLRP3 assembly and downstream signaling [113,114]. The bacterial toxin nigericin also promotes activation of NLRP3 by inducing K^+ efflux in a pannexin-1-dependent manner [115]. In addition to ATP and pore-forming toxins, alum, silica, and calcium pyrophosphate crystals also induce K^+ efflux. Moreover, the complement cascade component membrane attack complex (MAC) activates NLRP3 [116]. Apart from K^+ efflux, mobilization of Ca^{+2} in the cytosol through the opening of plasma membrane channels or the release of endoplasmic reticulum (ER)-linked Ca^{+2} stores represents another upstream event in NLRP3 activation [117]. It should be emphasized that K^+ efflux regulates Ca^{+2} flux and these two channels act cooperatively to activate NLRP3. In fact, NLRP3 activation induced by nigericin, alum, MSU crystals, and the MAC depends on Ca^{+2} flux along with K^+ efflux [118]. Cl^- efflux through chloride intracellular channel proteins (CLICs) enhances NLRP3 activation via the polymerization of ASC [119]. Translocation of CLIC1, CLIC4, and CLIC5 to the plasma membrane depends on the release of mitochondrial ROS (mtROS), whereas Cl^- efflux occurs downstream of K^+ efflux [119]. Lysosomal swelling and damage by phagocytosed but resistant to degradation crystals, such as silica, β-amyloid, liposomes, and asbestos, represents another mechanism of NLRP3 activation [120,121]. Briefly, the accumulation of crystals intracellulary destabilizes the lysophagosome and leads to the release of its components, including proteases, lipases, cathepsins, and Ca^{+2} in the cytosol, which, in turn, drive NLRP3 assembly and activation in a K^+ efflux-dependent manner [120,121] (Figure 1).

Numerous sources of ROS, such as, NADPH-oxidases, xanthine oxidase, cytochrome P450, cyclooxygenases, and lipoxygenases, induce NLRP3 activation [122] (Figure 1). The production of mtROS and mitochondrial DNA (mtDNA) also activate NLRP3. In fact, chemical inhibitors preventing ROS production inhibit NLRP3 inflammasome activation in response to several activators. Furthermore, factors that cause mitochondrial dysfunction increase the oxidation of mtDNA, which activates NLRP3 inflammasome. Increased mtROS production oxidizes thioredoxin (TRX), leading to its dissociation from the thioredoxin (TRX)-interacting protein (TXNIP). The dissociated TXNIP directly binds to NLRP3, leading to its activation [123]. Mitochondria also act as docking sites for NLRP3 inflammasome assembly. For example, the mitochondrial antiviral signalling protein (MAVS), an adaptor protein in RNA sensing, is critical for NLRP3 inflammasome activation during infections with RNA viruses and stimulation with the synthetic RNA polyinosinic-polycytidylic acid. MAVS recruits NLRP3, directing its localization to the mitochondria [124]. Still, MAVS is not essential for NLRP3 inflammation induced by other NLRP3 stimuli. Recently, it was shown that trans-Golgi network disassembly into vesicles, known as dispersed trans-Golgi network (dTGN), is another process that leads to NLRP3 inflammasome activation. More specifically, the phospholipid phosphatidylinositol-4-phosphate on dTGN drives NLRP3 aggregation, ASC oligomerization and caspase-1 activation, and downstream signaling [125].

Interestingly, recent studies have implicated cellular metabolic events in the activation of the NLRP3 inflammasome. Indeed, aerobic glycolysis and the mitochondrial electron transport chain (ETC) enhance NLRP3-driven responses [126–129] (Figure 1). In LPS-stimulated macrophages, activation of mammalian target of rapamycin complex 1 (mTORC1) promotes hexokinase (HK1)-dependent glycolysis which, in turn, induces NLRP3 activation [126–129]. Consequently, inhibition of mTORC1 or deficiency of Raptor, an mTORC1-binding partner, decreases HK1-dependent glycolysis and suppresses NLRP3 signaling [126–129]. Moreover, glucose deprivation, 2-deoxyglucose (2-DG) treatment, or HK-1 knockdown suppresses ATP-driven NLRP3 activation and inhibits IL-1β secretion by macrophages [126–129]. Additionally, saturated fatty acids, such as palmitate, suppress the activation of the anti-inflammatory AMP-activated kinase, leading to increased ROS production and NLRP3 activation [130].

Altogether, these secondary activating signals lead to IL-1β and IL-18 secretion downstream of NLRP3 activation and also to pyroptosis (Figure 1). Still, despite extensive research in understanding the upstream events during NLRP3 activation, there is still no single unifying model, and further studies using genetic approaches, rather than pharmacological inhibition that could lead to indirect and off-target effects, need to be performed.

7. Role of the Noncanonical and Alternative Nlrp3 Activation Pathways

The noncanonical pathway of NLRP3 activation is associated with the detection of intracellular LPS generated following infection by Gram-negative bacteria, such as *Escherichia coli, Salmonella typhimurium, Shigella flexneri,* and *Burkholderia thailandensis* [131–133]. As such, the noncanonical NLRP3 pathway induces pyroptotic cell death and restricts the growth of intracellular bacteria in myeloid and nonmyeloid cells. The noncanonical NLRP3 pathway requires signaling through caspase-11 in mice and caspases 4 and 5 in humans. The binding of LPS to caspases 11, 4, and 5 results in their autoactivation and cleavage of GSDMD, triggering pyroptosis and the secretion of IL-1α [134]. Pyroptosis enhances K^+ efflux which activates the canonical NLRP3 pathway and the release of IL-1β and IL-18. Hence, caspases 4, 5, and 11 do not cleave IL-1β and IL-18, but only lead to pyroptosis, and the subsequent canonical NLRP3 inflammasome activation pathway is responsible for caspase-1 activation and cytokine secretion. Activated caspase-11 also cleaves pannexin-1, a membrane ATP channel, which induces K^+ efflux and activates the canonical NLRP3 pathway [131–133].

The cytosolic accessibility of LPS is driven by Guanylate-Binding Proteins (GBPs) and the Immunity Related GTPase family member 10 (IRGB10) which lyse the Gram-negative bacterium-containing vacuoles, releasing bacterial LPS into the cytoplasm [134,135]. Bacterial outer membrane vesicles (OMVs) also deliver LPS into the cytoplasm through endocytosis. Another process through which extracellular LPS activates the nonconontical NLRP3 pathway is the binding and activating of its receptor, TLR4. TLR4 induces TRIF and MyD88 signaling, and drives the production of type I IFNs which, in turn, enhance the expression of the noncanonical inflammasome components, caspase-11, GBPs and IRGB10 [135,136]. In fact, type I IFNs, along with the complement C3-C3aR axis, upregulate caspase-11 expression. In neutrophils, the activation of the noncanonical NLRP3 pathway through detection of cytosolic LPS induces the release of neutrophil extracellular traps (NETs) that, in turn, activate the canonical NLRP3 pathway [137]. Reciprocally, IL-18 released upon NLRP3 inflammasome assembly induces NETosis [137].

An alternative NLRP3 inflammasome pathway was recently discovered in human and porcine monocytes and does not require a secondary signal [106]. LPS recognition by TLR4 induces the intracellular activation of the TIR-domain-containing adapter-inducing interferon-β - Receptor-interacting serine/threonine-protein kinase 1 - Fas-associated protein with death domain - Caspase-8 (TRIF-RIPK1-FADD-CASP8) cascade. Cleavage of caspase-8 induces NLRP3 activation and the maturation of IL-1β and IL-18, through an as yet unknown mechanism. This alternative pathway of NLRP3 activation occurs independently of K^+ efflux and ASC speck formation. An additional unique feature is that it does not trigger pyroptosis, and the secretion of IL-1β is independent of GSDM [106]. Notably, in mouse bone marrow-derived macrophages (BMDM), simultaneous TLR and NLRP3 stimulation leads to rapid inflammasome activation independent of de novo gene transcription [138]. This type of NLRP3 activation does not promote IL-1β secretion and pyroptosis, but enhances IL-18 production and provides a fast protective response against intracellular pathogen burden.

8. Regulation of Nlrp3 Functions

The activation of the NLRP3 inflammasome is associated with a diverse range of human diseases. Mutations in the *NLRP3* gene are associated with the dominantly inherited autoinflammatory diseases known as cryopyrin-associated periodic syndromes (CAPS), including familial cold autoinflammatory syndrome, Muckle–Wells syndrome, and chronic infantile neurological cutaneous and articular syndrome [139–141]. Single nucleotide polymorphisms in the genes encoding NLRP3 inflammasome components have been also associated with the pathophysiology of Crohn's disease and rheumatoid arthritis. Other studies have revealed that excessive NLRP3 activation is implicated in diseases driven by metabolic dysfunction such as type 2 diabetes and nonalcoholic steatohepatitis, in neurodegenerative diseases including Alzheimer's disease and Parkinson's disease, and in cancer [142–145]. Notably, NLRP3 activation through exposure to crystals and protein aggregates is associated with silicosis and fibrosis in the lung, atherosclerosis, gout flares, and kidney dysfunction [142]. Hence, stringent regulation of NLRP3 responses is essential for the control of overactive inflammatory processes and the prevention of tissue damage.

NLRP3 regulation takes place both at the transcriptional and the post-transcriptional levels. Type I-IFNs repress the expression of pro-IL-1β through the secretion of IL-10 [146] (Figure 1). Type-I IFNs also induce the expression of iNOS, which inhibits NLRP3 activation through the production of Nitric oxide (NO) and TRIM that reduces ROS release [147]. Post-transcriptional regulation of NLRP3 involves signaling through the microRNA, mir-223, which binds to the 3′ untranslated region UTR of NLRP3 and inhibits its expression [148] (Figure 1). PTMs can also negatively regulate NLRP3 responses. Indeed, the ubiquitylation of the LLR domain of NLRP3 by the membrane-associated Ring finger protein 7 (MARCH-7), and the phosphorylation of its Ser291 residue, negatively regulates NLRP3 activation [149,150].

One of the most important mechanisms that restrain NLRP3 functions is autophagy (Figure 1). Autophagy is an endogenous recycling process utilized by the host to maintain cell homeostasis in response to stress [151]. In autophagy, dysfunctional or unnecessary cellular components become degraded. In addition, mitophagy promotes the clearance of damaged mitochondria from the cytoplasm and reduces mtROS [151]. Recent studies have shown that activation of NLRP3 in macrophages deficient in autophagy components, such as *Beclin* or *Lc3b*, leads to increased secretion of mtDNA and ROS, and increased activation of caspase-1 and release of IL-1β and IL-18 [152,153]. Furthermore, in vitro treatment of monocytes with rapamycin, an autophagy inducer, reduces IL-1β secretion in response to LPS [154]. In addition, induction of mitophagy through activation of the receptor-interacting serine/threonine-protein kinase 2 (RIP2) limits virus-induced NLRP3 activation [155]. Moreover, infection with influenza A virus in mice deficient in *Nod2* and *Ripk2* results in defective mitophagy, leading to excessive activation of NLRP3 and increased IL-18 production [155].

Signaling through metabolic regulators can also inhibit NLRP3 activation. Dimethyl fumarate (DMF) activates the transcription factor NF-E2-related factor 2 (NRF2) that represses IL-1β and NLRP3 gene expression in LPS-treated microglia and in the human acute monocytic leukemia cell line (THP-1) [156]. NRF2 also regulates levels of antioxidant genes to support cell survival during oxidative stress, and through limiting ROS levels, it inhibits NLRP3 activation [157]. DMF also decreases mtROS release and suppresses NLRP3 assembly [156]. In addition, nicotinamide adenine dinucleotide (NAD^+) activates sirtuins (Sirt2) which inhibit NLRP3 inflammasome activation and decrease pro-IL-1β production [158] (Figure 1). Some metabolites of fatty acids, including β-hydroxybutyrate and α-linolenic acid, suppress NLRP3 activation via inhibiting K^+ efflux and the oligomerization of ASC, and by reducing ROS levels [159,160]. Interestingly, cholesterol metabolism is also associated with the regulation of NLRP3 responses. Of note, a recent report documented that bile acids through the TGR5-cAMP-protein kinase A axis inhibit NLRP3 activation and prevent LPS-induced systemic inflammation, alum-mediated peritoneal inflammation, and type 2 diabetes in mouse models [161]. Other studies in human primary monocyte-derived macrophages showed that PGE2 treatment following LPS stimulation inhibits NLRP3 activation through increasing intracellular cAMP levels [162]. In support, inhibition of cyclooxygenase 2, resulting in PGE2 blockade, enhances NLRP3 activation in human macrophages. In response to PGE2, protein kinase A is also upregulated, phosphorylates Ser295 of NLRP3, and attenuates its ATPase function [150]. Conversely, treatment of

BMDM with PGE2 prior stimulation with LPS and ATP increased IL-1β and active caspase-1 release in culture supernatants, highligting species-specific differences as well as differences dependent on the timing of PGE2 administration [163].

Several small-molecule compounds have been described as potent inhibitors of NLRP3 activation, including MCC950 [164], β-hydroxybutyrate (BHB) [159], Bay 11-7082 [165], dimethyl sulfoxide (DMSO) [166], and type I IFN [167]. Seminal studies by Coll et al. have documented that MCC950 inhibits both the canonical and the noncanonical pathways of NLRP3 activation, while it does not affect other inflammasomes. MCC950 prevents NLRP3-induced ASC oligomerization without affecting NLRP3 priming, and inhibits IL-1β secretion by human and mouse macrophages [164]. Subsequent studies demonstrated that MCC950 blocks nigericin-induced NLRP3 activation via inhibition of Cl^- efflux in LPS-primed BMDMs [168]. Moreover, MCC950 inhibits NLRP3 inflammasome formation through blocking ATP hydrolysis [169]. Of relevance, preclinical studies have shown that MCC950 alleviates the severity of experimental autoimmune encephalomyelitis and prevents neonatal lethality in a model of CAPS [164]. Pharmacological inhibition of NLRP3 with MCC950 also protected against dopaminergic degeneration in a mouse model of Parkinson's disease (PD), and reduced total leukocytes and inflammatory macrophages in the BAL of mice infected with influenza A virus [170,171].

The aforementioned paragraphs highlight crucial functions for NLRP3 inflammasome activation in the eradication of pathogens, the protection against damaged and/or dying cells, and the maintenance of tissue homeostasis. However, several gaps in our understanding of the precise molecular pathways involved in the initiation and regulation of NLRP3-driven inflammatory responses remain, and represent promising avenues for future research. In the next section, we describe current knowledge on the role of NLRP3 activation in the initiation and propagation of allergic airway inflammation and human asthma, and discuss the implications of excessive NLRP3 responses in the pathogenesis of allergic diseases.

9. Role of Nlrp3 Signaling in Allergic Airway Inflammation

NLRP3 inflammasome activation is involved in the initiation and the propagation of allergen-driven inflammatory responses in the airways. Studies using mouse models of allergic asthma induced by adjuvant-free ovalbumin (OVA) and adjuvant (aluminum hydroxide)-coupled OVA, demonstrate enhanced protein levels of NLRP3 and caspase-1, along with elevated IL-1β and TNF-α release by epithelial cells and macrophages in the airways, compared to Phosphate-buffered saline (PBS)-treated mice [172]. Moreover, in mice sensitized with OVA and LPS and challenged with OVA (OVA_{LPS}-OVA), as well as in HDM-instilled mice, increased ROS and mtROS production in BAL cells and in primary tracheal epithelial cells was detected, inducing augmented NLRP3, caspase-1, and IL-1β protein expression in the airways [173]. Interestingly, recent studies using three distinct HDM-induced mouse models of allergic airway inflammation (AAI), corresponding to eosiniphilic, mixed granulocytic, and neutrophilic asthma subtypes, documented increased expression of Nlrp3, Nlrc4, Nlrc5, Pycard, Casp-1 genes, and pro-IL-1β protein levels in the lungs, especially in the neutrophilic asthma model, while mature IL-1β was not shown, suggesting that although inflammasome molecules are upregulated, they do not form functional complexes without an additional trigger [174]. Moreover, increasing inflammasome sensor, caspase-1, and pro-IL-1β expression was documented from eosinophilic to neutrophilic asthma, illuminating an association of inflammasome signaling pathways with the type of airway inflammation [174]. Notably, induction of neutrophilic airway inflammation in mice challenged with HDM and polyinosinic-polycytidylic acid increased the concentration of Apolipoprotein E (APOE) in the epithelial lining fluid and enhanced IL-1β levels in the BAL, pointing to a potential role of APOE in IL-1β production [175].

Pertinent to the role of NLRP3 activation in allergic responses, studies using mice deficient in *NLRP3* and *ASC* in a model of OVA-induced AAI demonstrated decreased eosinophil influx, dampened AHR and reduced airway inflammation, and goblet cell accumulation, accompanied by decreased IL-1β expression in the airway, compared to wild type (WT) littermates [176]. Other studies also in a model of OVA-AAI, revealed that *NLRP3*$^{-/-}$ mice exhibit decreased pulmonary inflammation with suppressed mucus secretion, Th2 cytokine and chemokine production, and IgE levels [177]. Interestingly, in a model of OVA-AAI, production of IL-1α and IL-1β in the airways propagated Th2 cell-driven allergic responses and exacerbated pulmonary eosinophilia in a process mediated by caspase-8 activation [178]. These studies highlighted a novel role for caspase-8 in NLRP3 activation in the allergic airway, which was independent of caspase-1 and 11 signaling [178]. Other reports using a model of serum amyloid A (SAA)-induced AAI documented that the secretion of IL-1β in response to SAA is dependent on NLRP3 activation [179]. In fact, using mice deficient in *NLRP3* and *caspase-1*, the authors demonstrated a reduction in infiltrating neutrophils in the lung and decreased inflammatory cytokine/chemokine release (IL-1β, IL-6, and MCP-1 or CCL2) in the BAL compared to WT controls [179]. Another study using a complete Freund's adjuvant (CFA)/HDM-induced mouse model of AAI showed that administration of CRID3, an NLRP3 inhibitor, reduced IL1-β and Th2 cytokine production in the BAL and inhibited AHR [180]. Interestingly, a recent report demonstrated that NLRP3, along with IRF4, transactivates the *Il4* promoter, enhances Th2 cell differentiation, and exacerbates asthma symptoms in a mouse model [181]. Moreover, studies by Kim et al., in an experimental model of high fat diet-induced obesity, demonstrated that obese mice had increased AHR driven by aberrant NLRP3 inflammasome-dependent responses in the adipose tissue, which contributed to the activation of ILCs and increased IL-17 responses in the lung, in the absence of allergic sensitisation [182]. These studies highlighted a novel NLRP3-IL-1β-Th17 link in AHR development in obesity-associated allergic airway disease.

Notably, sensitization with OVA-alum or *Aspergillus fumigates* followed by challenge with OVA or *A. fumigates*, respectively, increased ROS production in lung homogenates mediated by mitochondrial Ca^{2+}/calmodium-dependent protein kinase II (CaMK II), which induced NLRP3, active caspase-1 and mature IL-18 at the mRNA, and protein levels in allergic lungs, as well as exacerbated OVA-AAI [183]. In contrast, inhibition of mitochondrial CaMK II reduced AHR, Th2 cytokine production and NLRP3 activation in the lungs [183]. Further studies in a mouse model of OVA-AAI, accompanied by infection with *Chlamydia muridarum* or *Haemofilus influenza*, demonstrated an increased expression of NLRP3 in airway epithelial and infiltrating immune cells, as well as enhanced IL-1β and caspase-1 mRNA levels in the lungs of infected mice [184]. Notably, in vivo administration of MCC950 decreased AHR and neutrophil accumulation in the airways of infected mice [184]. Furthermore, using mice deficient in *NLRP3* and *IL-1β*, another study documented reduced airway inflammation and cytokine release following rhinovirus (RV) infection in HDM-challenged mice, highlighting the implication of NLRP3 activation in RV-induced disease exacerbations [185]. Notably, subepithelial macrophages were the major source of IL-1β in response to RV, with low IL-1β expression by the airway epithelium, suggesting that NLRP3 activation mainly occurred in macrophages. Moreover, no induction of IL-18, either at the mRNA or the protein levels, was observed in airway epithelial cells upon RV infection. It should be emhpasized that, in contrast to the airway epithelium, the gut epithelium is characterized by increased IL-18 and low IL-1β production in response to NLRP3 signaling. Indeed, IL-1β levels remained unaltered in colonic intestinal epithelial cells from mice treated with a high-fibre diet, while active caspase-1 and IL-18 were increased [186]. Notably, using *NLRP3*$^{-/-}$ mice, the authors showed that the protective effects of a high-fibre diet against colitis were mediated through NLRP3 activation in colonic epithelial cells. Altogether, these studies suggest that epithelial cells at distinct sites respond differently to inflammasome activation, not only in terms of cytokine secretion but also in the inflammasome sensor utilized, and propose a key role of the tissue micromilieu in governing epithelial cell-induced inflammatory responses.

Contradictory data have been generated by studies showing that NLRP3 activation is not essential for allergic disease development in OVA and HDM induced AAI. Allen et al. showed that the adjuvant effects of aluminum hydroxide in the OVA-AAI model were not affected in *NLRP3*$^{-/-}$, *Casp*$^{-/-}$, or *PYCARD*$^{-/-}$ mice [187]. In another study, *NLRP3*$^{-/-}$ mice did not exhibit significant differences in airway eosinophilia, mucus production, AHR, and Th2 cell responses upon exposure to uric acid crystals compared to their WT counterparts [188]. Similar findings were observed in a combined particular matter (PM)/Ova-induced mouse model of experimental asthma [189]. Finally, Madouri et al. demonstrated that mice deficient in *NLRP3*$^{-/-}$, *Casp*$^{-/-}$, or *PYCARD*$^{-/-}$ exhibited enhanced lung inflammation and pathology, including eosinophilic inflitration and Th2 cytokine release, upon exposure to HDM, supporting the notion that NLRP3 activation exerts protective functions against HDM-induced allergic lung inflammation [190].

10. Nlrp3 Signaling in Human Asthma

A series of recent studies suggest that NLRP3 activation is involved in human asthma pathogenesis. Hirota et al. was among the first to describe NLRP3 and caspase-1 protein expression in human lung sections and in primary airway epithelial cells from healthy volunteers following exposure to PM_{10}. In fact, they demonstrated that NLRP3 silencing using short hairpin (sh) NLRP3 attenuated PM_{10}-induced release of IL-1β by human airway epithelial cells [191]. In other studies, in vitro RV infection of HBECs upregulated NLRP3, NLRC5, and caspase-1 protein levels that triggered IL-1β secretion [192]. Knock down of NLRP3 or NLRC5, using shRNA, decreased IL-1β secretion by HBECs, while simultaneous knock down of NLRP3 and NLRC5 abrogated IL-1β secretion. Moreover, HBEC from asthmatics exhibited enhanced co-localization of caspase-1 and ASC and increased mRNA expression of caspase-4 after IAV infection compared to healthy controls [193] (Figure 2). Still, it should be emphasized that the previous studies were using human bronchial epithelial cells cultured in a monolayer, and NLRP3 activation in airway epithelial cells cultured in an air–liquid interface (ALI), which is a more physiologically relevant model, remains incompletely defined. Increased NLRP3 and IL-18 protein levels were observed in airway epithelial cells in lung biopsies from asthmatics compared to healthy individuals [183]. Notably, individuals with neutrophilic asthma had elevated mRNA levels of NLRP3, caspase-1, and IL-1β, as well as NLRP3 and caspase-1 protein expression in sputum macrophages and neutrophils, compared to eosinophilic and paucigranulocytic asthmatics [180,194] (Figure 2). Increased expression of NLRP3 and IL-1β was also detected in the sputum of patients with SA compared to MMA, and correlated with clinical parameters of disease, such as neutrophilic airway inflammation, Asthma Control Questionnaire (ACQ) score, and Forced Expiratory Volume in 1 second (FEV1)% [184]. In another study, increased extracellular DNA (eDNA) sputum levels in SA correlated with sputum neutrophilic inflammation, increased NETs formation, caspase-1 activity, and IL-1β levels [195]. NLRP3 gene expression and IL-1β protein levels were also increased in sputum inflammatory cells from obese asthmatics compared to non-obese asthmatics, and correlated with body mass index [196] (Figure 2). Kim et al. showed higher expression of NLRP3 and caspase-1 in the BAL of asthmatics compared to healthy subjects [173] (Figure 2). BAL macrophages from asthmatics treated ex vivo with HDM also upregulated *NLRP3* and pro-IL-1β expression, resulting in increased IL-1β secretion in an APOE-dependent manner [174]. Lui et al. also showed that macrophages isolated from the PB of patients with Th2/Th17-predominant asthma had higher mRNA and protein levels of NLRP3 components and IL-1β compared to healthy controls [197].

Pertinent to inflammasome related-cytokines, most studies have shown that IL-1β is increased in the sputum and BAL of patients with neutrophilic asthma [198], and in the serum of asthmatic patients with or without steroid treatment, compared to controls [199] (Figure 2). Contradictory findings were observed regarding IL-18 release, with some studies showing increased IL-18 in the serum [200,201] and sputum from SA patients [202,203], and others reporting decreased levels in induced sputum [204]. Considering the increased activation of the NLRP3 pathways, along with excessive IL-1β release, in asthmatic patients, the concept of IL-1β blocking as a therapeutic approach in SA appears promising. Therapeutic administration of canakinumab, a fully human anti-IL-1β monoclоncal antibody, has been widely used in conditions ranging from CAPS to rheumatoid arthritis, atherosclerosis, and lung cancer [205–208]. Pertinent to asthma, there was only one randomized double-blind placebo-controlled study that evaluated the safety and tolerability of canakinumab in mild asthmatic patients, as well as its effects on the attenuation of the late asthmatic response (LAR) following allergen challenge [209].

Canakinumab appeared to be safe and attenuated LAR compared to pretreatment values. Despite these positive results, no further studies have been conducted since [209], and canakinumab is no longer under investigation as a treatment for asthma (searched on clinicaltrials.org on 11/09/2019).

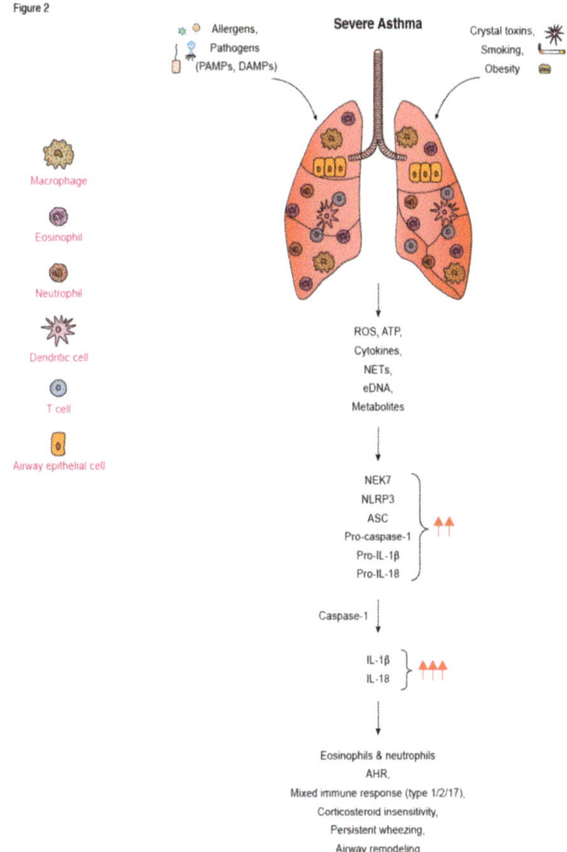

Figure 2. The role of NLRP3 inflammasome in the development of severe asthma. Exposure to pathogens, allergens, cigarette smoke, and other noxious stimuli in the asthmatic airway triggers the production of ROS, cytokines, and NETs which, in turn, can activate the NLRP3 inflammasome in infiltrating eosinophils, neutrophils, and macrophages, as well as in airway epithelial cells. This results in the enhanced release of IL-1β and IL-18, which leads to increased Th1 Th2 and/or Th17 cell infiltration and associated pathological consequences, such as mucus hypersecretion, AHR, and airway remodelin. eDNA, extracellular DNA; NETs, neutrophil extracellular traps; AHR, airway hyperresponsiveness.

In summary, a growing body of evidence suggests that NLRP3-induced inflammasome responses are implicated in AAI both in experimental models and human asthma (Figure 2). Still, certain controversial results obtained in animal studies are mainly associated with variations in the experimental models utilized, including type and concentration of allergen, route and time of administration, as well as mouse strain differences. The observed differences could be also associated with the distinct housing conditions affecting the microbiota composition. Hence, further mechanistic studies are warranted to resolve these disparities. More importantly, the precise role of NLRP3 activation in experimental models of SA remains elusive and deserves investigation. Of note, certain findings observed in animal studies were not observed in human asthmatics. For example, in human airway epithelial cells, it seems that other than NLRP3 inflammasome sensors become activated and trigger IL-1β release. Moreover, the precise factors that initate inflammasome assembly and activation in asthmatics remain incompletely defined. Mechanistic studies using animal models that more closely resemble SA need to be performed to clarify the type of cells in which NLRP3 signaling is activated, as well as its upstream regulators. In addition, functional studies using human primary airway epithelial cells in ALI cultures are essential for the elucidation of the differences in NLRP3-induced signaling in humans and mice. Finally, elucidation of the role of NLRP3 activation in the functional crosstalk between airway epithelial cells and other lung structural cells, such as ASMs, may shed new light on the mechanisms underlying tissue remodelling in SA.

11. Concluding Remarks

The past decade has witnessed a burgeoning appreciation of the existence of a wide range of SA endotypes. Still, and particularly in the type 2 low asthma endotypes, there is a considerable gap in our understanding of the cellular and molecular mechanisms involved and a remarkable scarcity of relevant biomarkers. More importantly, no effective treatments targeted at these endotypes have emerged. Growing evidence has illuminated a key role for NLRP3 inflammasome activation in the development and exacerbation of allergic responses. Hence, targeting NLRP3 inflammasome pathways in the airways of allergen-challenged mice, particularly in the context of SA, will improve our understanding of how NLRP3 signaling contributes to the development of specific aspects of disease severity. In fact, the direct comparison of the expression and activation of NLRP3 in mouse models and patients with distinct asthma severities is essential for the identification of novel biomarkers pertinent to the diverse asthma endotypes.

Current treatment modalities of NLRP3-related inflammatory human diseases target IL-1β with IL-1β antibodies or recombinant IL-1βR antagonists, such as canakinumab and anakinra, respectively. Nevertheless, most of these inhibitors are relatively nonspecific and have low efficacy. Thus, the development of targeted NLRP3 inflammasome site-specific therapeutics may be more beneficial in suppressing inflammasome-associated disease whilst not predisposing to infection. However, a deeper understanding of the NLRP3 inflammasome assembly and activation is needed before translation of these findings into therapies in clinical practice, especially in the context of SA. To achieve this, we need the development and use of better in vivo models of SA, along with complementary human studies using physiologically relevant in vitro models. Ultimately, this will facilitate the development of personalized medicine for the growing numbers of patients with SA.

Author Contributions: E.T. and M.S. searched the literature and wrote the manuscript; E.T. and J.M. designed the figures; G.X. wrote the manuscript.

Funding: General Secretariat for Research and Technology: 5035; General Secretariat for Research and Technology: 09-12-1074; Hellenic Foundation for Research and Innovation: 1030.

Conflicts of Interest: The authors declare no conflict of interest.

References

1. Holgate, S.T.; Holloway, J.; Wilson, S.; Howarth, P.H.; Haitchi, H.M.; Babu, S.; Davies, D.E. Understanding the pathophysiology of severe asthma to generate new therapeutic opportunities. *J. Allergy Clin. Immunol.* **2006**, *117*, 496–506. [CrossRef] [PubMed]
2. Wenzel, S. Severe asthma: From characteristics to phenotypes to endotypes. *Clin. Exp. Allergy* **2012**, *42*, 650–658. [CrossRef] [PubMed]
3. Wenzel, S.E. Asthma phenotypes: The evolution from clinical to molecular approaches. *Nat. Med.* **2012**, *18*, 716–725. [CrossRef] [PubMed]
4. Edwards, M.R.; Saglani, S.; Schwarze, J.; Skevaki, C.; Smith, J.A.; Ainsworth, B.; Almond, M.; Andreakos, E.; Belvisi, M.G.; Chung, K.F.; et al. Addressing unmet needs in understanding asthma mechanisms: From the European Asthma Research and Innovation Partnership (EARIP) Work Package (WP) 2 collaborators. *Eur. Respir. J.* **2017**, *49*, 1602448. [CrossRef]

5. Ray, A.; Raundhal, M.; Oriss, T.B.; Ray, P.; Wenzel, S.E. Current concepts of severe asthma. *J. Clin. Investig.* **2016**, *126*, 2394–2403. [CrossRef] [PubMed]
6. Chung, K.F. Managing severe asthma in adults: Lessons from the ERS/ATS guidelines. *Curr. Opin. Pulm. Med.* **2015**, *21*, 8–15. [CrossRef]
7. King, G.G.; James, A.; Harkness, L.; Wark, P.A.B. Pathophysiology of severe asthma: We've only just started. *Respirology* **2018**, *23*, 262–271. [CrossRef]
8. Medzhitov, R.; Janeway, C.A. Innate immunity: The virtues of a nonclonal system of recognition. *Cell* **1997**, *91*, 295–298. [CrossRef]
9. Matzinger, P. Tolerance, danger, and the extended family. *Annu. Rev. Immunol.* **1994**, *12*, 991–1045. [CrossRef]
10. Lamkanfi, M. Emerging inflammasome effector mechanisms. *Nat. Rev. Immunol.* **2011**, *11*, 213–220. [CrossRef]
11. Pinkerton, J.W.; Kim, R.Y.; Robertson, A.A.B.; Hirota, J.A.; Wood, L.G.; Knight, D.A.; Cooper, M.A.; O'Neill, L.A.J.; Horvat, J.C.; Hansbro, P.M. Inflammasomes in the lung. *Mol. Immunol.* **2017**, *86*, 44–55. [CrossRef] [PubMed]
12. Wu, W.; Bang, S.; Bleecker, E.R.; Castro, M.; Denlinger, L.; Erzurum, S.C.; Fahy, J.V.; Fitzpatrick, A.M.; Gaston, B.M.; Hastie, A.T.; et al. Multiview Cluster Analysis Identifies Variable Corticosteroid Response Phenotypes in Severe Asthma. *Am. J. Respir. Crit. Care Med.* **2019**, *199*, 1358–1367. [CrossRef] [PubMed]
13. Moore, W.C.; Meyers, D.A.; Wenzel, S.E.; Teague, W.G.; Li, H.; Li, X.; D'Agostino, R., Jr.; Castro, M.; Curran-Everett, D.; Fitzpatrick, A.M.; et al. National Heart, Lung, and Blood Institute's Severe Asthma Research Program. Identification of asthma phenotypes using cluster analysis in the Severe Asthma Research Program. *Am. J. Respir. Crit. Care Med.* **2010**, *181*, 315–323. [CrossRef] [PubMed]
14. Wu, W.; Bleecker, E.; Moore, W.; Busse, W.W.; Castro, M.; Chung, K.F.; Calhoun, W.J.; Erzurum, S.; Gaston, B.; Israel, E.; et al. Unsupervised phenotyping of Severe Asthma Research Program participants using expanded lung data. *J. Allergy Clin. Immunol.* **2014**, *133*, 1280–1288. [CrossRef] [PubMed]
15. Robinson, D.; Humbert, M.; Buhl, R.; Cruz, A.A.; Inoue, H.; Korom, S.; Hanania, N.A.; Nair, P. Revisiting Type 2-high and Type 2-low airway inflammation in asthma: Current knowledge and therapeutic implications. *Clin. Exp. Allergy* **2017**, *47*, 161–175. [CrossRef] [PubMed]
16. Santus, P.; Saad, M.; Damiani, G.; Patella, V.; Radovanovic, D. Current and future targeted therapies for severe asthma: Managing treatment with biologics based on phenotypes and biomarkers. *Pharmacol. Res.* **2019**, *146*, 104296. [CrossRef]
17. Samitas, K.; Delimpoura, V.; Zervas, E.; Gaga, M. Anti-IgE treatment, airway inflammation and remodelling in severe allergic asthma: Current knowledge and future perspectives. *Eur. Respir. Rev.* **2015**, *24*, 594–601. [CrossRef] [PubMed]
18. Kubo, M. Innate and adaptive type 2 immunity in lung allergic inflammation. *Immunol. Rev.* **2017**, *278*, 162–172. [CrossRef] [PubMed]
19. Lloyd, C.M.; Saglani, S. Epithelial cytokines and pulmonary allergic inflammation. *Curr. Opin. Immunol.* **2015**, *34*, 52–58. [CrossRef]
20. Angkasekwinai, P.; Chang, S.H.; Thapa, M.; Watarai, H.; Dong, C. Regulation of IL-9 expression by IL-25 signaling. *Nat. Immunol.* **2010**, *11*, 250–256. [CrossRef]
21. Angkasekwinai, P. Th9 Cells in Allergic Disease. *Curr. Allergy Asthma Rep.* **2019**, *19*, 29. [CrossRef]
22. Moretti, S.; Renga, G.; Oikonomou, V.; Galosi, C.; Pariano, M.; Iannitti, R.G.; Borghi, M.; Puccetti, M.; De Zuani, M.; Pucillo, C.E.; et al. A mast cell-ILC2-Th9 pathway promotes lung inflammation in cystic fibrosis. *Nat. Commun.* **2017**, *8*, 14017. [CrossRef]
23. Jones, C.P.; Gregory, L.G.; Causton, B.; Campbell, G.A.; Lloyd, C.M. Activin an and TGF-beta promote T(H)9 cell-mediated pulmonary allergic pathology. *J. Allergy Clin. Immunol.* **2012**, *129*, 1000–1010.e3. [CrossRef]
24. Erpenbeck, V.J.; Hohlfeld, J.M.; Volkmann, B.; Hagenberg, A.; Geldmacher, H.; Braun, A.; Krug, N. Segmental allergen challenge in patients with atopic asthma leads to increased IL-9 expression in bronchoalveolar lavage fluid lymphocytes. *J. Allergy Clin. Immunol.* **2003**, *111*, 1319–1327. [CrossRef]
25. Barlow, J.L.; McKenzie, A.N. Type-2 innate lymphoid cells in human allergic disease. *Curr. Opin. Allergy Clin. Immunol.* **2014**, *14*, 397–403. [CrossRef]
26. Chang, J.E.; Doherty, T.A.; Baum, R.; Broide, D. Prostaglandin D2 regulates human type 2 innate lymphoid cell chemotaxis. *J. Allergy Clin. Immunol.* **2014**, *133*, 899–901. [CrossRef]

27. Fahy, J.V. Type 2 inflammation in asthma–present in most, absent in many. *Nat. Rev. Immunol.* **2015**, *15*, 57–65. [CrossRef]
28. Matsumoto, H. Serum periostin: A novel biomarker for asthma management. *Allergol. Int.* **2014**, *63*, 153–160. [CrossRef]
29. Takayama, G.; Arima, K.; Kanaji, T.; Toda, S.; Tanaka, H.; Shoji, S.; McKetnzie, A.N.; Nagai, H.; Hotokebuchi, T.; Izuhara, K. Periostin: A novel component of subepithelial fibrosis of bronchial asthma downstream of IL-4 and IL-13 signals. *J. Allergy Clin. Immunol.* **2006**, *118*, 98–104. [CrossRef]
30. Modena, B.D.; Tedrow, J.R.; Milosevic, J.; Bleecker, E.R.; Meyers, D.A.; Wu, W.; Bar-Joseph, Z.; Erzurum, S.C.; Gaston, B.M.; Busse, W.W.; et al. Gene expression in relation to exhaled nitric oxide identifies novel asthma phenotypes with unique biomolecular pathways. *Am. J. Respir. Crit. Care Med.* **2014**, *190*, 1363–1372. [CrossRef]
31. Raundhal, M.; Morse, C.; Khare, A.; Oriss, T.B.; Milosevic, J.; Trudeau, J.; Huff, R.; Pilewski, J.; Holguin, F.; Kolls, J.; et al. High IFN-γ and low SLPI mark severe asthma in mice and humans. *J. Clin. Investig.* **2015**, *125*, 3037–3050. [CrossRef]
32. Shannon, J.; Ernst, P.; Yamauchi, Y.; Olivenstein, R.; Lemiere, C.; Foley, S.; Cicora, L.; Ludwig, M.; Hamid, Q.; Martin, J.G. Differences in airway cytokine profile in severe asthma compared to moderate asthma. *Chest* **2008**, *133*, 420–426. [CrossRef]
33. Truyen, E.; Coteur, L.; Dilissen, E.; Overbergh, L.; Dupont, L.J.; Ceuppens, J.L.; Bullens, D.M. Evaluation of airway inflammation by quantitative Th1/Th2 cytokine mRNA measurement in sputum of asthma patients. *Thorax* **2006**, *61*, 202–208. [CrossRef]
34. Dahlberg, P.E.; Busse, W.W. Is intrinsic asthma synonymous with infection? *Clin. Exp. Allergy* **2009**, *39*, 1324–1329. [CrossRef]
35. Bhakta, N.R.; Woodruff, P.G. Human asthma phenotypes: From the clinic, to cytokines, and back again. *Immunol. Rev.* **2011**, *242*, 220–232. [CrossRef]
36. Park, H.; Li, Z.; Yang, X.O.; Chang, S.H.; Nurieva, R.; Wang, Y.H.; Wang, Y.; Hood, L.; Zhu, Z.; Tian, Q.; et al. A distinct lineage of CD4 T cells regulates tissue inflammation by producing interleukin 17. *Nat. Immunol.* **2005**, *6*, 1133–1141. [CrossRef]
37. Pène, J.; Chevalier, S.; Preisser, L.; Vénéreau, E.; Guilleux, M.H.; Ghannam, S.; Molès, J.P.; Danger, Y.; Ravon, E.; Lesaux, S.; et al. Chronically inflamed human tissues are infiltrated by highly differentiated Th17 lymphocytes. *J. Immunol.* **2008**, *180*, 7423–7430. [CrossRef]
38. Laan, M.; Cui, Z.H.; Hoshino, H.; Lötvall, J.; Sjöstrand, M.; Gruenert, D.C.; Skoogh, B.E.; Lindén, A. Neutrophil recruitment by human IL-17 via C-X-C chemokine release in the airways. *J. Immunol.* **1999**, *162*, 2347–2352.
39. Bullens, D.M.; Truyen, E.; Coteur, L.; Dilissen, E.; Hellings, P.W.; Dupont, L.J.; Ceuppens, J.L. IL-17 mRNA in sputum of asthmatic patients: Linking T cell driven inflammation and granulocytic influx? *Respir. Res.* **2006**, *7*, 135. [CrossRef]
40. Agache, I.; Ciobanu, C.; Agache, C.; Anghel, M. Increased serum IL-17 is an independent risk factor for severe asthma. *Respir. Med.* **2010**, *1049*, 1131–1137. [CrossRef]
41. Massoud, A.H.; Charbonnier, L.M.; Lopez, D.; Pellegrini, M.; Phipatanakul, W.; Chatila, T.A. An asthma-associated IL4R variant exacerbates airway inflammation by promoting conversion of regulatory T cells to TH17-like cells. *Nat. Med.* **2016**, *22*, 1013–1022. [CrossRef]
42. Busse, W.W.; Holgate, S.; Kerwin, E.; Chon, Y.; Feng, J.; Lin, J.; Lin, S.L. Randomized, double-blind, placebo-controlled study of brodalumab, a human anti-IL-17 receptor monoclonal antibody, in moderate to severe asthma. *Am. J. Respir. Crit. Care Med.* **2013**, *188*, 1294–1302. [CrossRef]
43. Agalioti, T.; Villablanca, E.J.; Huber, S.; Gagliani, N. TH17 cell plasticity: The role of dendritic cells and molecular mechanisms. *J. Autoimmun.* **2018**, *87*, 50–60. [CrossRef]
44. Hastie, A.T.; Moore, W.C.; Li, H.; Rector, B.M.; Ortega, V.E.; Pascual, R.M.; Peters, S.P.; Meyers, D.A.; Bleecker, E.R.; National Heart, Lung, and Blood Institute's Severe Asthma Research Program. Biomarker surrogates do not accurately predict sputum eosinophil and neutrophil percentages in asthmatic subjects. *J. Allergy Clin. Immunol.* **2013**, *132*, 72–80. [CrossRef]
45. Zhang, X.Y.; Simpson, J.L.; Powell, H.; Yang, I.A.; Upham, J.W.; Reynolds, P.N.; Hodge, S.; James, A.L.; Jenkins, C.; Peters, M.J.; et al. Full blood count parameters for the detection of asthma inflammatory phenotypes. *Clin. Exp. Allergy* **2014**, *44*, 1137–1145. [CrossRef]

46. D'silva, L.; Cook, R.J.; Allen, C.J.; Hargreave, F.E.; Parameswaran, K. Changing pattern of sputum cell counts during successive exacerbations of airway disease. *Respir. Med.* **2007**, *101*, 2217–2220. [CrossRef]
47. Chupp, G.L.; Lee, C.; Jarjour, N.; Shim, Y.M.; Holm, C.T.; He, S.; Dziura, J.D.; Reed, J.; Coyle, A.J.; Kiener, P.; et al. A chitinase-like protein in the lung and circulation of patients with severe asthma. *N. Engl. J. Med.* **2007**, *357*, 2016–2027. [CrossRef]
48. Adner, M.; Rose, A.C.; Zhang, Y.; Swärd, K.; Benson, M.; Uddman, R.; Shankley, N.P.; Cardell, L.O. An assay to evaluate the long-term effects of inflammatory mediators on murine airway smooth muscle: Evidence that TNFαup-regulates 5-HT 2A-mediated contraction. *Br. J. Pharmacol.* **2002**, *137*, 971–982. [CrossRef]
49. Howarth, P.H.; Babu, K.S.; Arshad, H.S.; Lau, L.; Buckley, M.; McConnell, W.; Beckett, P.; Al Ali, M.; Chauhan, A.; Wilson, S.J.; et al. Tumour necrosis factor (TNFalpha) as a novel therapeutic target in symptomatic corticosteroid dependent asthma. *Thorax* **2005**, *60*, 1012–1018. [CrossRef]
50. Thomas, P.S.; Yates, D.H.; Barnes, P.J. Tumor necrosis factor-alpha increases airway responsiveness and sputum neutrophilia in normal human subjects. *Am. J. Respir. Crit. Care Med.* **1995**, *152*, 76–80. [CrossRef]
51. Thomas, P.S.; Heywood, G. Effects of inhaled tumour necrosis factor alpha in subjects with mild asthma. *Thorax* **2002**, *57*, 774–778. [CrossRef]
52. Brightling, C.; Berry, M.; Amrani, Y. Targeting TNF-alpha: A novel therapeutic approach for asthma. *J. Allergy Clin. Immunol.* **2008**, *121*, 5–10. [CrossRef]
53. Tliba, O.; Panettieri, R.A., Jr. Paucigranulocytic asthma: Uncoupling of airway obstruction from inflammation. *J. Allergy Clin. Immunol.* **2019**, *143*, 1287–1294. [CrossRef]
54. Ntontsi, P.; Loukides, S.; Bakakos, P.; Kostikas, K.; Papatheodorou, G.; Papathanassiou, E.; Hillas, G.; Koulouris, N.; Papiris, S.; Papaioannou, A.I. Clinical, functional and inflammatory characteristics in patients with paucigranulocytic stable asthma: Comparison with different sputum phenotypes. *Allergy* **2017**, *72*, 1761–1767. [CrossRef]
55. Haldar, P.; Pavord, I.D. Noneosinophilic asthma: A distinct clinical and pathologic phenotype. *J. Allergy Clin. Immunol.* **2007**, *119*, 1043–1052. [CrossRef]
56. Zhang, J.Y.; Wenzel, S.E. Tissue and BAL based biomarkers in asthma. *Immunol. Allergy Clin. N. Am.* **2007**, *27*, 623–632. [CrossRef]
57. Kuipers, I.; Louis, R.; Manise, M.; Dentener, M.A.; Irvin, C.G.; Janssen-Heininger, Y.M.; Brightling, C.E.; Wouters, E.F.; Reynaert, N.L. Increased glutaredoxin-1 and decreased protein S-glutathionylation in sputum of asthmatics. *Eur. Respir. J.* **2013**, *41*, 469–472. [CrossRef]
58. Gao, P.; Gibson, P.G.; Baines, K.J.; Yang, I.A.; Upham, J.W.; Reynolds, P.N.; Hodge, S.; James, A.L.; Jenkins, C.; Peters, M.J.; et al. Anti-inflammatory deficiencies in neutrophilic asthma: Reduced galectin-3 and IL-1RA/IL-1β. *Respir. Res.* **2015**, *16*, 5. [CrossRef]
59. Simpson, J.L.; Scott, R.J.; Boyle, M.J.; Gibson, P.G. Differential proteolytic enzyme activity in eosinophilic and neutrophilic asthma. *Am. J. Respir. Crit. Care Med.* **2005**, *172*, 559–565. [CrossRef]
60. Porsbjerg, C.; Lund, T.K.; Pedersen, L.; Backer, V. Inflammatory subtypes in asthma are related to airway hyperresponsiveness to mannitol and exhaled NO. *J. Asthma* **2009**, *46*, 606–612. [CrossRef]
61. Wang, F.; He, X.Y.; Baines, K.J.; Gunawardhana, L.P.; Simpson, J.L.; Li, F.; Gibson, P.G. Different inflammatory phenotypes in adults and children with acute asthma. *Eur. Respir. J.* **2011**, *38*, 567–574. [CrossRef]
62. Schleich, F.; Demarche, S.; Louis, R. Biomarkers in the Management of Difficult Asthma. *Curr. Top. Med. Chem.* **2016**, *16*, 1561–1573. [CrossRef]
63. Cox, C.; Kjarsgaard, M.; Surette, M.G.; Cox, P.G.; Nair, P. A multidimensional approach to the management of severe asthma: Inflammometry, molecular microbiology and bronchial thermoplasty. *Can. Respir J.* **2015**, *22*, 221–224. [CrossRef]
64. Fitzpatrick, A.M.; Higgins, M.; Holguin, F.; Brown, L.A.; Teague, W.G.; National Institutes of Health/National Heart, Lung, and Blood Institute's Severe Asthma Research Program. The molecular phenotype of severe asthma in children. *J. Allergy Clin. Immunol.* **2010**, *125*, 851–857. [CrossRef]
65. De Blic, J.; Tillie-Leblond, I.; Tonnel, A.B.; Jaubert, F.; Scheinmann, P.; Gosset, P. Difficult asthma in children: An analysis of airway inflammation. *J. Allergy Clin. Immunol.* **2004**, *113*, 94–100. [CrossRef]
66. Lex, C.; Payne, D.N.R.; Zacharasiewicz, A.; Li, A.M.; Wilson, N.M.; Hansel, T.T.; Bush, A. Sputum induction in children with difficult asthma: Safety, feasibility, and inflammatory cell pattern. *Pediatric Pulmonol.* **2005**, *39*, 318–324. [CrossRef]

67. Hauk, P.; Krawiec, M.; Murphy, J.; Boguniewicz, J.; Schiltz, A.; Goleva, E.; Liu, A.H.; Leung, D.Y. Neutrophilic airway inflammation and association with bacterial lipopolysaccharide in children with asthma and wheezing. *Pediatric Pulmonol.* **2008**, *43*, 916–923. [CrossRef]
68. Gibson, P.G.; Simpson, J.L.; Hankin, R.; Powell, H.; Henry, R.L. Relationship between induced sputum eosinophils and the clinical pattern of childhood asthma. *Thorax* **2003**, *58*, 116–121. [CrossRef]
69. Guilbert, T.W.; Bacharier, L.B.; Fitzpatrick, A.M. Severe asthma in children. *J. Allergy Clin. Immunol. Pract.* **2014**, *2*, 489–500. [CrossRef]
70. Fleming, L.; Tsartsali, L.; Wilson, N.; Regamey, N.; Bush, A. Sputum inflammatory phenotypes are not stable in children with asthma. *Thorax* **2012**, *67*, 675–681. [CrossRef]
71. Jochmann, A.; Artusio, L.; Robson, K.; Nagakumar, P.; Collins, N.; Fleming, L.; Bush, A.; Saglani, S. Infection and inflammation in induced sputum from preschool children with chronic airways diseases. *Pediatric Pulmonol.* **2016**, *51*, 778–786. [CrossRef] [PubMed]
72. Andersson, C.K.; Adams, A.; Nagakumar, P.; Bossley, C.; Gupta, A.; De Vries, D.; Adnan, A.; Bush, A.; Saglani, S.; Lloyd, C.M. Intraepithelial neutrophils in pediatric severe asthma are associated with better lung function. *J. Allergy Clin. Immunol.* **2017**, *139*, 1819–1829. [CrossRef] [PubMed]
73. Licari, A.; Castagnoli, R.; Brambilla, I.; Marseglia, A.; Tosca, M.A.; Marseglia, G.L.; Ciprandi, G. Asthma Endotyping and Biomarkers in Childhood Asthma. *Pediatric Allergy Immunol. Pulmonol.* **2018**, *31*, 44–55. [CrossRef] [PubMed]
74. Corren, J. New Targeted Therapies for Uncontrolled Asthma. *J. Allergy Clin. Immunol. Pract.* **2019**, *5*, 1394–1403. [CrossRef]
75. Holgate, S.T.; Djukanović, R.; Casale, T.; Bousquet, J. Anti-immunoglobulin E treatment with omalizumab in allergic diseases: An update on anti-inflammatory activity and clinical efficacy. *Clin. Exp. Allergy* **2005**, *35*, 408–416. [CrossRef] [PubMed]
76. Hanania, N.A.; Alpan, O.; Hamilos, D.L.; Condemi, J.J.; Reyes-Rivera, I.; Zhu, J.; Rosen, K.E.; Eisner, M.D.; Wong, D.A.; Busse, W. Omalizumab in severe allergic asthma inadequately controlled with standard therapy: A randomized trial. *Ann. Intern. Med.* **2011**, *154*, 573–582. [CrossRef]
77. U.S. Food and Drug Administration. FDA Drug Safety Communication: FDA Approves Label Changes for Asthma Drug Xolair (omalizumab), Including Describing Slightly Higher Risk of Heart and Brain Adverse Events. Available online: http://www.fda.gov/Drugs/DrugSafety/ucm414911.htm (accessed on 9 November 2017).
78. Thompson, C.A. Mepolizumab approved as add-on long-term therapy for severe asthma. *Am. J. Health Pharm.* **2015**, *72*, 2125. [CrossRef]
79. Castro, M.; Mathur, S.; Hargreave, F.; Boulet, L.P.; Xie, F.; Young, J.; Wilkins, H.J.; Henkel, T.; Nair, P.; Res-5-0010 Study Group. Reslizumab for poorly controlled, eosinophilic asthma: A randomized, placebo-controlled study. *Am. J. Respir. Crit. Care Med.* **2011**, *184*, 1125–1132. [CrossRef]
80. Tan, L.D.; Bratt, J.M.; Godor, D.; Louie, S.; Kenyon, N.J. Benralizumab: A unique IL-5 inhibitor for severe asthma. *J. Asthma Allergy* **2016**, *9*, 71–81. [CrossRef]
81. Kartush, A.G.; Schumacher, J.K.; Shah, R.; Patadia, M.O. Biologic Agents for the Treatment of Chronic Rhinosinusitis with Nasal Polyps. *Am. J. Rhinol. Allergy* **2019**, *33*, 203–211. [CrossRef]
82. Brubaker, S.W.; Bonham, K.S.; Zanoni, I.; Kagan, J.C. Innate immune pattern recognition: A cell biological perspective. *Annu. Rev. Immunol.* **2015**, *33*, 257–290. [CrossRef] [PubMed]
83. Kawai, T.; Akira, S. The role of pattern-recognition receptors in innate immunity: Update on Toll-like receptors. *Nat. Immunol.* **2010**, *11*, 373–384. [CrossRef] [PubMed]
84. Ting, J.P.; Lovering, R.C.; Alnemri, E.S.P.; Bertin, J.; Boss, J.M.; Davis, B.K.; Flavell, R.A.; Girardin, S.E.; Godzik, A.; Harton, J.A.; et al. The NLR gene family: A standard nomenclature. *Immunity* **2008**, *28*, 285–287. [CrossRef] [PubMed]
85. Schroder, K.; Tschopp, J. The inflammasomes. *Cell* **2010**, *140*, 821–832. [CrossRef] [PubMed]
86. Sutterwala, F.S.; Haasken, S.; Cassel, S.L. Mechanism of NLRP3 inflammasome activation. *Ann. N. Y. Acad. Sci.* **2014**, *1319*, 82–95. [CrossRef] [PubMed]
87. Brodsky, I.E.; Monack, D. NLR-mediated control of inflammasome assembly in the host response against bacterial pathogens. *Semin. Immunol.* **2009**, *21*, 199–207. [CrossRef] [PubMed]
88. Barbé, F.; Douglas, T.; Saleh, M. Advances in Nod -like receptors (NLR) biology. *Cytokine Growth Factor Rev.* **2014**, *25*, 681–697. [CrossRef] [PubMed]

89. Elliott, E.I.; Sutterwala, F.S. Initiation and perpetuation of NLRP3 inflammasome activation and assembly. *Immunol. Rev.* **2015**, *265*, 35–52. [CrossRef]
90. Schmidt, F.I.; Lu, A.; Chen, J.W.; Ruan, J.; Tang, C.; Wu, H.; Ploegh, H.L. A single domain antibody fragment that recognizes the adaptor ASC defines the role of ASC domains in inflammasome assembly. *J. Exp. Med.* **2016**, *213*, 771–790. [CrossRef]
91. Boucher, D.; Monteleone, M.; Coll, R.C.; Chen, K.W.; Ross, C.M.; Teo, J.L.; Gomez, G.A.; Holley, C.L.; Bierschenk, D.; Stacey, K.J.; et al. Caspase-1 self- cleavage is an intrinsic mechanism to terminate inflammasome activity. *J. Exp. Med.* **2018**, *215*, 827–840. [CrossRef]
92. He, Y.; Zeng, M.Y.; Yang, D.; Motro, B.; Núñez, G. NEK7 is an essential mediator of NLRP3 activation downstream of potassium efflux. *Nature* **2016**, *530*, 354. [CrossRef]
93. Broz, P.; Dixit, V.M. Inflammasomes: Mechanism of assembly, regulation and signalling. *Nat. Rev. Immunol.* **2016**, *16*, 407. [CrossRef] [PubMed]
94. Franklin, B.S.; Bossaller, L.; De Nardo, D.; Ratter, J.M.; Stutz, A.; Engels, G.; Brenker, C.; Nordhoff, M.; Mirandola, S.R.; Mangan, M.S.; et al. The adaptor ASC has extracellular and 'prionoid' activities that propagate inflammation. *Nat. Immunol.* **2014**, *15*, 727–737. [CrossRef] [PubMed]
95. Franklin, B.S.; Latz, E.; Schmidt, F.I. The intra- and extracellular functions of ASC specks. *Immunol. Rev.* **2018**, *281*, 74–87. [CrossRef] [PubMed]
96. Basiorka, A.A.; McGraw, K.L.; Eksioglu, E.A.; Chen, X.; Johnson, J.; Zhang, L.; Zhang, Q.; Irvine, B.A.; Cluzeau, T.; Sallman, D.A.; et al. The NLRP3 inflammasome functions as a driver of the myelodysplastic syndrome phenotype. *Blood* **2016**, *128*, 2960–2975. [CrossRef]
97. Basu, R.; Whitley, S.K.; Bhaumik, S.; Zindl, C.L.; Schoeb, T.R.; Benveniste, E.N.; Pear, W.S.; Hatton, R.D.; Weaver, C.T. IL-1 signaling modulates activation of STAT transcription factors to antagonize retinoic acid signaling and control the TH17 cell-iTreg cell balance. *Nat. Immunol.* **2015**, *16*, 286–295. [CrossRef] [PubMed]
98. Sims, J.E.; March, C.J.; Cosman, D.; Widmer, M.B.; MacDonald, H.R.; McMahan, C.J.; Grubin, C.E.; Wignall, J.M.; Jackson, J.L.; Call, S.M.; et al. cDNA expression cloning of the IL-1 receptor, a member of the immunoglobulin superfamily. *Science* **1988**, *241*, 585–589. [CrossRef]
99. Greenfeder, S.A.; Nunes, P.; Kwee, L.; Labow, M.; Chizzonite, R.A.; Ju, G. Molecular cloning and characterization of a second subunit of the interleukin 1 receptor complex. *J. Biol. Chem.* **1995**, *270*, 13757–13765. [CrossRef]
100. Martin, R.A.; Ather, J.L.; Lundblad, L.K.; Suratt, B.T.; Boyson, J.E.; Budd, R.C.; Alcorn, J.F.; Flavell, R.A.; Eisenbarth, S.C.; Poynter, M.E. Interleukin-1 receptor and caspase-1 are required for the Th17 response in nitrogen dioxide-promoted allergic airway disease. *Am. J. Respir. Cell Mol. Biol.* **2013**, *48*, 655–664. [CrossRef]
101. Kroeger, K.M.; Sullivan, B.M.; Locksley, R.M. IL-18 and IL-33 elicit Th2 cytokines from basophils via a MyD88- and p38alpha-dependent pathway. *J. Leukoc. Biol.* **2009**, *86*, 769–778. [CrossRef]
102. Wiener, Z.; Pocza, P.; Racz, M.; Nagy, G.; Tolgyesi, G.; Molnar, V.; Jaeger, J.; Buzas, E.; Gorbe, E.; Papp, Z.; et al. IL-18 induces a marked gene expression profile change and increased Ccl1 (I-309) production in mouse mucosal mast cell homologs. *Int. Immunol.* **2008**, *20*, 1565–1573. [CrossRef] [PubMed]
103. Liu, X.; Zhang, Z.; Ruan, J.; Pan, Y.; Magupalli, V.G.; Wu, H.; Lieberman, J. Inflammasome-activated gasdermin D causes pyroptosis by forming membrane pores. *Nature* **2016**, *535*, 153–158. [CrossRef] [PubMed]
104. He, W.T.; Wan, H.; Hu, L.; Chen, P.; Wang, X.; Huang, Z.; Yang, Z.H.; Zhong, C.Q.; Han, J. Gasdermin D is an executor of pyroptosis and required for interleukin-1β secretion. *Cell Res.* **2015**, *25*, 1285–1298. [CrossRef] [PubMed]
105. Kayagaki, N.; Stowe, I.B.; Lee, B.L.; O'Rourke, K.; Anderson, K.; Warming, S.; Liu, P.S. Caspase-11 cleaves gasdermin D for non-canonical inflammasome signalling. *Nature* **2015**, *526*, 666–671. [CrossRef] [PubMed]
106. Gaidt, M.M.; Ebert, T.S.; Chauhan, D.; Schmidt, T.; Schmid-Burgk, J.L.; Rapino, F.; Robertson, A.A.; Cooper, M.A.; Graf, T.; Hornung, V. Human monocytes engage an alternative inflammasome pathway. *Immunity* **2016**, *44*, 833–846. [CrossRef] [PubMed]
107. Man, S.M.; Kanneganti, T.D. Regulation of inflammasome activation. *Immunol. Rev.* **2015**, *265*, 6–21. [CrossRef] [PubMed]
108. Bauernfeind, F.G.; Horvath, G.; Stutz, A.; Alnemri, E.S.; MacDonald, K.; Speert, D.; Fernandes-Alnemri, T.; Wu, J.; Monks, B.G.; Fitzgerald, K.A.; et al. Cutting edge: NF- kappaB activating pattern recognition and cytokine receptors license NLRP3 inflammasome activation by regulating NLRP3 expression. *J. Immunol.* **2009**, *183*, 787–791. [CrossRef] [PubMed]

109. Franchi, L.; Eigenbrod, T.; Núñez, G. Cutting edge: TNF- alpha mediates sensitization to ATP and silica via the NLRP3 inflammasome in the absence of microbial stimulation. *J. Immunol.* **2009**, *183*, 792–796. [CrossRef]
110. Swanson, K.V.; Deng, M.; Ting, J.P. The NLRP3 inflammasome: Molecular activation and regulation to therapeutics. *Nat. Rev. Immunol.* **2019**, *19*, 477–489. [CrossRef]
111. He, Y.; Hara, H.; Núñez, G. Mechanism and Regulation of NLRP3 Inflammasome Activation. *Trends Biochem. Sci.* **2016**, *41*, 1012–1021. [CrossRef]
112. Muñoz-Planillo, R.; Kuffa, P.; Martínez-Colón, G.; Smith, B.L.; Rajendiran, T.M.; Núñez, G. K^+ efflux is the common trigger of NLRP3 inflammasome activation by bacterial toxins and particulate matter. *Immunity* **2013**, *38*, 1142–1153. [CrossRef] [PubMed]
113. Pétrilli, V.; Papin, S.; Dostert, C.; Mayor, A.; Martinon, F.; Tschopp, J. Activation of the NALP3 inflammasome is triggered by low intracellular potassium concentration. *Cell Death Differ.* **2007**, *14*, 1583–1589. [CrossRef] [PubMed]
114. Piccini, A.; Carta, S.; Tassi, S.; Lasiglié, D.; Fossati, G.; Rubartelli, A. ATP is released by monocytes stimulated with pathogen-sensing receptor ligands and induces IL-1beta and IL-18 secretion in an autocrine way. *Proc. Natl. Acad. Sci. USA* **2008**, *105*, 8067–8072. [CrossRef] [PubMed]
115. Pelegrin, P.; Surprenant, A. Pannexin-1 couples to maitotoxin- and nigericin-induced interleukin-1beta release through a dye uptake-independent pathway. *J. Biol Chem.* **2007**, *282*, 2386–2394. [CrossRef] [PubMed]
116. Triantafilou, K.; Hughes, T.R.; Triantafilou, M.; Morgan, B.P. The complement membrane attack complex triggers intracellular Ca2+ fluxes leading to NLRP3 inflammasome activation. *J. Cell Sci.* **2013**, *126*, 2903–2913. [CrossRef] [PubMed]
117. Lemasters, J.J.; Theruvath, T.P.; Zhong, Z.; Nieminen, A.L. Mitochondrial calcium and the permeability transition in cell death. Biochim Biophys. *Acta Bioenerg.* **2009**, *1787*, 1395–1401. [CrossRef] [PubMed]
118. Wolf, A.J.; Reyes, C.N.; Liang, W.; Becker, C.; Shimada, K.; Wheeler, M.L.; Cho, H.C.; Popescu, N.I.; Coggeshall, K.M.; Arditi, M.; et al. Hexokinase is an innate immune receptor for the detection of bacterial peptidoglycan. *Cell* **2016**, *166*, 624–636. [CrossRef] [PubMed]
119. Tang, T.; Lang, X.; Xu, C.; Wang, X.; Gong, T.; Yang, Y.; Cui, J.; Bai, L.; Wang, J.; Jiang, W.; et al. CLICs-dependent chloride efflux is an essential and proximal upstream event for NLRP3 inflammasome activation. *Nat. Commun.* **2017**, *8*, 202. [CrossRef]
120. Hornung, V.; Bauernfeind, F.; Halle, A.; Samstad, E.O.; Kono, H.; Rock, K.L.; Fitzgerald, K.A.; Latz, E. Silica crystals and aluminum salts activate the NALP3 inflammasome through phagosomal destabilization. *Nat. Immunol.* **2008**, *9*, 847–856. [CrossRef] [PubMed]
121. Dostert, C.; Pétrilli, V.; Van Bruggen, R.; Steele, C.; Mossman, B.T.; Tschopp, J. Innate immune activation through Nalp3 inflammasome sensing of asbestos and silica. *Science* **2008**, *320*, 674–677. [CrossRef]
122. Zhou, R.; Yazdi, A.S.; Menu, P.; Tschopp, J. A role for mitochondria in NLRP3 inflammasome activation. *Nature* **2011**, *469*, 221–225. [CrossRef] [PubMed]
123. Kim, S.; Joe, Y.; Jeong, S.O.; Zheng, M.; Back, S.H.; Park, S.W.; Ryter, S.W.; Chung, H.T. Endoplasmic reticulum stress is sufficient for the induction of IL-1β production via activation of NF-κB and inflammasome pathways. *Innate Immun.* **2014**, *20*, 799–815. [CrossRef] [PubMed]
124. Franchi, L.; Eigenbrod, T.; Muñoz-Planillo, R.; Ozkurede, U.; Kim, Y.G.; Arindam, C.; Gale, M., Jr.; Silverman, R.H.; Colonna, M.; Akira, S.; et al. Cytosolic double-stranded RNA activates the NLRP3 inflammasome via MAVS-induced membrane permeabilization and K+ efflux. *J. Immunol.* **2014**, *193*, 4214–4222. [CrossRef] [PubMed]
125. Chen, J.; Chen, Z.J. PtdIns4P on dispersed *trans*-Golgi network mediates NLRP3 inflammasome activation. *Nature* **2018**, *564*, 71–76. [CrossRef] [PubMed]
126. Hughes, M.M.; O'Neill, L.A.J. Metabolic regulation of NLRP3. *Immunol. Rev.* **2018**, *281*, 88–98. [CrossRef] [PubMed]
127. Jiang, D.; Chen, S.; Sun, R.; Zhang, X.; Wang, D. The NLRP3 inflammasome: Role in metabolic disorders and regulation by metabolic pathways. *Cancer Lett.* **2018**, *419*, 8–19. [CrossRef] [PubMed]
128. Moon, J.S.; Hisata, S.; Park, M.A.; DeNicola, G.M.; Ryter, S.W.; Nakahira, K.; Choi, A.M.K. mTORC1-Induced HK1-Dependent Glycolysis Regulates NLRP3 Inflammasome Activation. *Cell Rep.* **2015**, *12*, 102–115. [CrossRef]
129. Yang, Q.; Liu, R.; Yu, Q.; Bi, Y.; Liu, G. Metabolic regulation of inflammasomes in inflammation. *Immunology* **2019**, *157*, 95–109. [CrossRef]

130. Wen, H.; Gris, D.; Lei, Y.; Jha, S.; Zhang, L.; Huang, M.T.; Brickey, W.J.; Ting, J.P. Fatty acid-induced NLRP3-ASC inflammasome activation interferes with insulin signaling. *Nat. Immunol.* **2011**, *12*, 408–415. [CrossRef]
131. Rathinam, V.A.K.; Zhao, Y.; Shao, F. Innate immunity to intracellular LPS. *Nat. Immunol.* **2019**, *20*, 527–533. [CrossRef]
132. Mathur, A.; Hayward, J.A.; Man, S.M. Molecular mechanisms of inflammasome signaling. *J. Leukoc. Biol.* **2018**, *103*, 233–257. [CrossRef] [PubMed]
133. Kayagaki, N.; Wong, M.T.; Stowe, I.B.; Ramani, S.R.; Gonzalez, L.C.; Akashi-Takamura, S.; Miyake, K.; Zhang, J.; Lee, W.P.; Muszynski, A.; et al. Noncanonical inflammasome activation by intracellular LPS independent of TLR4. *Science* **2013**, *341*, 1246–1249. [CrossRef]
134. Kim, B.H.; Chee, J.D.; Bradfield, C.J.; Park, E.S.; Kumar, P.; MacMicking, J.D. Interferon-induced guanylate-binding proteins in inflammasome activation and host defense. *Nat. Immunol.* **2016**, *17*, 481–489. [CrossRef] [PubMed]
135. Man, S.M.; Place, D.E.; Kuriakose, T.; Kanneganti, T.D. Interferon-inducible guanylate-binding proteins at the interface of cell-autonomous immunity and inflammasome activation. *J. Leukoc. Biol.* **2017**, *101*, 143–150. [CrossRef] [PubMed]
136. Man, S.M.; Karki, R.; Sasai, M.; Place, D.E.; Kesavardhana, S.; Temirov, J.; Frase, S.; Zhu, Q.; Malireddi, R.K.S.; Kuriakose, T.; et al. IRGB10 liberates bacterial ligands for sensing by the AIM2 and caspase-11-NLRP3 inflammasomes. *Cell* **2016**, *167*, 382–396. [CrossRef] [PubMed]
137. Kahlenberg, J.M.; Carmona- Rivera, C.; Smith, C.K.; Kaplan, M.J. Neutrophil extracellular trap–associated protein activation of the NLRP3 inflammasome is enhanced in lupus macrophages. *J. Immunol.* **2012**, *190*, 1217–1226. [CrossRef] [PubMed]
138. Lin, K.M.; Hu, W.; Troutman, T.D.; Jennings, M.; Brewer, T.; Li, X.; Nanda, S.; Cohen, P.; Thomas, J.A.; Pasare, C. IRAK-1 bypasses priming and directly links TLRs to rapid NLRP3 inflammasome activation. *Proc. Natl Acad. Sci. USA* **2014**, *111*, 775–780. [CrossRef] [PubMed]
139. Hoffman, H.M.; Wanderer, A.A.; Broide, D.H. Familial cold autoinflammatory syndrome. *J. Allergy Clin. Immunol.* **2001**, *108*, 615–620. [CrossRef]
140. Shinkai, K.; Mccalmont, T.H.; Leslie, K.S. Cryopyrin-associated periodic syndromes and autoinflammation. *Clin. Exp. Dermatol.* **2008**, *33*, 1–9. [CrossRef]
141. Heneka, M.T.; Kummer, M.P.; Latz, E. Innate immune activation in neurodegenerative disease. *Nat. Rev. Immunol.* **2014**, *14*, 463–477. [CrossRef]
142. Mangan, M.S.J.; Olhava, E.J.; Roush, W.R.; Seidel, H.M.; Glick, G.D.; Latz, E. Targeting the NLRP3 inflammasome in inflammatory diseases. *Nat. Rev. Drug Discov.* **2018**, *17*, 588–606. [CrossRef] [PubMed]
143. Martinon, F.; Pétrilli, V.; Mayor, A.; Tardivel, A.; Tschopp, J. Gout-associated uric acid crystals activate the NALP3 inflammasome. *Nature* **2006**, *440*, 237–241. [CrossRef] [PubMed]
144. Vandanmagsar, B.; Youm, Y.-H.; Ravussin, A.; Galgani, J.E.; Stadler, K.; Mynatt, R.L.; Ravussin, E.; Stephens, J.M.; Dixit, V.D. The NALP3/NLRP3 inflammasome instigates obesity-induced autoinflammation and insulin resistance. *Nat. Med.* **2011**, *17*, 179–188. [CrossRef] [PubMed]
145. Youm, Y.-H.; Grant, R.W.; McCabe, L.R.; Albarado, D.C.; Nguyen, K.Y.; Ravussin, A.; Pistell, P.; Newman, S.; Carter, R.; Laque, A.; et al. Canonical Nlrp3 inflammasome links systemic low grade inflammation to functional decline in aging. *Cell Metab.* **2013**, *18*, 519–532. [CrossRef] [PubMed]
146. Guarda, G.; Braun, M.; Staehli, F.; Tardivel, A.; Mattmann, C.; Förster, I.; Farlik, M.; Decker, T.; Du Pasquier, R.A.; Romero, P.; et al. Type I interferon inhibits interleukin-1 production and inflammasome activation. *Immunity* **2011**, *34*, 213–223. [CrossRef] [PubMed]
147. Mishra, B.B.; Rathinam, V.A.; Martens, G.W.; Martinot, A.J.; Kornfeld, H.; Fitzgerald, K.A.; Sassetti, C.M. Nitric oxide controls the immunopathology of tuberculosis by inhibiting NLRP3 inflammasome-dependent processing of IL-1β. *Nat. Immunol.* **2013**, *14*, 52–60. [CrossRef] [PubMed]
148. Bauernfeind, F.; Rieger, A.; Schildberg, F.A.; Knolle, P.A.; Schmid-Burgk, J.L.; Hornung, V. NLRP3 inflammasome activity is negatively controlled by miR-223. *J. Immunol.* **2012**, *189*, 4175–4181. [CrossRef] [PubMed]
149. Yan, Y.; Jiang, W.; Liu, L.; Wang, X.; Ding, C.; Tian, Z.; Zhou, R. Dopamine controls systemic inflammation through inhibition of NLRP3 inflammasome. *Cell* **2015**, *160*, 62–73. [CrossRef]

150. Mortimer, L.; Moreau, F.; MacDonald, J.A.; Chadee, K. NLRP3 inflammasome inhibition is disrupted in a group of auto-inflammatory disease CAPS mutations. *Nat. Immunol.* **2016**, *17*, 1176–1186. [CrossRef]
151. He, C.; Klionsky, D.J. Regulation mechanisms and signaling pathways of autophagy. *Annu. Rev. Genet.* **2009**, *43*, 67–93. [CrossRef]
152. Deretic, V.; Saitoh, T.; Akira, S. Autophagy in infection, inflammation and immunity. *Nat. Rev. Immunol.* **2013**, *13*, 722–737. [CrossRef] [PubMed]
153. Nakahira, K.; Haspel, J.A.; Rathinam, V.A.; Lee, S.J.; Dolinay, T.; Lam, H.C.; Englert, J.A.; Rabinovitch, M.; Cernadas, M.; Kim, H.P.; et al. Autophagy proteins regulate immune responses by inhibiting the release of mitochondrial DNA mediated by the NALP3 inflammasome. *Nat. Immunol.* **2011**, *12*, 222–230. [CrossRef] [PubMed]
154. Van der Burgh, R.; Nijhuis, L.; Pervolaraki, K.; Compeer, E.B.; Jongeneel, L.H.; van Gijn, M.; Coffer, P.J.; Murphy, M.P.; Mastroberardino, P.G.; Frenkel, J.; et al. Defects in mitochondrial clearance predispose human monocytes to interleukin-1 hypersecretion. *J. Biol. Chem.* **2014**, *289*, 5000–5012. [CrossRef] [PubMed]
155. Lupfer, C.; Thomas, P.G.; Anand, P.K.; Vogel, P.; Milasta, S.; Martinez, J.; Huang, G.; Green, M.; Kundu, M.; Chi, H.; et al. Receptor interacting protein kinase 2-mediated mitophagy regulates inflammasome activation during virus infection. *Nat. Immunol.* **2013**, *14*, 480–488. [CrossRef] [PubMed]
156. Liu, X.; Zhou, W.; Zhang, X.; Lu, P.; Du, Q.; Tao, L.; Ding, Y.; Wang, Y.; Hu, R. Dimethyl fumarate ameliorates dextran sulfate sodium-induced murine experimental colitis by activating Nrf2 and suppressing NLRP3 inflammasome activation. *Biochem. Pharm.* **2016**, *112*, 37–49. [CrossRef]
157. Liu, X.; Zhang, X.; Ding, Y.; Zhou, W.; Tao, L.; Lu, P.; Wang, Y.; Hu, R. Nuclear factor E2-related factor-2 negatively regulates NLRP3 inflammasome activity by inhibiting reactive oxygen species-induced NLRP3 priming. *Antioxid. Redox Signal.* **2017**, *26*, 28–43. [CrossRef] [PubMed]
158. Misawa, T.; Takahama, M.; Kozaki, T.; Lee, H.; Zou, J.; Saitoh, T.; Akira, S. Microtubule-driven spatial arrangement of mitochondria promotes activation of the NLRP3 inflammasome. *Nat. Immunol.* **2013**, *14*, 454–460. [CrossRef]
159. Youm, Y.H.; Nguyen, K.Y.; Grant, R.W.; Goldberg, E.L.; Bodogai, M.; Kim, D.; D'Agostino, D.; Planavsky, N.; Lupfer, C.; Kanneganti, T.-D.; et al. The ketone metabolite beta-hydroxybutyrate blocks NLRP3 inflammasome-mediated inflammatory disease. *Nat. Med.* **2015**, *21*, 263–269. [CrossRef]
160. Kumar, N.; Gupta, G.; Anilkumar, K.; Fatima, N.; Karnati, R.; Reddy, G.V.; Giri, P.V.; Reddanna, P. 15-Lipoxygenase metabolites of alpha-linolenic acid, [13-(S)-HPOTrE and 13-(S)-HOTrE], mediate anti-inflammatory effects by inactivating NLRP3 inflammasome. *Sci Rep.* **2016**, *6*, 31649. [CrossRef]
161. Guo, C.; Xie, S.; Chi, Z.; Zhang, J.; Liu, Y.; Zhang, L.; Zheng, M.; Zhang, X.; Xia, D.; Ke, Y.; et al. Bile Acids Control Inflammation and Metabolic Disorder through Inhibition of NLRP3 Inflammasome. *Immunity* **2016**, *45*, 802–816. [CrossRef]
162. Sokolowska, M.; Chen, L.Y.; Liu, Y.; Martinez-Anton, A.; Qi, H.Y.; Logun, C.; Alsaaty, S.; Park, Y.H.; Kastner, D.L.; Chae, J.J.; et al. Prostaglandin E2 inhibits NLRP3 inflammasome activation through EP4 receptor and intracellular cyclic AMP in human macrophages. *J. Immunol.* **2015**, *194*, 5472–5487. [CrossRef] [PubMed]
163. Zaslona, Z.; Palsson-McDermott, E.M.; Menon, D.; Haneklaus, M.; Flis, E.; Prendeville, H.; Corcoran, S.E.; Peters-Golden, M.; O'Neill, L.A.J. The induction of Pro-IL- 1beta by lipopolysaccharide requires endogenous prostaglandin E2 production. *J. Immunol.* **2017**, *198*, 3558–3564. [CrossRef] [PubMed]
164. Coll, R.C.; Robertson, A.A.; Chae, J.J.; Higgins, S.C.; Muñoz-Planillo, R.; Inserra, M.C.; Vetter, I.; Dungan, L.S.; Monks, B.G.; Stutz, A.; et al. A small-molecule inhibitor of the NLRP3 inflammasome for the treatment of inflammatory diseases. *Nat. Med.* **2015**, *21*, 248. [CrossRef] [PubMed]
165. Juliana, C.; Fernandes-Alnemri, T.; Wu, J.; Datta, P.; Solorzano, L.; Yu, J.W.; Meng, R.; Quong, A.A.; Latz, E.; Scott, C.P.; et al. Anti-inflammatory compounds parthenolide and Bay 11-7082 are direct inhibitors of the inflammasome. *J. Biol. Chem.* **2010**, *285*, 9792–9802. [CrossRef] [PubMed]
166. Ahn, H.; Kim, J.; Jeung, E.B.; Lee, G.S. Dimethyl sulfoxide inhibits NLRP3 inflammasome activation. *Immunobiology* **2014**, *219*, 315–322. [CrossRef] [PubMed]
167. Inoue, M.; Williams, K.L.; Oliver, T.; Vandenabeele, P.; Rajan, J.V.; Miao, E.A.; Shinohara, M.L. Interferon-β therapy against EAE is effective only when development of the disease depends on the NLRP3 inflammasome. *Sci. Signal.* **2012**, *5*, 38. [CrossRef] [PubMed]

168. Jiang, H.; He, H.; Chen, Y.; Huang, W.; Cheng, J.; Ye, J.; Wang, A.; Tao, J.; Wang, C.; Liu, Q.; et al. Identification of a selective and direct NLRP3 inhibitor to treat inflammatory disorders. *J. Exp. Med.* **2017**, *214*, 3219–3238. [CrossRef] [PubMed]
169. Coll, R.C.; Hill, J.R.; Day, C.J.; Zamoshnikova, A.; Boucher, D.; Massey, N.L.; Chitty, J.L.; Fraser, J.A.; Jennings, M.P.; Robertson, A.A.B.; et al. MCC950 directly targets the NLRP3 ATPhydrolysis motif for inflammasome inhibition. *Nat. Chem. Biol.* **2019**, *15*, 556–559. [CrossRef]
170. Gordon, R.; Albornoz, E.A.; Christie, D.C.; Langley, M.R.; Kumar, V.; Mantovani, S.; Robertson, A.A.B.; Butler, M.S.; Rowe, D.B.; O'Neill, L.A.; et al. Inflammasome inhibition prevents α-synuclein pathology and dopaminergic neurodegeneration in mice. *Sci. Transl. Med.* **2018**, *10*, 4066. [CrossRef]
171. Tate, M.D.; Ong, J.D.H.; Dowling, J.K.; McAuley, J.L.; Robertson, A.B.; Latz, E.; Drummond, G.R.; Cooper, M.A.; Hertzog, P.J.; Mansell, A. Reassessing the role of the NLRP3 inflammasome during pathogenic influenza A virus infection via temporal inhibition. *Sci. Rep.* **2016**, *6*, 2791. [CrossRef]
172. Eisenbarth, S.C.; Colegio, O.R.; O'Connor, W.; Sutterwala, F.S.; Flavell, R.A. Crucial role for the Nalp3 inflammasome in the immunostimulatory properties of aluminium adjuvants. *Nature* **2008**, *453*, 1122–1126. [CrossRef] [PubMed]
173. Kim, S.R.; Kim, D.I.; Kim, S.H.; Lee, H.; Lee, K.S.; Cho, S.H.; Lee, Y.C. NLRP3 inflammasome activation by mitochondrial ROS in bronchial epithelial cells is required for allergic inflammation. *Cell Death Dis.* **2014**, *5*, 1498. [CrossRef] [PubMed]
174. Tan, H.T.; Hagner, S.; Ruchti, F.; Radzikowska, U.; Tan, G.; Altunbulakli, C.; Eljaszewicz, A.; Moniuszko, M.; Akdis, M.; Akdis, C.A.; et al. Tight junction, mucin, and inflammasome-related molecules are differentially expressed in eosinophilic, mixed, and neutrophilic experimental asthma in mice. *Allergy* **2019**, *74*, 294–307. [CrossRef] [PubMed]
175. Gordon, E.M.; Yao, X.; Xu, H.; Karkowsky, W.; Kaler, M.; Kalchiem-Dekel, O.; Barochia, A.V.; Gao, M.; Keeran, K.J.; Jeffries, K.R.; et al. Apolipoprotein E is a concentration-dependent pulmonary danger signal that activates the NLRP3 inflammasome and IL-1β secretion by bronchoalveolar fluid macrophages from asthmatic subjects. *J. Allergy Clin. Immunol.* **2019**. [CrossRef] [PubMed]
176. Ritter, M.; Straubinger, K.; Schmidt, S.; Busch, D.H.; Hagner, S.; Garn, H.; Prazeres da Costa, C.; Layland, L.E. Functional relevance of NLRP3 inflammasome-mediated interleukin (IL)-1β during acute allergic airway inflammation. *Clin. Exp. Immunol.* **2014**, *178*, 212–223. [CrossRef] [PubMed]
177. Besnard, A.G.; Guillou, N.; Tschopp, J.; Erard, F.; Couillin, I.; Iwakura, Y.; Quesniaux, V.; Ryffel, B.; Togbe, D. NLRP3 inflammasome is required in murine asthma in the absence of aluminum adjuvant. *Allergy* **2011**, *66*, 1047–1057. [CrossRef] [PubMed]
178. Qi, X.; Gurung, P.; Malireddi, R.K.; Karmaus, P.W.; Sharma, D.; Vogel, P.; Chi, H.; Green, D.R.; Kanneganti, T.D. Critical role of caspase-8-mediated IL-1 signaling in promoting Th2 responses during asthma pathogenesis. *Mucosal Immunol.* **2017**, *10*, 128–138. [CrossRef]
179. Ather, J.L.; Ckless, K.; Martin, R.; Foley, K.L.; Suratt, B.T.; Boyson, J.E.; Fitzgerald, K.A.; Flavell, R.A.; Eisenbarth, S.C.; Poynter, M.E. Serum amyloid A activates the NLRP3 inflammasome and promotes Th17 allergic asthma in mice. *J. Immunol.* **2011**, *187*, 64–73. [CrossRef]
180. Rossios, C.; Pavlidis, S.; Hoda, U.; Kuo, C.H.; Wiegman, C.; Russell, K.; Sun, K.; Loza, M.J.; Baribaud, F.; Durham, A.L.; et al. Sputum transcriptomics reveal upregulation of IL-1 receptor family members in patients with severe asthma. *J. Allergy Clin. Immunol.* **2018**, *141*, 560–570. [CrossRef]
181. Bruchard, M.; Rebé, C.; Derangère, V.; Togbé, D.; Ryffel, B.; Boidot, R.; Humblin, E.; Hamman, A.; Chalmin, F.; Berger, H.; et al. The receptor NLRP3 is a transcriptional regulator of TH2 differentiation. *Nat. Immunol.* **2015**, *16*, 859–870. [CrossRef]
182. Kim, H.Y.; Lee, H.J.; Chang, Y.J.; Pichavant, M.; Shore, S.A.; Fitzgerald, K.A.; Iwakura, Y.; Israel, E.; Bolger, K.; Faul, J.; et al. IL-17 producing innate lymphoid cells and the NLRP3 inflammasome facilitate obesity-associated airway hyperreactivity. *Nat. Med.* **2014**, *20*, 54–61. [CrossRef] [PubMed]
183. Sebag, S.C.; Koval, O.M.; Paschke, J.D.; Winters, C.J.; Jaffer, O.A.; Dworski, R.; Sutterwala, F.S.; Anderson, M.E.; Grumbach, I.M. Mitochondrial CaMKII inhibition in airway epithelium protects against allergic asthma. *JCI Insight* **2017**, *2*, e88297. [CrossRef] [PubMed]
184. Kim, R.Y.; Pinkerton, J.W.; Essilfie, A.T.; Robertson, A.A.B.; Baines, K.J.; Brown, A.C.; Mayall, J.R.; Ali, M.K.; Starkey, M.R.; Hansbro, N.G. Role for NLRP3 Inflammasome-mediated, IL-1β-dependent Responses in Severe, Steroid-resistant Asthma. *Am. J. Respir. Crit. Care Med.* **2017**, *196*, 283–297. [CrossRef] [PubMed]

185. Han, M.; Bentley, J.K.; Rajput, C.; Lei, J.; Ishikawa, T.; Jarman, C.R.; Lee, J.; Goldsmith, A.M.; Jackson, W.T.; Hoenerhoff, M.J.; et al. Inflammasome activation is required for human rhinovirus-induced airway inflammation in naïve and allergen-sensitizes mice. *Mucosal Immunol.* **2019**. [CrossRef] [PubMed]
186. Macia, L.; Tan, J.; Vieira, A.T.; Leach, K.; Stanley, D.; Luong, S.; Maruya, M.; McKenzie, C.I.; Hijikata, A.; Wong, C.; et al. Metabolite-sensing receptors GPR43 and GPR109A facilitate dietary fibre-induced gut homeostasis through regulation of the inflammasome. *Nat. Commun.* **2015**, *6*, 6734. [CrossRef] [PubMed]
187. Allen, I.C.; Jania, C.M.; Wilson, J.E.; Tekeppe, E.M.; Hua, X.; Brickey, W.J.; Kwan, M.; Koller, B.H.; Tilley, S.L.; Ting, J.P. Analysis of NLRP3 in the development of allergic airway disease in mice. *J. Immunol.* **2012**, *6*, 2884–2893. [CrossRef]
188. Kool, M.; Willart, M.A.; van Nimwegen, M.; Bergen, I.; Pouliot, P.; Virchow, J.C.; Rogers, N.; Osorio, F.; Reis e Sousa, C.; Hammad, H.; et al. An unexpected role for uric acid as an inducer of T helper 2 cell immunity to inhaled antigens and inflammatory mediator of allergic asthma. *Immunity* **2011**, *4*, 527–540. [CrossRef] [PubMed]
189. Hirota, J.A.; Gold, M.J.; Hiebert, P.R.; Parkinson, L.G.; Wee, T.; Smith, D.; Hansbro, P.M.; Carlsten, C.; VanEeden, S.; Sin, D.D.; et al. The Nucleotide-Binding Domain, Leucine-Rich Repeat Protein 3 Inflammasome/IL-1 Receptor I Axis Mediates Innate, but Not Adaptive, Immune Responses after Exposure to Particulate Matter under 10 μm. *Am. J. Respir. Cell Mol. Biol.* **2015**, *52*, 96–105. [CrossRef]
190. Madouri, F.; Guillou, N.; Fauconnier, L.; Marchiol, T.; Rouxel, N.; Chenuet, P.; Ledru, A.; Apetoh, L.; Ghiringhelli, F.; Chamaillard, M.; et al. Caspase-1 activation by NLRP3 inflammasome dampens IL-33-dependent p-induced allergic lung inflammation. *J. Mol. Cell Biol.* **2015**, *7*, 351–365. [CrossRef]
191. Hirota, J.A.; Hirota, S.A.; Warner, S.M.; Stefanowicz, D.; Shaheen, F.; Beck, P.L.; Macdonald, J.A.; Hackett, T.L.; Sin, D.D.; Van Eeden, S.; et al. The airway epithelium nucleotide -binding domain and leucine -rich repeat protein 3 inflammasome is activated by urban particulate matter. *J. Allergy Clin. Immunol.* **2012**, *129*, 1116–1125. [CrossRef]
192. Triantafilou, K.; Kar, S.; van Kuppeveld, F.J.; Triantafilou, M. Rhinovirus-induced calcium flux triggers NLRP3 and NLRC5 activation in bronchial cells. *Am. J. Respir. Cell Mol. Biol.* **2013**, *49*, 923–934. [CrossRef] [PubMed]
193. Bauer, R.N.; Brighton, L.E.; Mueller, L.; Xiang, Z.; Rager, J.E.; Fry, R.C.; Peden, D.B.; Jaspers, I. Influenza enhances caspase-1 in bronchial epithelial cells from asthmatic volunteers and is associated with pathogenesis. *J. Allergy Clin. Immunol.* **2012**, *130*, 958–967. [CrossRef] [PubMed]
194. Simpson, J.L.; Phipps, S.; Baines, K.J.; Oreo, K.M.; Gunawardhana, L.; Gibson, P.G. Elevated expression of the NLRP3 inflammasome in neutrophilic asthma. *Eur. Respir. J.* **2014**, *43*, 1067–1076. [CrossRef] [PubMed]
195. Lachowicz, M.E.; Dunican, E.M.; Charbit, A.R.; Raymond, W.; Looney, M.R.; Peters, M.C.; Gordon, E.D.; Woodruff, P.G.; Lefrançais, E.; Phillips, B.R.; et al. Extracellular DNA, Neutrophil Extracellular Traps, and Inflammasome Activation in Severe Asthma. *Am. J. Respir. Crit. Care Med.* **2019**, *199*, 1076–1085. [CrossRef] [PubMed]
196. Wood, L.G.; Li, Q.; Scott, H.A.; Rutting, S.; Berthon, B.S.; Gibson, P.G.; Hansbro, P.M.; Williams, E.; Horvat, J.; Simpson, J.L.; et al. Saturated fatty acids, obesity, and the nucleotide oligomerization domain-like receptor 3 (NLRP3) inflammasome in asthmatic patients. *J. Allergy Clin. Immunol.* **2019**, *143*, 305–315. [CrossRef] [PubMed]
197. Liu, W.; Liu, S.; Verma, M.; Zafar, I.; Good, J.T.; Rollins, D.; Groshong, S.; Gorska, M.M.; Martin, R.J.; Alam, R. Mechanism of Th2/Th17-predominant and neutrophilic Th2/Th17- low subtypes of asthma. *J. Allergy Clin. Immunol.* **2017**, *139*, 1548–1558. [CrossRef] [PubMed]
198. Hastie, A.T.; Moore, W.C.; Meyers, D.A.; Vestal, P.L.; Li, H.; Peters, S.P.; Bleecker, E.R. Analyses of asthma severity phenotypes and inflammatory proteins in subjects stratified by sputum granulocytes. *J. Allergy Clin. Immunol.* **2010**, *125*, 1028–1036. [CrossRef]
199. Chu, M.; Chu, I.M.; Yung, E.C.; Lam, C.W.; Leung, T.F.; Wong, G.W.; Wong, C.K. Aberrant Expression of Novel Cytokine IL-38 and Regulatory Lymphocytes in Childhood Asthma. *Molecules* **2016**, *21*, 933. [CrossRef] [PubMed]
200. Wong, C.K.; Ho, C.Y.; Ko, F.W.; Chan, C.H.; Ho, A.S.; Hui, D.S.; Lam, C.W. Proinflammatory cytokines (IL17, IL-6, IL-18 and IL-12) and Th cytokines (IFN-gamma, IL-4, IL-10 and IL-13) in patients with allergic asthma. *Clin. Exp. Immunol.* **2001**, *125*, 177–183. [CrossRef] [PubMed]

201. Tanaka, H.; Miyazaki, N.; Oashi, K.; Teramoto, S.; Shiratori, M.; Hashimoto, M.; Ohmichi, M.; Abe, S. IL-18 might reflect disease activity in mild and moderate asthma exacerbation. *J. Allergy Clin. Immunol.* **2001**, *107*, 331. [CrossRef]
202. Rovina, N.; Dima, E.; Gerassimou, C.; Kollintza, A.; Gratziou, C.; Roussos, C. IL-18 in induced sputum and airway hyperresponsiveness in mild asthmatics: Effect of smoking. *Respir. Med.* **2009**, *103*, 1919–1925. [CrossRef] [PubMed]
203. McKay, A.; Komai-Koma, M.; MacLeod, K.J.; Campbell, C.C.; Kitson, S.M.; Chaudhuri, R.; Thomson, L.; McSharry, C.; Liew, F.Y.; Thomson, N.C. Interleukin-18 levels in induced sputum are reduced in asthmatic and normal smokers. *Clin. Exp. Allergy* **2004**, *34*, 904–910. [CrossRef] [PubMed]
204. Rovina, N.; Dima, E.; Bakakos, P.; Tseliou, E.; Kontogianni, K.; Papiris, S.; Koutsoukou, A.; Koulouris, N.G.; Loukides, S. Low interleukin (IL)-18 levels in sputum supernatants of patients with severe refractory asthma. *Respir. Med.* **2015**, *109*, 580–587. [CrossRef] [PubMed]
205. Ridker, P.M.; Everett, B.M.; Thuren, T.; MacFadyen, J.G.; Chang, W.H.; Ballantyne, C.; Fonseca, F.; Nicolau, J.; Koenig, W.; Anker, S.D.; et al. Antiinflammatory Therapy with Canakinumab for Atherosclerotic Disease. *N. Engl. J. Med.* **2017**, *377*, 1119–1131. [CrossRef] [PubMed]
206. Lachmann, H.J.; Lachmann, H.J.; Kone-Paut, I.; Kuemmerle-Deschner, J.B.; Leslie, K.S.; Hachulla, E.; Quartier, P.; Gitton, X.; Widmer, A.; Patel, N.; et al. Canakinumab in CAPS Study Group. Use of Canakinumab in the Cryopyrin-Associated Periodic Syndrome. *N. Engl. J. Med.* **2009**, *360*, 2416–2425. [CrossRef] [PubMed]
207. Pascoe, S.; Kanniess, F.; Bonner, J.; Lloyd, P.; Lowe, P.; Beier, J. A monoclonal antibody to IL-1β attenuates the late asthmatic response to antigen challenge in patients with mild asthma. *Annu. Congr. Eur. Resp. Soc.* **2016**, *48* Suppl. 60, 752. Available online: http://www.ersnet.org/learning_resources_player/abstract_print_06/files/51.pdf (accessed on 8 June 2016).
208. Church, L.D.; McDermott, M.F. Canakinumab, a fully-human mAb against IL-1beta for the potential treatment of inflammatory disorders. *Curr. Opin. Mol. Ther.* **2009**, *11*, 81–89. [PubMed]
209. Menzella, F.; Lusuardi, M.; Galeone, C.; Zucchi, L. Tailored therapy for severe asthma. *Multidis. Respir. Med.* **2015**, *10*, 1. [CrossRef] [PubMed]

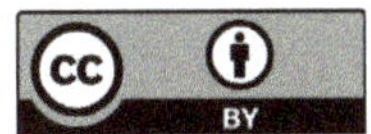

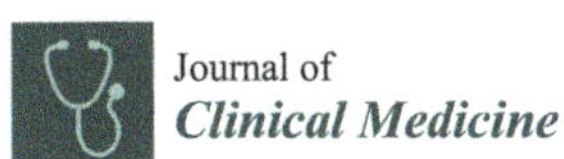
Journal of
Clinical Medicine

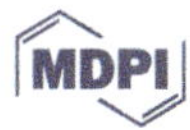

Article

The Enhanced Adhesion of Eosinophils Is Associated with Their Prolonged Viability and Pro-Proliferative Effect in Asthma

Andrius Januskevicius [1,*], Ieva Janulaityte [1], Virginija Kalinauskaite-Zukauske [2], Reinoud Gosens [3] and Kestutis Malakauskas [1,2]

1 Laboratory of Pulmonology, Department of Pulmonology, Lithuanian University of Health Sciences, LT-44307 Kaunas, Lithuania
2 Department of Pulmonology, Lithuanian University of Health Sciences, LT-44307 Kaunas, Lithuania
3 Department of Molecular Pharmacology, University of Groningen, 9713 AV Groningen, The Netherlands
* Correspondence: andrius.januskevicius@lsmuni.lt

Received: 29 July 2019; Accepted: 20 August 2019; Published: 22 August 2019

Abstract: Before eosinophils migrate into the bronchial lumen, they promote airway structural changes after contact with pulmonary cells and extracellular matrix components. We aimed to investigate the impact of eosinophil adhesion to their viability and pro-proliferative effect on airway smooth muscle (ASM) cells and pulmonary fibroblasts during different asthma phenotypes. A total of 39 individuals were included: 14 steroid-free non-severe allergic asthma (AA) patients, 10 severe non-allergic eosinophilic asthma (SNEA) patients, and 15 healthy control subjects (HS). For AA patients and HS groups, a bronchial allergen challenge with *Dermatophagoides pteronysinnus* was performed. Individual combined cells cultures were prepared between isolated peripheral blood eosinophils and ASM cells or pulmonary fibroblasts. Eosinophil adhesion was measured by evaluating their peroxidase activity, cell viability was performed by annexin V and propidium iodide staining, and proliferation by Alamar blue assay. We found that increased adhesion of eosinophils was associated with prolonged viability ($p < 0.05$) and an enhanced pro-proliferative effect on ASM cells and pulmonary fibroblasts in asthma ($p < 0.05$). However, eosinophils from SNEA patients demonstrated higher viability and inhibition of pulmonary structural cell apoptosis, compared to the AA group ($p < 0.05$), while their adhesive and pro-proliferative properties were similar. Finally, in the AA group, in vivo allergen-activated eosinophils demonstrated a higher adhesion, viability, and pro-proliferative effect on pulmonary structural cells compared to non-activated eosinophils ($p < 0.05$).

Keywords: eosinophil; adhesion; viability; proliferation; airway smooth muscle cell; pulmonary fibroblast; phenotype; asthma

---

1. Introduction

Chronic eosinophilic inflammation is a major factor in the development of airway remodeling in asthma [1]. The contribution of various cytokine networks makes asthma pathophysiology very complex, and these mechanisms vary between patients with different asthma phenotypes. Eosinophils are a significant source of cytokines, chemokines, growth factors, and enzymes [2], therefore, their increased infiltration into asthmatic lungs leads to the disturbance of normal lung homeostasis [3].

Eosinophils develop from bone marrow progenitors under the control of a dedicated set of transcription factors and the cytokines interleukin (IL)-3, IL-5, and granulocyte-macrophage colony-stimulating factor (GM-CSF) [4]. Eosinophils' half-life is between 3 to 24 h in peripheral blood [5], while being in the lungs prolongs their half-life up to 36 h [6]. Survivability-promoting signals can be different. IL-5 is the most important and specific survival factor for eosinophils [7], but important mediators also include GM-CSF and IL-3 [8], tumor necrosis factor-α [9], leptin [10], and cluster of differentiation 40 engagement [11]. It is known that combined culturing with pulmonary structural cells promotes eosinophils survival [12–15], however, the precise mechanisms remain unknown. Integrins as transmembrane molecular mechanosensors may change their activation states under asthmatic conditions and transduce the signal through the cytoskeleton, thus regulating eosinophil activity and viability [16,17].

In addition to chronic inflammation, both allergic and non-allergic phenotypes of asthma are characterized by structural changes in the lungs, which is called airway remodeling [18]. Airway remodeling in asthma includes epithelial changes, subepithelial and airway smooth muscle (ASM) thickening, as well as bronchial neoangiogenesis that develops after repetitive cycles of tissue injury and abnormal repair processes because of chronic inflammation [19]. Airway remodeling develops mainly because of disturbed ASM cells and pulmonary fibroblast proliferation that determine the increase in tissue mass due to enhanced cell numbers and the release of the extracellular matrix (ECM) [20]. Studies demonstrate that direct interaction with eosinophils promotes pulmonary fibroblasts and ASM cell proliferation [21–24]. Eosinophil-released mediators, such as transforming growth factor β-1 and cysteinyl leukotrienes, are the main ASM cells, as well as being pulmonary fibroblast proliferation- and differentiation-promoting factors [25,26]; however, more research is needed to understand increased eosinophil activity or prolonged viability dominates in their pro-proliferative effect.

Asthma severity correlates with peripheral blood and sputum eosinophils count [27]. However, as major symptoms and airway structural changes between allergic and non-allergic asthma phenotypes overlap, the pathways through which the disease develops and how eosinophils are involved in the disease pathogenesis are different [28]. This highlights the hypothesis that further course of the disease during different asthma phenotypes or during disease exacerbation can be predicted not only by increased eosinophil count but also by their different biological properties.

We hypothesized that adhesion of eosinophils may determine their survivability properties and further effect on pulmonary structural changes in asthma. Isolated blood eosinophils demonstrate the biological role closely related to lung eosinophil functions because they are mainly activated in the bone marrow under the maturation and in peripheral blood by inflammatory mediators [29,30]. Therefore, our use of a combined cell culture model between blood eosinophils and pulmonary structural cells allows for imitation of in vivo processes. We evaluated the effect of adhesion to pulmonary structural cells on eosinophil viability and pro-proliferative effects for different asthma phenotypes. Moreover, we investigated, in vivo, how a provoked acute allergic asthma episode after a bronchial allergen challenge affects eosinophil activity.

2. Experimental Section

2.1. Ethics Statement

The study protocol was approved by the Regional Biomedical Research Ethics Committee of the Lithuanian University of Health Sciences (BE-2-13). Each participant was informed about the ongoing investigation and gave his/her written consent. Trial registration: ClinicalTrials.gov Identifier NCT03388359.

2.2. Study Population

The study population consists of only newly recruited, not studied individuals.

The study included steroid-free allergic asthma (AA) patients, severe non-allergic eosinophilic asthma (SNEA) patients with high doses of inhaled steroids, and healthy non-smoking subjects (HS) who comprised the control group. The participants were men and women between the ages of

18–50 years old who signed written informed consent. The patients were recruited from the Department of Pulmonology at the Hospital of the Lithuanian University of Health Sciences Kaunas Clinics.

The AA group were newly-established and untreated non-severe patients, approved with symptoms and medical history for at least a 12 month period, having a positive skin prick test to *Dermatophagoides pteronyssinus* allergen and positive bronchial challenge with methacholine.

The SNEA group was a non-allergic phenotype, approved by negative skin prick tests, and with asthma diagnosis for at least 1 year. Peripheral eosinophil counts were $\geq 0.3 \times 10^9$/L during the screening visit or $\geq 0.15 \times 10^9$/L if there was a documented eosinophil count $\geq 0.3 \times 10^9$/L in the 12 month period before the screening. A severe course of the disease was approved with at least 12 month treatment of high doses of inhaled steroids combined with long-acting beta-agonist ± long-acting antimuscarinic agent ± episodic use of oral corticosteroids.

The HS group was without allergic and other chronic respiratory diseases.

Exclusion criteria for all groups were clinically significant permanent allergy symptoms, active airway infection 1 month prior the study, exacerbation ≤ 1 month prior to study, use of oral steroids ≤ 1 month prior to study, and smoking.

2.3. Study Design

Initially, all study subjects underwent physical examination, spirometry, a methacholine challenge test, and a skin prick test to verify the inclusion and exclusion criteria. If individuals matched the criteria, they were informed about the requirements for participation and informed written consent was obtained.

At the first visit of the study, peripheral blood was collected and measured for exhaled fractional exhaled nitric oxide (FeNO). Isolated peripheral blood eosinophils were counted, assessed in their viability, and immediately prepared in combined cell cultures with ASM cells and pulmonary fibroblasts. Additionally, AA patients and HS after primary collection of peripheral blood underwent a bronchial allergen challenge with *D. pteronyssinus* allergen.

The second visit was 24 h after a bronchial allergen challenge for subjects whom this test was performed, and all procedures were repeated according to the first visit. The experimental study design is represented in Figure 1.

Eosinophil count ($<1.5 \times 10^6$/20 mL blood), viability (<98%), and purity (<96%) after their isolation processes, as well as eosinophil adhesion intensity (equal to control value) was used as experimental exclusion criteria for all investigated subjects. All data provided in the manuscript were from subjects who passed these criteria.

We performed the unblinded type of experiments, as well-planned preparation before the recruitment of each study subjects was required, and the whole experimental plan was performed in the same week.

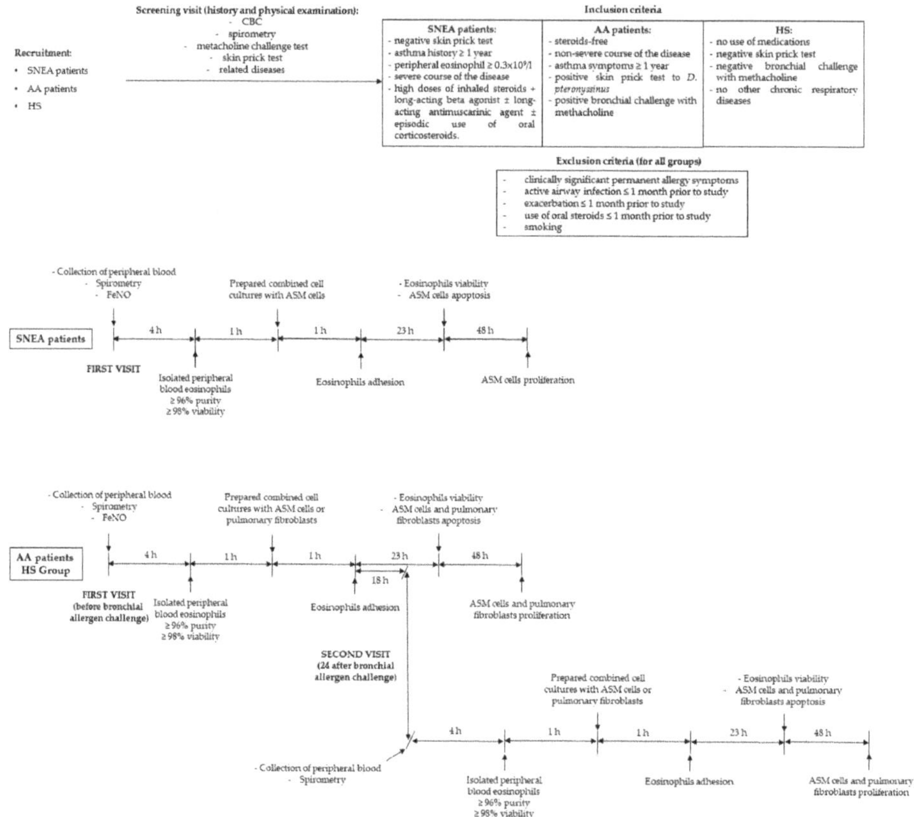

Figure 1. Experimental study design. CBC—Complete blood count; SNEA—Severe non-allergic eosinophilic asthma; AA—Allergic asthma; HS—Healthy subjects; FeNO—Fractional exhaled nitric oxide; ASM—Airway smooth muscle.

2.4. Lung Function Testing

Pulmonary function was tested by using an ultrasonic spirometer (Ganshorn Medizin Electronic, Niederlauer, Germany). Baseline forced expiratory volume in 1 s (FEV_1), forced vital capacity (FVC), and FEV_1/FVC ratio were recorded as the highest of three reproducible measurements. The results were compared with the predicted values matched for age, body height, and sex according to the standard methodology.

Airway responsiveness was assessed using inhaled methacholine via pressure dosimeter (ProvoX, Ganshorn Medizin Electronic, Niederlauer, Germany). Aerosolized methacholine was inhaled at 2 min intervals, starting with a 0.0101 mg methacholine dose, and increasing it by steps up to 0.121, 0.511, and 1.31 mg of the total cumulative dose was achieved, or until a 20% decrease in FEV_1 from the baseline. The bronchoconstriction effect of each dose of methacholine was expressed as a percentage of decrease in FEV_1 from the baseline value. The provocative dose of methacholine causing a ≥20% fall in FEV_1 (PD_{20M}) was calculated from the log dose-response curve by linear interpolation of two adjacent data points.

2.5. Skin Prick Testing

All patients were screened for allergy by the skin prick test using standardized allergen extracts (Stallergenes, S.A., France) for the following allergens: *D. pteronyssinus*, *Dermatophagoides farinae*, cat and dog dandruff, five mixed grass pollens, birch pollen, mugwort, *Alternaria*, *Aspergillus*, and *Cladosporium*. Diluent (saline) was used for the negative control, and histamine hydrochloride (10 mg/mL) was used for the positive control. Skin testing was read 15 min after application. The results of the skin prick test were considered positive if the mean wheal diameter was higher than 3 mm.

2.6. FeNO Measurement

All study subjects underwent fractional exhaled nitric oxide (FeNO) analysis with an on-line method using a single breath exhalation and an electrochemical assay (NIOX VERO, Circassia, UK), according to European Respiratory Society—American Thoracic Society guidelines. Patients made an inspiration of FeNO-free air via a mouthpiece, immediately followed by full exhalation at a constant rate (50 mL/s) for at least 10 s. The mean of three readings at the end of the expiration (plateau phase) was taken as the representative value for each measurement. Values that were 12 ppb or more were considered elevated values, according to ATS-ERS criteria.

2.7. Bronchial Allergen Challenge Test

Inhaled *D. Pteronyssinus* allergen (DIATER, Spain) was delivered via pressure dosimeter (ProvoX, Ganshorn Medizin Electronic, Niederlauer, Germany). The starting point for the assessment of bronchoconstriction effect was 2 min after nebulized saline inhalation. The aerosolized allergen was inhaled at 10 min intervals, starting with 0.1 histamine equivalent prick (HEP)/mL allergen concentration, increasing it by steps up to 1.0, 10.0, 20.0, 40.0, 60.0 HEP/mL, or if a 20% decrease in FEV_1 from the baseline was achieved. The provocative dose of allergen causing a ≥20% fall in FEV_1 (PD_{20A}) was calculated from the log dose-response curve by linear interpolation of two adjacent data points.

2.8. Analysis of Peripheral Blood Cells

The peripheral blood analysis for the complete blood count test was performed on an automated hematology analyzer XE-5000™ (Sysmex, Kobe, Japan).

2.9. Granulocyte Isolation from Human Peripheral Blood and Eosinophil Enrichment

Approximately 24 mL of peripheral blood was collected into sterile Ethylenediaminetetraacetic acid-containing vacutainers (BD Bioscience, San Jose, CA, USA). The whole blood was then diluted with 1x phosphate-buffered saline (PBS) (GIBCO, Paisley, UK) up to 50 mL and mixed thoroughly. The whole blood was layered on Ficoll-Paque PLUS (GE Healthcare, Helsinki, Finland) and centrifuged at 400× *g* force for 30 min at room temperature. The supernatant was removed and the bottom-most layer comprising the granulocyte fraction of cells and erythrocytes was collected. Then, hypotonic lysis of erythrocytes was performed. Into the tubes with cells, half volume of sterile water was added and gently mixed for no longer than 10 s, immediately supplementing the mixture with an equal volume of 2x concentrated PBS and centrifuged at 300× *g* force for 10 min. The procedure was repeated until no red blood cells were left. Then, cells were counted and viability evaluated using an ADAM automatic cell counter (Witec AG, Switzerland). Eosinophil enrichment was performed by negative selection from the granulocyte fraction using Magnetic-activated cell sorting (MACS)magnetically-labeled MicroBeads (Miltenyi Biotec, Somerville, MA, USA). The manufacturer confirms that eosinophil separation kits do not influence eosinophil viability, and that separation efficiency is more than 96%. MACS buffer (containing 0.5% bovine serum albumin (BSA) and 2 mM EDTA in PBS, with a pH of 7.2) was prepared by diluting MACS BSA stock solution 1:20 in autoMACS rinsing solution. The granulocyte pellet was resuspended in cold MACS buffer (40 μL per 1×10^7 cells) and incubated with biotin antibody cocktail (biotin-conjugated monoclonal antibodies against CD2, CD14, CD16, CD19, CD56, CD123, and CD235a (glycophorin A)) (10 μL per 1×10^7 cells) for 10 min. After incubation, 20 μL of anti-biotin microbeads (microbeads conjugated to monoclonal mouse anti-biotin immunoglobulin(Ig)-G1 per 1×10^7 cells were added, mixed, and incubated for an additional 15 min at 4 °C. An large separation column (Miltenyi Biotec, USA) was prepared during this time by placing the column in the magnetic field of a MACS separator and washing it with 2 mL of MACS buffer. A pre-separation filter (30 µm; Miltenyi Biotec) was rinsed with MACS buffer and placed on top of the column. The cells were then applied to the pre-separation filter/LS column, and the magnetically labeled non-eosinophils were retained on the column in the magnetic field of the separator while the unlabeled eosinophils passed through the column. Cells were eluted with 5 mL of MACS buffer and centrifuged (300× *g*, 10 min, 4 °C), and the pellet was resuspended in 5 mL of PBS. Eosinophils were counted using an ADAM automatic cell counter. To check eosinophil purity after magnetic separation, a diluted eosinophil suspension was analyzed by flow cytometer FacsCalibur (BD, USA) according to forward and side light scattering to determine whether there were any other cells in the suspension (Figure 2). As an internal control, after usage of the new isolation kit, eosinophil purity was tested with alternative May-Grunwald Giemsa staining and inspected by light microscopy.

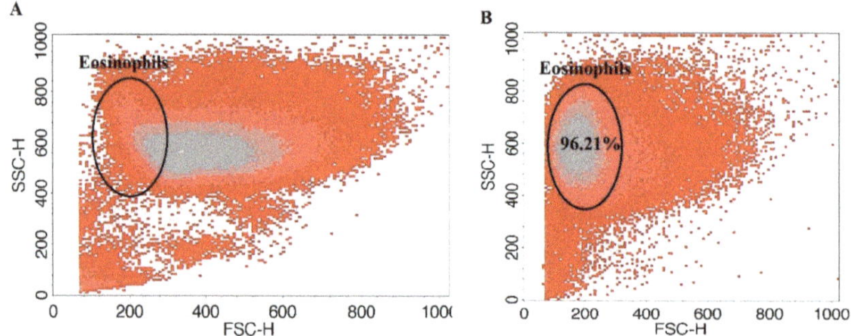

Figure 2. Eosinophil enrichment. (**A**) peripheral blood granulocytes after high-density centrifugation and erythrocyte lysis. (**B**) peripheral blood eosinophils after negative magnetic labeling and separation. Collected cell number—1×10^5. Eosinophil quantity expressed from total collected cells counts rejecting debris.

2.10. Combined Cell Cultures between Isolated Eosinophils and ASM Cells or Pulmonary Fibroblasts

Individual combined cell cultures (co-cultures) of eosinophils and pulmonary structural cells were prepared for all experiments. We used healthy human ASM cells, immortalized by stable expression of human telomerase reverse transcriptase as described in [31] and a commercial MRC-5 (Sigma, Ronkonkoma, NY, USA) lung fibroblast line. The main cell line was cultivated under standard culture conditions of 5% CO_2 in air at 37 °C with medium renewal every 3 days. For all experiments, passaged ASM cells were grown on plastic dishes in Dulbecco's modified Eagle's medium (DMEM) (GIBCO by Life Technologies, UK) and MRC-5 pulmonary fibroblasts in minimum essential Eagle's medium (EMEM) (GIBCO, Paisley, UK), supplemented with streptomycin/penicillin (2% *v/v*; Pen-Strep, GIBCO by Life Technologies, Paisley, UK), amphotericin B (1% *v/v*; GIBCO, Paisley, UK), and fetal bovine serum (10% *v/v*; GIBCO by Life Technologies). After reaching sufficient confluence, cells were passaged by trypsinization. Cells were serum-deprived in respective medium, supplemented with antibiotics and insulin, transferrin, and selenium reagent (GIBCO by Life Technologies) before each experiment to stop cell proliferation and avoid possible errors due to the effect of mediators in serum. The same lines of ASM and MRC-5 cells were used for whole investigating subjects. Avoiding a decrease in cell activity and viability after repeated times of passage, the new cells of the mainline were unfrozen every time after six passages.

ASM and MRC-5 cells were grown in six-well (confluency approximately 16×10^4 cells) or 24-well (confluency approximately 4×10^4 cells) culture plates (CytoOne, StarLab, Brussels, Belgium.). Co-cultures with isolated eosinophils were prepared by adding 5×10^4 or 1.25×10^4 of eosinophils, respectively. For observing and visualization of cell growth and co-cultures, we used an inverted microscope (CETI Inverso TC100, Medline Scientific, Chalgrove, UK) with a 10×/22 mm wide-field eyepiece and phase contrast 10×/0.25 objective and an installed XM10-IR-2 camera (Olympus, Tokyo, Japan) (Figure 3).

At the study day, experiments were divided into different groups, according to the growth medium supplements. Investigated individual blood serum—2% of *v*/*v*—was used to maintain further eosinophil activation after isolation processes and to verify if the eosinophils were isolated in their most activated form, whilst 25 nm of vitamin C (ascorbic acid) was used as the most accessible natural antioxidant to eliminate eosinophil-released reactive oxygen species and verify its effect on the proliferation of pulmonary structural cells.

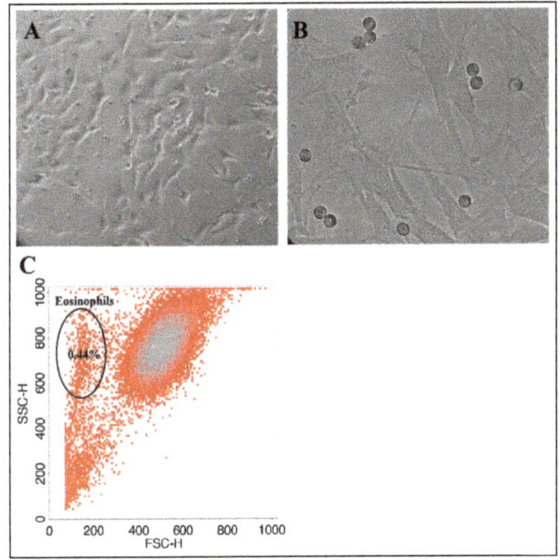

Figure 3. Combined cell cultures between eosinophils and ASM cells. (**A**) the picture at 10× objective. (**B**) the picture at 40× objective. (**C**) remaining eosinophil number after combined cell culture separation. Collected cell number—1×10^5. Eosinophil number is expressed from total collected cell count, rejecting cell debris.

2.11. Eosinophils Adhesion Assay

ASM or MRC-5 cells were seeded in 24-well plates and grown for 3 days in 5% CO_2 at 37 °C until a confluency of approximately 4×10^4 cells. Then, the medium was removed, and wells were washed twice with warm PBS. The medium was changed 24 h before the experiments by adding serum-free medium, supplemented with 1% insulin-transferrin-selenium reagent. Eosinophil adhesion was measured after 1 h of incubation, which is a sufficient period for eosinophils to adhere in co-culture [22]. After incubation, non-adhered eosinophils were removed, and the remaining cells were washed twice with warm PBS. Eosinophil adhesion was determined by measuring residual eosinophil peroxidase (EPO) activity as described [32]. Because intercellular EPO levels were identified as being decreased in eosinophils from asthmatic individuals owing to degranulation [33], we normalized it by preparing a calibration curve of fixed eosinophil count EPO activity for each experiment. To assay EPO activity, 116 μL of DMEM medium without phenol red and 116 μL of EPO substrate (1 mM H_2O_2, 1 mM *o*-phenylenediamine, and 0.1% Triton X-100 in Tris buffer, pH 8.0) were added to each well. After 30 min at 37 °C, 68 μL of 4 M H_2SO_4 was added to each well to stop the reaction and the absorbance was measured at 490 nm by a microplate reader. Results were expressed as % of adhered eosinophil number from max added, calculated from a calibration curve. Added eosinophil number—1.25×10^4 (double amount—2.5×10^4).

2.12. Cell Viability Assay

Viability of ASM cells, pulmonary fibroblasts, and eosinophils were performed by fluorescent staining with annexin V for apoptotic cells and propidium iodide (PI) for necrotic cells.

ASM cells and pulmonary fibroblasts were grown in six-well plates until confluency of approximately 16×10^4 cells. On the day of experiments, a co-culture with 5×10^4 of isolated eosinophils was prepared in the serum-free growth medium, or medium supplemented with 2% (*v*/*v*) of investigated subjects' blood serum. After 24 h of co-culturing, used eosinophils were collected into 15mL centrifuge tubes (Corning Inc., New York, NY, USA), together with eosinophils incubated alone at the same conditions. Then, ASM cells and pulmonary fibroblasts were trypsinized, collected and, together with eosinophils, centrifuged at 400× *g* for 10 min.

For the cell viability assay, we used an fluorescein isothiocyanate (FITC) Annexin V Apoptosis Detection Kit II (BD Bioscience, San Jose, CA, USA) and adapted the method according to the manufacturer's recommendation. Before every experiment, we used additional controls of unstained cells, cells stained with FITC annexin V (no PI), and cells stained with PI (no FITC annexin V). For the viability assay of structural cells as a control, we used ASM cells or pulmonary fibroblasts without co-culturing with eosinophils. Eosinophil's effect was compared with normal ASM and pulmonary fibroblast apoptosis in the serum-free growth medium, but was supplemented with an insulin-transferrin-selenium compound to maintain normal conditions.

For the viability assay of eosinophils, we normalized the data according to the results received from the centrifuged growth medium, which was used in the control structural cell cultures without co-culturing with eosinophils and excluding possible errors from cellular debris. Eosinophils and structural cells significantly differ in size and granularity, therefore, appropriate gating on forward and side scattering excludes any remaining culture heterogeneity.

2.13. Alamar Blue Proliferation Assay

Cells for proliferation measurements were grown in 24-well plates in conditions described previously in fetal bovine serum-supplemented growth medium until confluency of approximately 4×10^4 cells/well. Growth medium was changed into the serum-free medium 24 h before the experiments. ASM cells or pulmonary fibroblasts were co-cultured with a respective group of eosinophils isolated from AA patients, SNEA patients, or the HS for 72 h. Thereafter, all cells were washed twice with warm PBS, plates were gently smashed in the middle of the plate to detach residual eosinophils who were significantly more weakly adhered compared with structural cells, and again were washed twice with warm PBS. Proliferation was evaluated by incubating wells with Hank's balanced salt solution containing Alamar blue solution (10% *v*/*v*; Invitrogen by Life Technologies, Paisley, UK). Conversion of Alamar blue to the reduced form was dependent on the metabolic activity of structural cells and was assayed by dual-wavelength spectrophotometry at wavelengths of 570 nm and 600 nm. As indicated by the manufacturer, the degree of Alamar blue conversion is proportional to the number of viable cells. The data are expressed as the percent increase or decrease in Alamar blue conversion by ASM cells or pulmonary fibroblasts compared with control cells (without co-culturing with eosinophils), which did not proliferate during the culturing period because serum-free growth medium were used. Added eosinophils number—1.25×10^4; 2x amount—2.5×10^4; 1/2x amount—0.6×10^4. Used investigated subjects blood serum volume—2% *v*/*v*; ascorbic acid concentration—25 nM.

2.14. Statistical Analysis

Statistical analysis was performed with GraphPad Prism 6 for Windows (ver. 6.05, 2014; GraphPad Software Inc., San Diego, CA, USA). Significant differences between two independent groups were determined using the Mann–Whitney two-sided U-test. The Wilcoxon matched-pairs signed-rank two-sided test was used for dependent groups. Minimum limit for statistically significant values—$p < 0.05$.

3. Results

3.1. Characteristics of the Studied Participants

We investigated 39 nonsmoking adults (14 men and 25 women): 14 steroid-free non-severe allergic asthma (AA) patients, 10 severe non-allergic eosinophilic asthma (SNEA) patients, and 15 healthy non-smoking control subjects (HS). The main characteristics of the study participants are shown in Table 1. The highest eosinophils count was observed in the SNEA group, however, in AA patients, it was also increased compared with HS. The IgE levels were significantly increased in AA and SNEA patients, compared with HS, but the highest level was in the AA group. FeNO was equally increased in both the AA and SNEA groups, compared with HS. Moreover, at the baseline, significant deterioration of lung function was observed only in SNEA patients.

Table 1. Demographic and clinical characteristics of the study population.

	Healthy Subjects	SNEA Patients	AA Patients
Number, n	15	10	14
Sex, M/F	3/12	4/6	7/7
Age, years	28.4 ± 1.8	46.5 ± 3.0 $^{\#,*}$	28.0 ± 2.3
BMI, kg/m^2	23.2 ± 1.2	26.9 ± 2.2	24.7 ± 1.6
PD_{20M}, geometric mean (range), mg	NR	ND	0.08 (0.02–0.26)
PD_{20A}, geometric mean (range), HEP/mL	NR	ND	0.84 (0.15–3.04)
IgE, IU/mL	29.5 ± 6.0	147.2 ± 30.7 *	202.8 ± 41.9 *
FEV_1, L	3.9 ± 0.18	2.0 ± 0.4 $^{\#,*}$	3.9 ± 0.2
FEV_1, % of predicted	106.6 ± 3.7	57.6 ± 8.6 $^{\#,*}$	95.9 ± 3.3
Blood eosinophil count, ×10^9/L	0.18 ± 0.02	0.52 ± 0.11 $^{\#,*}$	0.36 ± 0.07 *
FeNO, ppb	12.9 ± 1.5	44.9 ± 10.7 *	59.5 ± 11.5 *

AA—Allergic asthma; SNEA—Severe non-allergic eosinophilic asthma; F—Female; M—Male; FEV_1—Forced expiratory volume in 1s; PD_{20M}—The provocation dose of methacholine causing a 20% decrease in FEV_1; PD20A—the provocation dose of allergen D. pteronyssinus causing a 20% decrease in FEV1; BMI—Body mass index; FeNO—Fractional exhaled nitric oxide; IgE—Immunoglobulin E; NR—Not responded; ND—Not done. Data presented as the mean ± standard error of the mean, except PD_{20M} and PD_{20A} which are provided as geometric mean (range). * $p < 0.05$ compared with HS group; # $p < 0.05$ compared with AA group. Statistical analysis—Mann–Whitney two-sided U-test.

3.2. Eosinophil Adhesion and Survivability

We observed that 71.7% ± 3.5% of AA patients' and 66.6% ± 5.8% of SNEA patients' eosinophils adhere onto the surface of ASM cells after 1 h of incubation, and this count was significantly increased compared to healthy eosinophils (47.2% ± 3.7%, $p < 0.05$) (Figure 4A). Supplementing growth medium with investigated individuals' blood serum had a significant negative effect only in the SNEA group—the adhered eosinophils ratio decreased to 46.7% ± 7.9% of the added eosinophils count, $p < 0.05$. Moreover, by using double the amount of added eosinophils in the culture well, we received a significant ($p < 0.05$) decrease in the adhered eosinophils ratio in the AA and SNEA groups to 53.8% ± 5.0% and 50.5% ± 6.4% of the total added eosinophil count, respectively, with no differences in the HS group (Figure 4A). Similar results were obtained by measuring AA and HS eosinophil adhesion to pulmonary fibroblasts—adhered eosinophils' number in the AA group was 61.2% ± 4.6%, and 37.3% ± 3.7% in the HS group, $p < 0.05$. Significant differences after supplementing the medium with blood serum were not observed in both groups. Moreover, in the AA group, the adhered eosinophil ratio decreased to 43.8% ± 7.4% after using double the amount of added eosinophils ($p < 0.05$) (Figure 4B).

Moreover, we observed that AA and HS eosinophils' peroxidase activity, evaluated as the ability to oxidize o-phenylenediamine in the presence of their peroxidases, are similar—The average absolute value values of oxidized o-PD was 0.21 ± 0.04 optical density (O.D) and 0.2 ± 0.3 O.D, respectively. The average SNEA eosinophil peroxidase activity was only 0.12 ± 0.02 O.D; however, there was no statistical significance upon comparison with AA and HS groups, $p = 0.069$ and 0.073, respectively (Figure 4C).

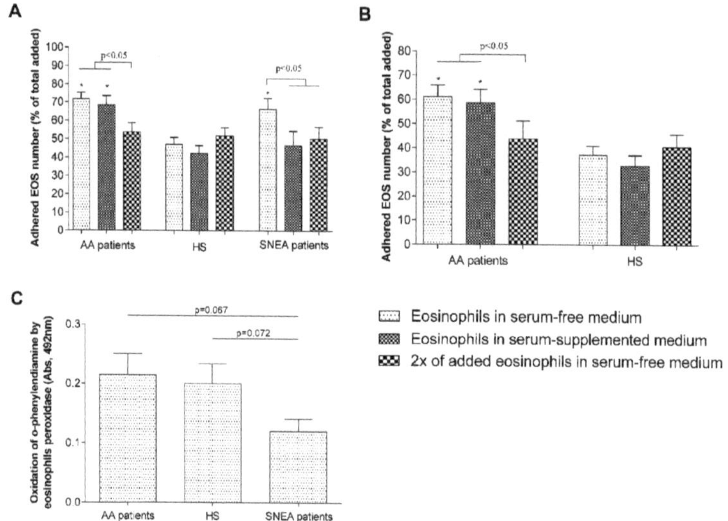

Figure 4. The efficiency of eosinophil adhesion. (**A**) Eosinophil adhesion in co-culture with airway smooth muscle (ASM) cells; (**B**) eosinophil adhesion in co-culture with pulmonary fibroblasts. (**C**) Eosinophil peroxidase (EPO) substrate activity of 12,500 eosinophils. EOS—eosinophils, AA—Allergic asthma, SNEA—Severe non-allergic eosinophilic asthma, HS—Healthy subjects. Results from independent experiments of AA—$n = 14$; HS—$n = 15$; SNEA—$n = 10$. * $p < 0.05$ compared with adhesion of the healthy eosinophil group. Added blood serum: 2% of V/V. Statistical analysis: between investigated groups—Mann–Whitney two-sided *U*-test; within one study group—Wilcoxon matched-pairs signed-rank two-sided test.

Furthermore, we investigated the eosinophil adhesion effect on their survivability. We observed that 71.5% ± 1.1% of HS eosinophils are still viable after 24 h of incubation in serum-free growth medium, and that this amount is significantly lower when compared with the viability of AA and SNEA patients' eosinophils at 74.6% ± 0.5% and 77.1 ± 0.5%, respectively. The number of viable eosinophils increased significantly to 82.3% ± 0.4% in the AA group and to 74.2% ± 0.5% in the HS group when the medium was supplemented with 2% of *v*/*v* of the investigated subjects' blood serum ($p < 0.01$), but it had no effect on the SNEA patient group. Making co-cultures with ASM cells in serum-free medium had the same effect as blood serum—In the AA group, the number of viable eosinophils increased to 83.6% ± 0.4%; in the SNEA group, to 84.2% ± 0.4%; in the HS group, to 75.1% ± 0.8% ($p < 0.05$), and this effect in AA and SNEA groups was significantly greater compared with HS ($p < 0.05$). A similar effect was obtained when co-cultures of eosinophils were taken from AA and HS groups with pulmonary fibroblasts–viability increased to 82.3% ± 0.4% and 73.0% ± 1.2%, respectively, ($p < 0.05$). Supplementing co-culture growth medium with investigated subjects' blood serum did not have any additional effect on the viability of eosinophils (Figure 5).

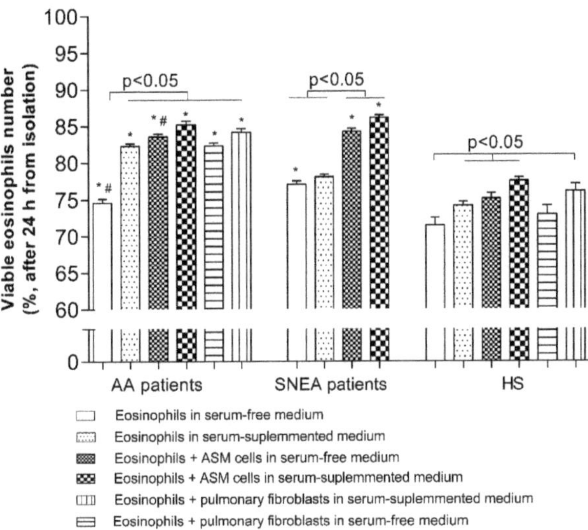

Figure 5. Eosinophil viability. Changes in the number of viable eosinophils during different incubation conditions. Results from independent experiments of AA—$n = 14$, HS—$n = 15$, SNEA—$n = 10$; AA—Allergic asthma, SNEA—Severe non-allergic eosinophilic asthma, HS—Healthy subjects. * $p < 0.05$ compared with the viability of the healthy eosinophil group; # $p < 0.05$ compared with the viability of the SNEA eosinophil group; Added blood serum—2% of v/v. Statistical analysis: between investigated groups—Mann–Whitney two-sided U-test; within one study group—Wilcoxon matched-pairs signed-rank two-sided test.

3.3. Eosinophil Effect on Pulmonary Structural Cell Proliferation and Apoptosis

After 72 h of co-culturing, eosinophils promoted ASM cell proliferation by 13.0% ± 2.4% in AA and 9.3% ± 3.2% in SNEA, and the effect was significantly higher compared to the HS group—proliferation increased by 4.0% ± 1.6% ($p < 0.05$). Supplementing growth medium with 2% of investigated subjects' blood serum had a positive effect on ASM cell proliferation. In the AA group, proliferation increased by 23.8% ± 7.0% if ASM cells were cultured alone in serum-supplemented medium and did not significantly different if they were cultured in serum-supplemented medium with eosinophils—proliferation increased by 27.2% ± 8.7%. The same results were received in the SNEA group (proliferation increased by 34.3% ± 10.8% and 28.1% ± 10.4%, $p < 0.05$) and the HS group (increased by 25.4% ± 5.7% and 30.8% ± 4.6%, $p < 0.05$). Moreover, supplementing serum-free growth medium with 25 nM of ascorbic acid significantly decreased ASM proliferation by 36.3% ± 11.6% in AA, 27.4% ± 17.6% in SNEA, and 22.3% ± 12.5% in the HS group. The combined cell culture with eosinophils did not change the ascorbic acid effect on ASM cell proliferation in the AA and SNEA groups (decreased by 33.9% ± 10.7% and 33.6% ± 14.8%, respectively) but removed its negative effect in the HS group (Figure 6A).

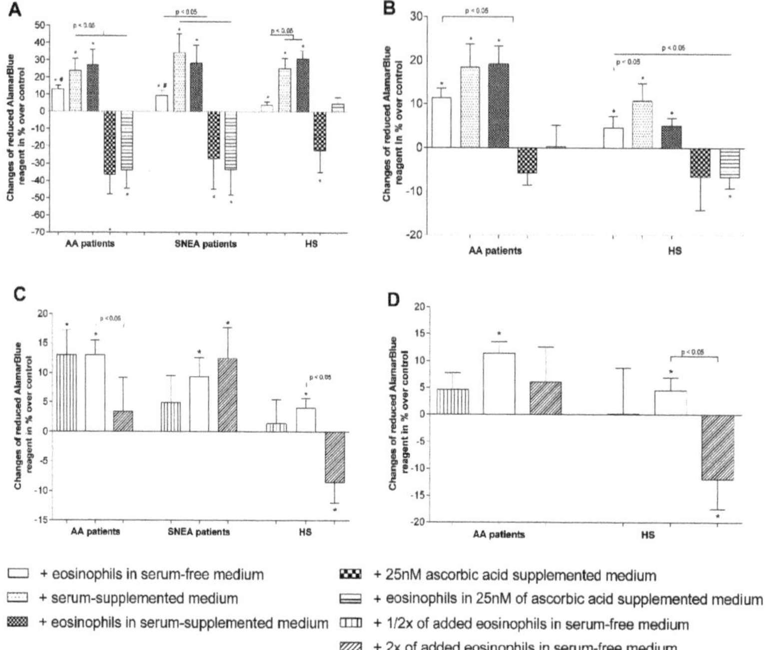

Figure 6. Eosinophils' effect on pulmonary structural cell proliferation. (**A**) Eosinophils' effect on ASM cell proliferation; (**B**) eosinophils' effect on pulmonary fibroblast proliferation; (**C**) the effect of adding a different eosinophil count on ASM cell proliferation; (**D**) the effect of adding a different eosinophil count on pulmonary fibroblast proliferation. Results from independent experiments of AA—$n = 14$, HS—$n = 15$, SNEA—$n = 10$. * $p < 0.05$ compared with control ASM cells or pulmonary fibroblasts without co-culturing with eosinophils, # $p < 0.05$ compared with the healthy subject group. Added eosinophils count—1/2x = 6,250, 1x = 12,500, 2x = 25,000. Added blood serum—2% of v/v. Ascorbic acid concentration—25 nM. Statistical analysis: between investigated groups—Mann-Whitney two-sided U-test; within one study group—Wilcoxon matched-pairs signed-rank two-sided test.

We measured the AA and HS eosinophil effect on the proliferation of another structural cell type—Pulmonary fibroblasts. We received similar results—Proliferation significantly increased by 11.4% ± 2.3% in AA and 4.6% ± 1.6% in HS groups after co-culturing with eosinophils. Supplementing growth medium with blood serum also had a positive effect—The pulmonary fibroblast cell number increased by 18.4% ± 5.3% and 10.8% ± 4% in the AA and HS groups, respectively. However, co-culturing with eosinophils in serum-supplemented growth medium increased proliferation by 19.2% ± 4.1% in the AA group, but in the HS group, the effect of eosinophils was the same as in serum-free medium. Different results, compared with co-cultures with ASM cells, were seen by evaluating the effect of ascorbic acid on the proliferation of pulmonary fibroblasts. In the AA group, fibroblasts did not lose their proliferative activity after supplementing growth medium with 25 nM of ascorbic acid; however, a significant decrease (6.5% ± 2.6%) was observed when measuring the effect of HS eosinophils on fibroblast proliferation in ascorbic acid-supplemented growth medium (Figure 6B).

Finally, we investigated how adding different quantities of eosinophils correlate with their effect on structural cell proliferation. We determined that in the AA group, half (1/2x) the number of eosinophils had a similar effect as a typically-used eosinophil number on ASM cell proliferation and increased it by 13.02% ± 4.2%; however, after using twice (2x) the number of eosinophils, the significant pro-proliferative effect was lost. By using pulmonary fibroblasts, the results were different—1/2x and 2x quantity of eosinophils had no positive effect on cell proliferation. In the SNEA group, we used only co-cultures with ASM cells and observed that a 1/2x quantity of eosinophils had no significant proliferative effect, but a 2x quantity increased ASM proliferation by 12.4% ± 5.2% ($p < 0.05$), without significant differences to the effect of a typically-used eosinophil number. In the HS group, we determined that a 1/2x quantity of eosinophils had no effect on ASM cells or pulmonary fibroblast proliferation; however, for a 2x eosinophil quantity, both cases significantly decreased the eosinophil proliferation by 8.5% ± 3.4% and 12.0% ± 5.5%, respectively ($p < 0.05$) (Figure 6C,D).

We investigated the mechanisms through which eosinophils affect pulmonary structural cell proliferation. We measured the eosinophil effect on pulmonary structural cell apoptosis after 24 h of co-culturing. Approximately 9.2% ± 0.6% of ASM cells and 7.5% ± 0.4% of pulmonary fibroblasts in culture are apoptotic after culturing and detachment procedures. After co-culturing with eosinophils, the apoptotic ASM cell number significantly ($p < 0.05$) decreased to 5.3% ± 0.5% in the AA patients group, to 4.0 ± 0.3 in the SNEA patients group ($p < 0.05$ compared with AA), but had no significant effect ($p = 0.14$) in the HS group. Co-culturing with eosinophils reduced the number of apoptotic pulmonary fibroblasts in the AA patient group by 5.5% ± 0.4% ($p < 0.05$) but had no effect in the HS group. Supplementing growth medium with blood serum (2% of v/v) of the investigated individuals enhanced the effect of eosinophils, and the apoptotic ASM cell number decreased from 7.9% ± 0.9% in serum-free medium to 4.9% ± 0.7% in serum-supplemented medium ($p < 0.05$). Unlike in the ASM cells group, supplementing growth medium with blood serum enhanced the effect of eosinophils on pulmonary fibroblasts only in the AA patients group—the apoptotic number reduced from 5.5% ± 0.4% to 3.7% ± 0.5% of the total cell count in culture. Moreover, considering that ascorbic acid is a well-known antioxidant and can eliminate the effect of the released reactive oxygen species of eosinophils on ASM cells or pulmonary fibroblast apoptosis, we supplemented the growth medium with a minimum of 25 nM of final concentration of ascorbic acid and obtained the result that the apoptotic ASM cell number increased to 11.1% ± 0.9% in the AA group, to 12.3% ± 1.1% in the SNEA patient group, and 11.2% ± 1.1% in the HS group ($p < 0.05$), as well as the pulmonary fibroblast number to 13.0% ± 2.4% in the AA patient group and 11.5% ± 1.0% in the HS group ($p < 0.05$) (Figure 7).

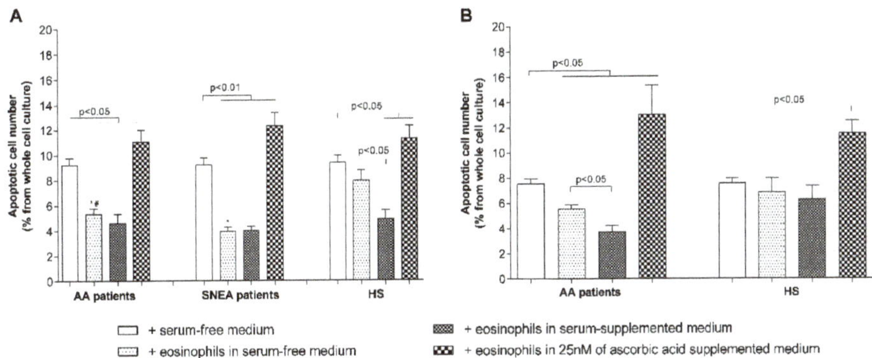

Figure 7. Eosinophils' effect on pulmonary structural cell apoptosis. (**A**) Apoptosis of ASM cells; (**B**) apoptosis of pulmonary fibroblasts. AA—Allergic asthma, SNEA—Severe non-allergic eosinophilic asthma, HS—Healthy subjects. Results from independent experiments of AA—n = 14, HS—n = 15, SNEA—n = 10. * $p < 0.05$ compared with the healthy eosinophils group; # $p < 0.05$ compared with the SNEA eosinophils group. Added blood serum—2% of v/v; ascorbic acid concentration—25 nM. Statistical analysis: between investigated groups—Mann–Whitney two-sided U-test; within one study group—Wilcoxon matched-pairs signed-rank two-sided test.

3.4. The Effect of Bronchial Allergen Challenge to Eosinophil Activity

The bronchial challenge with *D. pteronysinnus* allergen was performed for 11 individuals from the AA patient group and 11 individuals from the HS group. The effect of in vivo allergen provoked disease exacerbation to eosinophil activity and was evaluated by comparing the results before and 24 h after a bronchial allergen challenge of the same study subject. A significant increase was observed in the peripheral blood eosinophil count in the AA group following allergen exposure from $0.38 \pm 0.08 \times 10^9$/L to $0.45 \pm 0.06 \times 10^9$/L of cells, without significant changes in the HS group.

Eosinophil adhesion 24 h after a bronchial allergen challenge increased only in the AA group with no effect on HS eosinophils. The number of adhered eosinophils in co-cultures with ASM cells increased from 69.5% ± 5.4% to 87.06% ± 3.1% and in co-cultures with pulmonary fibroblasts from 59.4% ± 4.3% to 76.2% ± 4.2% of the total added eosinophil count ($p < 0.05$) (Figure 8).

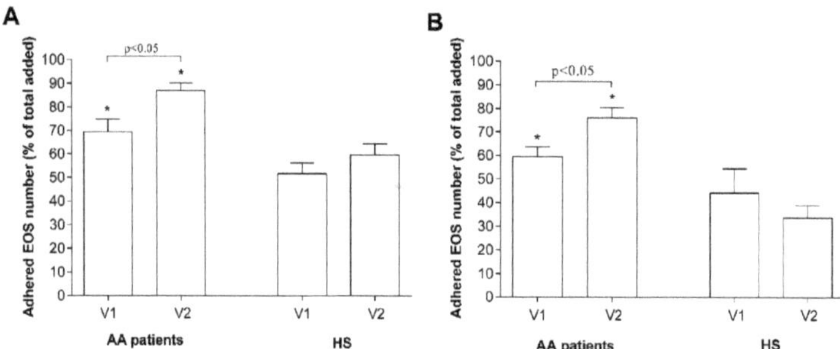

Figure 8. Bronchial allergen challenge effect on the efficiency of eosinophil adhesion. (**A**) Eosinophils adhesion in co-culture with ASM cells; (**B**) eosinophils adhesion in co-culture with pulmonary fibroblasts. Results from independent experiments of AA—n = 11, HS—n = 11; EOS—Eosinophils, AA—Allergic asthma, HS—Healthy subjects. * $p < 0.05$ compared with the adhesion of the healthy eosinophil group. V1—Visit 1 (before bronchial allergen challenge); V2—Visit 2 (24 h after bronchial allergen challenge). Statistical analysis: between investigated groups—Mann–Whitney two-sided U-test; within one study group—Wilcoxon matched-pairs signed-rank two-sided test.

A bronchial allergen challenge activated eosinophils in vivo and had a positive effect on AA patients eosinophils viability—The number of non-viable eosinophils decreased by 7.6% ± 1.8% if eosinophils were incubated alone or in serum-free growth medium ($p < 0.005$), but had no effect on healthy eosinophils. However, by using in vivo allergen-activated eosinophils and serum-supplemented growth medium, a positive effect was only obtained in the HS group (non-viable eosinophils number decreased by 6.3% ± 1.8%, $p < 0.01$), but had no effect on the AA patient group compared with non-activated eosinophils. Moreover, AA patients' allergen-activated eosinophil viability was increased if they were co-cultured with pulmonary structural cells in serum-free medium (non-viable eosinophils' number decreased by 7.6% ± 2.7% in co-culture with ASM cells, and by 8.3% ± 2.1% in co-culture with pulmonary fibroblasts, $p < 0.01$). Co-culturing in investigated subjects' blood serum-supplemented growth medium did not have any further effect on eosinophil viability (Figure 9).

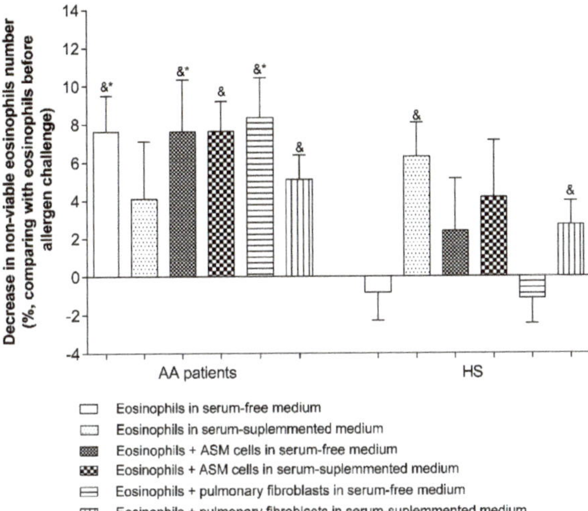

Figure 9. The bronchial allergen challenge effect on the number of non-viable eosinophils. Results from independent experiments of AA—$n = 11$, HS—$n = 11$; AA—Allergic asthma, HS—Healthy subjects. * $p < 0.05$ compared with the viability of the healthy eosinophil group; & $p < 0.05$ compared with the viability of eosinophils before the bronchial challenge. Added blood serum—2% of *v/v*. Statistical analysis: between investigated groups—Mann–Whitney two-sided U-test; within one study group—Wilcoxon matched-pairs signed-rank two-sided test.

Moreover, we evaluated in vivo the effect of activated AA and HS eosinophils on structural cell proliferation. We observed that eosinophils' pro-proliferative effect on ASM cells after a bronchial allergen challenge was enhanced by 11.6% ± 8.7% in the AA group and by 9.8% ± 4.1% in the HS group, compared with the effect of non-activated eosinophils. An enhanced pro-proliferative effect on pulmonary fibroblasts was only observed in the AA group (enhanced by 7.2% ± 2.5%), compared with the effect of non-activated eosinophils (Figure 10).

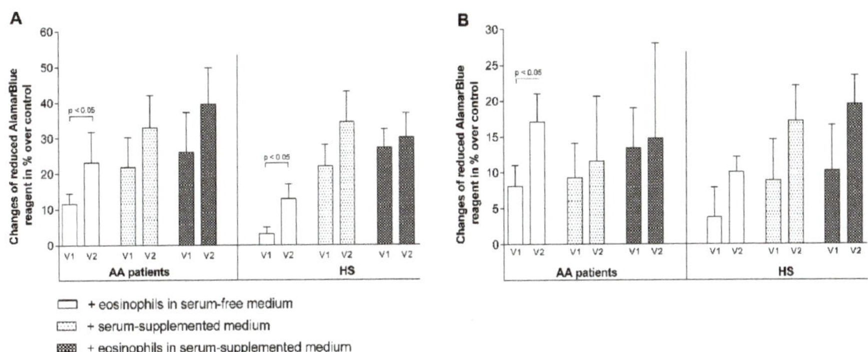

Figure 10. Bronchial allergen challenge effect on pulmonary structural cell proliferation. (**A**) The effect of a bronchial allergen challenge on eosinophil-promoted ASM cell proliferation; (**B**) the effect of a bronchial allergen challenge on eosinophil-promoted pulmonary fibroblast proliferation. Results from independent experiments of AA—$n = 11$, HS—$n = 11$; V1—Visit 1 (before the bronchial allergen challenge); V2—Visit 2 (24 h after the bronchial allergen challenge). Statistical analysis: between investigated groups—Mann–Whitney two-sided U-test; within one study group—Wilcoxon matched-pairs signed-rank two-sided test.

Finally, a bronchial allergen challenge enhanced the effect of eosinophils on the reduction of ASM cells and pulmonary fibroblast apoptosis. The apoptotic ASM cell number reduced from 5.5% ± 0.5% of the total cell count in culture, to 4.2% ± 0.4% in the AA patient group, and from 7.7% ± 0.7% to 5.8% ± 0.3% in the HS group. Meanwhile, the number of apoptotic pulmonary fibroblasts reduced from 5.3% ± 0.4% to 3.9% ± 0.4% in the AA patient group, and from 7.2% ± 1.3% to 4.7% ± 0.5% in the HS group. After supplementing growth medium with the blood serum of the investigated individuals—collected after the bronchial allergen challenge—the effect of eosinophils on the reduction of apoptosis in pulmonary fibroblasts was only enhanced in the AA patients group—the apoptotic cell number decreased from 3.7% ± 0.5% in serum-free medium to 1.8% ± 0.6% in serum-supplemented medium ($p < 0.05$) (Figure 11).

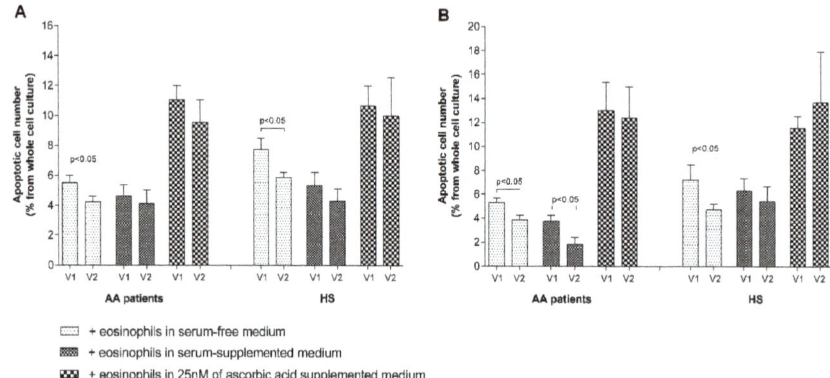

Figure 11. The effect of a bronchial allergen challenge on pulmonary structural cell apoptosis. (**A**) The effect of a bronchial allergen challenge on eosinophil-induced ASM cell apoptosis. (**B**) The effect of a bronchial allergen challenge on eosinophil-induced pulmonary fibroblast apoptosis. Results from independent experiments of AA—$n = 11$, HS—$n = 11$; V1—Visit 1 (before the bronchial allergen challenge); V2—Visit 2 (24 h after the bronchial allergen challenge). Added blood serum—2% of *v*/*v*; ascorbic acid concentration—25 nM. Statistical analysis: between investigated groups—Mann–Whitney two-sided U-test; within one study group—Wilcoxon matched-pairs signed-rank two-sided test.

4. Discussion

Increased eosinophil adhesion and prolonged viability in asthma could be the reason for the increased eosinophil number in asthmatic lungs because of their delayed migration to the bronchial lumen, which contributes to more intense development of airway remodeling. In this study, we found that adhesion of eosinophils of AA and SNEA patients to ASM cells or pulmonary fibroblasts was increased when compared to the HS group. Adhesion to pulmonary structural cells had a significant effect on prolonging the viability of eosinophils in all the investigated groups; however, the highest effect was observed in SNEA patients. Moreover, serum-activated eosinophils from AA and SNEA patients demonstrated an enhanced pro-proliferative effect on pulmonary structural cells. Furthermore, eosinophils from SNEA patients had a more pronounced effect on reducing apoptosis of ASM cells and pulmonary fibroblasts, however, with a similar pro-proliferative effect when compared with eosinophils from patients with AA. In the AA group, in vivo allergen-activated eosinophils demonstrated higher adhesion, viability, and pro-proliferative effects on pulmonary structural cells compared to non-activated eosinophils.

Airway eosinophilia is associated with more frequent exacerbations of asthma, which contributes to the development of airway remodeling [34–36]. Eosinophil infiltration from the circulation into the asthmatic airway depends on the activation sites of eosinophils, which leads to their arrest on activated endothelium, extravasation into the airway wall, and migration through airway tissues into the airway lumen. Airway eosinophils demonstrate increased activity of two main eosinophils integrins—$\alpha_4\beta_1$ and $\alpha_M\beta_2$ [37]; moreover, blood eosinophil integrins are found to be in a more-activated state during asthma [38]. Previously, we demonstrated that increased expression of eosinophil integrins in asthma leads to increased eosinophil adhesion and is associated with eosinophil-induced airway remodeling [22,23]. In the current study, we showed that in the bloodstream of the HS, between 40% and 50% of eosinophils exist, which could rapidly (within the hour) adhere onto other cell or ECM proteins, while during asthmatic conditions, this number increases to 60–70%, with no significant difference between AA and SNEA phenotypes (Figure 4A,B). Moreover, pre-activation of isolated eosinophils with mediators found in blood serum does not affect their adhesion properties; on the contrary, blood serum from SNEA patients reduced the maximum number of adhered eosinophils, probably because of the use of inhaled steroids. It demonstrates that eosinophils do not lose their activity during the isolation processes. Furthermore, eosinophil degranulation, assessed by EPO activity, did not statistically differ between the investigated groups; however, the EPO activity of eosinophils of SNEA patients is prone to decrease (Figure 4C).

Eosinophils adhere when their integrins recognize and connect to counter-receptors on other cells or ligands in the ECM proteins. However, there is a limited number of these counter-receptors that could restrict eosinophil adhesion. We showed that after increasing the number of more-adhesive eosinophils from AA and SNEA patients in the co-cultures, the ratio of adhered eosinophils to total added eosinophils significantly decreased and became the same as in the HS group (Figure 4A,B). We assumed that the management of pulmonary structural cell adhesion molecules and ECM component expression could play an important role by regulating eosinophil-induced airway structural changes. Increased eosinophil adhesion intensity could be explained by increased expression of outer membrane integrins [22] or by their different activation states [37,39]. Integrins exist in an inactive bent, an intermediate-activity extended closed, and a high-activity extended open conformation, and in that way modulate eosinophil adhesion and migration [40,41]. The severity of the disease or disease exacerbation could affect eosinophil's integrin expression and its activation states, contributing to eosinophil's further pro-inflammatory effect. However, it requires expanded investigation in a background of different asthma phenotypes and allergen-induced eosinophil activation.

Eosinophil's contribution to airway remodeling in asthma depends not only on its increased infiltration, but on its survivability in airways as well, which prolongs the effect of eosinophils on pulmonary structural cells. It was primarily described from several scientist teams, who revealed the importance of direct contact with pulmonary structural cells to their survivability, probably via signaling through GM-CSF and IL-1β [12–15]. Circulating eosinophils are contained in the mixture of various mediators found in peripheral blood, which regulates eosinophils' activation and survival. We found that AA and SNEA patients' eosinophils are characterized by greater survival compared with those of HS; moreover, the highest eosinophil viability was observed in the SNEA group (Figure 5). As eosinophils were incubated in serum-free growth medium, this demonstrated that SNEA patients' eosinophils had the strongest cytokine-induced survivability signals in peripheral blood. If eosinophils were incubated in investigated individual serum-supplemented medium, AA eosinophils' survival significantly increased and remained higher when compared with HS eosinophils. Blood serum enhanced eosinophils viability, thus demonstrating the healing process of isolated eosinophils if they are not pre-activated by mediators found in asthmatic blood serum. However, SNEA patients' blood serum had no effect on eosinophils' survival, probably due to fully-occupied survivability regulating receptors after eosinophil activation in vivo, or medications present in the blood serum (Figure 5).

Activation of eosinophilopoietin receptors [42] may not be the only factors regulating eosinophil viability. Adhesion through integrins can also be understood as a survival signal [43]. Incubation for 24 h with ASM cells or pulmonary fibroblasts significantly increased AA and SNEA patients' eosinophil viability, compared with eosinophils cultured alone, and the highest effect was observed in the SNEA patient group. This highlights the importance of contact with the opposite cell or their released extracellular matrix proteins on eosinophils' viability. Moreover, eosinophils equally adhere to ASM cells and pulmonary fibroblasts without preference for one cell type (Figure 4). However, more detailed research is needed to understand whether eosinophils adhere more to adhesion molecules on the surface of structural cells, or to specific sites on ECM proteins, and how this determines eosinophils' viability. Furthermore, a longer incubation period between eosinophils and structural cells should be used to find out how long eosinophils can stay viable for with or without an external stimulus in different asthma phenotypes.

Asthma-related airway remodeling mostly involves the airway epithelium, ASM, and extracellular matrix components [44]. As the number of eosinophils in asthmatic airways is enhanced, their role in disturbing local homeostasis is indisputable. It is known that ASM cells proliferate more during asthma; however, there is only minimal research showing that eosinophils influence this process [21–23]. Likewise, there is lack of information regarding the effect of eosinophils on pulmonary fibroblast proliferation [24], which could significantly contribute to ECM remodeling in asthma, as well as how eosinophils of SNEA patients affect pulmonary structural cell proliferation. When eosinophils migrate to the airways, the surrounding mediators might change, and further activation of eosinophils mostly depends on their activation in peripheral blood or pre-activation by released mediators of pulmonary structural cells. In the current study, we investigated the effect of eosinophils on ASM cells or pulmonary fibroblast proliferation in the context of individuals' blood serum that might maintain the initial activation of eosinophils. Our results demonstrated that eosinophils, isolated from SNEA patients, have the same effect on ASM cell proliferation as eosinophils isolated from AA patients. Moreover, both ASM cells and pulmonary fibroblasts respond similarly to the pro-proliferative effect of eosinophils (Figure 6A,B).

There are many mechanisms through which cell proliferation can be promoted [45]. One of the mechanisms revealed in this study demonstrated that eosinophils significantly inhibit pulmonary structural cell apoptosis in AA and SNEA groups, but not in HS (Figure 7A,B); however, the precise mechanism is unknown. Blood serum is important for structural cell proliferation and had a higher pro-proliferative effect compared with eosinophils in all the investigated groups. However, there is no exact information regarding the concentrations of mediators in the surrounding ASM cells and the pulmonary fibroblast environment in vivo, which could be different from those used in vitro. Apoptosis measurements also demonstrated that blood serum does not enhance the effect of eosinophils on reducing ASM cell apoptosis in the AA and SNEA groups, as these eosinophils did not lose their primary activity in peripheral blood after 24 h of incubation. However, less-activated eosinophils in the HS group were pre-activated by blood serum and demonstrated a more pronounced effect in reducing structural cell apoptosis (Figure 7A).

Eosinophils release not only remodeling-related mediators [1] but could also be toxic to many tissues because of released cytotoxic cationic proteins [46]. The best known and most accessible antioxidant is ascorbic acid, in which the blood levels are linked to asthma pathogenesis and its prevention [47,48]. A concentration of more than 100 nM ascorbic acid could be toxic to many cells while demonstrating a lower proliferative effect [49]. We used a concentration of only 25 nM ascorbic acid, avoiding possible changes in growth-medium pH levels. However, our data showed that ascorbic acid alone significantly reduced ASM cells, but not pulmonary fibroblast proliferation, which could be partially explained by the close interface between ascorbic acid and collagen synthesis [50]. In combination with eosinophils, a negative ascorbic acid effect on ASM cells was eliminated only in the HS group, but was evidenced for pulmonary fibroblasts. Moreover, eosinophils in ascorbic acid-supplemented medium significantly increased ASM cells and pulmonary fibroblast apoptosis in all the investigated groups (Figure 6A,B). However, there is no clear explanation of these results according to the literature data, and therefore more research should be done with different ascorbic acid concentrations and cell densities in co-cultures.

Eosinophils have two sides to their biological role that could be partly explained by existing distinct eosinophil phenotypes in peripheral blood and lung tissues [51] with different biological roles. One phenotype is inflammation-related, another one has a greater effect on the remodeling processes.

It shows that in the AA, SNEA, and HS groups there can exist different proportions of eosinophil phenotypes; therefore, an increased or decreased number of eosinophils in co-cultures disbalance the effect of the predominant phenotype effect (Figure 5C,D). In the AA group, a twofold reduced number of eosinophils had the same proliferative effect on ASM cells, but the effect was lost to pulmonary fibroblasts; however, a twofold increased number of eliminated eosinophils induced ASM cells and pulmonary fibroblast proliferation, probably due to an increased effect of the inflammation-related eosinophil phenotype. In the SNEA group, a reduced number of eosinophils had no effect on ASM proliferation, while normal and increased numbers of eosinophils had a similar positive effect. In the HS group, the reduced eosinophil number eliminated their effect on ASM cells and pulmonary fibroblast proliferation; however, a twofold increase in the number of eosinophils significantly reduced structural cell proliferation. Different ratios of eosinophil phenotypes in peripheral blood during AA, SNEA, and HS could explain these findings. In the HS group, as there should be less of specific disease-related signals for the attraction of homeostatic eosinophils, the predominant phenotype might be more inflammation-related eosinophils, which started to dominate after an increase in their count. With the SNEA group, the predominant phenotype was remodeling-related homeostatic eosinophils, and their proliferative effect correlated with their count, whereas in AA, the ratio should have been intermediate and increased the number of added eosinophils, eliminating the proliferation-promoting effect. However, the number of inflammatory eosinophils was not enough to reduce this effect (Figure 5C,D). Moreover, there is a lack of studies about different eosinophil phenotypes; therefore, more data is needed to confirm these results.

Asthma is a heterogeneous disease with multiple possible targets in its pathogenesis. AA severity is associated with the frequency of exacerbations after exposure to allergens that may contribute to the development of airway remodeling [52]. We sought to find out the role of eosinophils during an acute asthma episode, which is determined only by their quantitative differences or can be characterized by significant changes in their activity. During an allergen attack, released alarmins promote Th2 cells to produce eosinophilopoetins that may affect the number and functions of eosinophils [53]. Allergen-induced late asthmatic responses are mainly described by an increased number of airway inflammatory cells; however, the exact changes in eosinophil activity under allergen-induced disease exacerbation are mostly unknown. Our team previously demonstrated that during allergen-induced late-phase airway inflammation, peripheral blood eosinophils demonstrated further alterations of their functional activity, manifested by enhanced spontaneous reactive oxygen species production, increased chemotaxis, and diminished apoptosis in patients with AA [54]. Our findings show that the exposure of allergens activates AA patients' eosinophils in vivo, or they are released from bone marrow in a more activated state. They demonstrated increased adhesion and survivability properties and confirmed that after an acute episode, released eosinophils can survive in an asthmatic airway for a longer period (Figures 7 and 8). Moreover, allergen exposure had an effect on HS eosinophils, also promoting their viability, although subjects from the HS group were not sensitized to *D. pteronyssinus*. We used one of the most common home dust mite allergens with which the whole human population frequently comes into contact. It allowed us to assume that after a constant natural exposure of *D. pteronyssinus*, a memory of this allergen develops. The reaction of organisms to the high doses of inhaled concentrated allergen is too weak for bronchoconstriction; however, it is enough to slightly stimulate type-2 inflammation and activate eosinophils. This is important for future investigations, which should aim to understand possible AA development later in life.

More-enhanced eosinophil activity during allergen-induced asthma exacerbation required more intense disease treatment. Allergen-activated eosinophils demonstrated a twofold increased effect to ASM cells and pulmonary fibroblast proliferation via reduced apoptosis (Figures 9 and 10). It demonstrates that asthma exacerbation is associated with more intense development of airway remodeling via eosinophils' pro-proliferative effect. Tang and colleagues discovered that recruitment of eosinophils into asthmatic lungs during allergen-induced airway responses proceed via the IL-25/IL-25R axis and IL-25 neutralization and may be a potential therapeutic target for the attenuation of allergen-induced asthmatic responses mediated by airway eosinophilia [55]. However, there exists other well-known alarmins, such as IL-33 or thymic stromal lymphopoietin, that could also contribute to the recruitment of eosinophils into asthmatic lungs. Our findings suggest that eosinophil adhesion is important for their activity and effect on pulmonary structural cells; therefore, inhibiting their adhesion properties, together with chemotaxis, could be an effective way of attenuating their negative role during different asthma phenotypes and disease exacerbations.

5. Conclusions

Increased adhesion of eosinophils prolonged their viability, and might be related to enhancing their pro-proliferative effect on ASM cells and pulmonary fibroblasts in asthma. Moreover, eosinophils from SNEA patients demonstrated higher viability and inhibition of pulmonary structural cell apoptosis compared to the AA group, while the adhesive properties and pro-proliferative effects were similar for both. In the AA group, in vivo allergen-activated eosinophils presented enhanced adhesive properties, viability, and a pro-proliferative effect on pulmonary structural cells compared to non-activated eosinophils. These results could be important in the development of new therapeutic tools for the suppression of eosinophil functions in asthma, focusing not only on eosinophils' depletion but also on their survivability.

Author Contributions: Conceiving and designing the experiments: A.J., I.J., R.G., and K.M.; performing of the experiments: A.J. and I.J.; analyzing the experimental data: A.J. and K.M.; taking care of patients and analyzing clinical data: V.K.Z. and K.M.; contributing reagent/material/analysi tools: A.J. and I.J.; revising the manuscript for intellectual content: A.J., R.G., I.J., V.K.Z. and K.M.

Funding: This research received no external funding.

Acknowledgments: We are grateful to Airidas Rimkunas, Beatrice Tamasauskaite, Egle Jurkeviciute and Greta Gabuzeviciute for assistance in the experimental examination of study subjects.

Conflicts of Interest: The authors declare no conflict of interest.

References

1. McBrien, C.N.; Menzies-Gow, A. The biology of eosinophils and their role in asthma. *Front. Med.* **2017**, *4*, 93. [CrossRef] [PubMed]
2. Ravin, K.A.; Loy, M. The eosinophil in infection. *Clin. Rev. Allergy Immunol.* **2016**, *50*, 214–227. [CrossRef] [PubMed]
3. Marichal, T.; Mesnil, C.; Bureau, F. Homeostatic eosinophils: Characteristics and functions. *Front. Med.* **2017**, *4*, 101. [CrossRef] [PubMed]
4. Shearer, W.T.; Rosenwasser, L.J.; Bochner, B.S.; Martinez-Moczygemba, M.; Huston, D.P. Biology of common β receptor-signaling cytokines: IL-3, IL-5, and GM-CSF. *J. Allergy Clin. Immunol.* **2003**, *112*, 653–665. [CrossRef]
5. Farahi, N.; Singh, N.R.; Heard, S.; Loutsios, C.; Summers, C.; Solanki, C.K.; Solanki, K.; Balan, K.K.; Ruparelia, P.; Peters, A.M. Use of 111-Indium-labeled autologous eosinophils to establish the in vivo kinetics of human eosinophils in healthy subjects. *Blood* **2012**, *120*, 4068–4071. [CrossRef] [PubMed]
6. Carlens, J.; Wahl, B.; Ballmaier, M.; Bulfone-Paus, S.; Förster, R.; Pabst, O. Common γ-chain-dependent signals confer selective survival of eosinophils in the murine small intestine. *J. Immunol.* **2009**, *183*, 5600–5607. [CrossRef] [PubMed]
7. Bagley, C.J.; Lopez, A.F.; Vadas, M.A. New frontiers for IL-5. *J. Allergy Clin. Immunol.* **1997**, *99*, 725–728. [CrossRef]
8. Valerius, T.; Repp, R.; Kalden, J.R.; Platzer, E. Effects of IFN on human eosinophils in comparison with other cytokines. A novel class of eosinophil activators with delayed onset of action. *J. Immunol.* **1990**, *145*, 2950–2958. [PubMed]
9. Smith, C.A.; Farrah, T.; Goodwin, R.G. The TNF receptor superfamily of cellular and viral proteins: Activation, costimulation, and death. *Cell* **1994**, *76*, 959–962. [CrossRef]
10. Conus, S.; Bruno, A.; Simon, H.U. Leptin is an eosinophil survival factor. *J. Allergy Clin. Immunol.* **2005**, *116*, 1228–1234. [CrossRef]

11. Bureau, F.; Seumois, G.; Jaspar, F.; Vanderplasschen, A.; Detry, B.; Pastoret, P.P.; Louis, R.; Lekeux, P. CD40 engagement enhances eosinophil survival through induction of cellular inhibitor of apoptosis protein 2 expression: Possible involvement in allergic inflammation. *J. Allergy Clin. Immunol.* **2002**, *110*, 443–449. [CrossRef] [PubMed]
12. Zhang, S.; Mohammed, Q.; Burbidge, A.; Morland, C.; Roche, W. Cell cultures from bronchial subepithelial myofibroblasts enhance eosinophil survival in vitro. *Eur. Respir. J.* **1996**, *9*, 1839–1846. [CrossRef] [PubMed]
13. Vancheri, C.; Gauldie, J.; Bienenstock, J.; Cox, G.; Scicchitano, R.; Stanisz, A.; Jordana, M. Human lung fibroblast-derived granulocyte-macrophage colony stimulating factor (GM-CSF) mediates eosinophil survival in vitro. *Am. J. Respir. Cell Mol. Biol.* **1989**, *1*, 289–295. [CrossRef] [PubMed]
14. Solomon, A.; Shmilowich, R.; Shasha, D.; Frucht–Pery, J.; Pe'er, J.; Bonini, S.; Levi–Schaffer, F. Conjunctival fibroblasts enhance the survival and functional activity of peripheral blood eosinophils in vitro. *Investig. Ophthalmol. Vis. Sci.* **2000**, *41*, 1038–1044.
15. Hallsworth, M.P.; Soh, C.P.; Twort, C.H.; Lee, T.H.; Hirst, S.J. Cultured human airway smooth muscle cells stimulated by interleukin-1 β enhance eosinophil survival. *Am. J. Respir. Cell Mol. Biol.* **1998**, *19*, 910–919. [CrossRef] [PubMed]
16. Ahmadzai, M.; Small, M.; Sehmi, R.; Gauvreau, G.; Janssen, L.J. Integrins are mechanosensors that modulate human eosinophil activation. *Front. Immunol.* **2015**, *6*, 525. [CrossRef]
17. Meerschaert, J.; Vrtis, R.F.; Shikama, Y.; Sedgwick, J.B.; Busse, W.W.; Mosher, D.F. Engagement of α4β7 integrins by monoclonal antibodies or ligands enhances survival of human eosinophils in vitro. *J. Immunol.* **1999**, *163*, 6217–6227.
18. Postma, D.S.; Timens, W. Remodeling in asthma and chronic obstructive pulmonary disease. *Proc. Am. Thorac. Soc.* **2006**, *3*, 434–439. [CrossRef]
19. Trejo Bittar, H.E.; Yousem, S.A.; Wenzel, S.E. Pathobiology of severe asthma. *Ann. Rev. Pathol. Mech. Dis.* **2015**, *10*, 511–545. [CrossRef]
20. Murphy, D.M.; O'Byrne, P.M. Recent advances in the pathophysiology of asthma. *Chest* **2010**, *137*, 1417–1426. [CrossRef]
21. Halwani, R.; Vazquez-Tello, A.; Sumi, Y.; Pureza, M.A.; Bahammam, A.; Al-Jahdali, H.; Soussi-Gounni, A.; Mahboub, B.; Al-Muhsen, S.; Hamid, Q. Eosinophils induce airway smooth muscle cell proliferation. *J. Clin. Immunol.* **2013**, *33*, 595–604. [CrossRef] [PubMed]
22. Januskevicius, A.; Gosens, R.; Sakalauskas, R.; Vaitkiene, S.; Janulaityte, I.; Halayko, A.J.; Hoppenot, D.; Malakauskas, K. Suppression of eosinophil integrins prevents remodeling of airway smooth muscle in asthma. *Front. Physiol.* **2017**, *7*, 680. [CrossRef] [PubMed]
23. Januskevicius, A.; Vaitkiene, S.; Gosens, R.; Janulaityte, I.; Hoppenot, D.; Sakalauskas, R.; Malakauskas, K. Eosinophils enhance WNT-5a and TGF-β 1 genes expression in airway smooth muscle cells and promote their proliferation by increased extracellular matrix proteins production in asthma. *BMC Pulm. Med.* **2016**, *16*, 94. [CrossRef] [PubMed]
24. Shock, A.; Rabe, K.; Dent, G.; Chambers, R.; Gray, A.; Chung, K.; Barnes, P.; Laurent, G. Eosinophils adhere to and stimulate replication of lung fibroblasts 'in vitro'. *Clin. Exp. Immunol.* **1991**, *86*, 185–190. [CrossRef] [PubMed]
25. Boyce, J.A.; Barrett, N.A. Cysteinyl leukotrienes: An innate system for epithelial control of airway smooth muscle proliferation? *Am. Thorac. Soc.* **2015**, *191*, 496–497. [CrossRef] [PubMed]
26. Cheng, W.; Yan, K.; Xie, L.Y.; Chen, F.; Yu, H.C.; Huang, Y.X.; Dang, C.X. MiR-143-3p controls TGF-β1-induced cell proliferation and extracellular matrix production in airway smooth muscle via negative regulation of the nuclear factor of activated T cells 1. *Mol. Immunol.* **2016**, *78*, 133–139. [CrossRef] [PubMed]
27. Westerhof, G.A.; Korevaar, D.A.; Amelink, M.; de Nijs, S.B.; de Groot, J.C.; Wang, J.; Weersink, E.J.; ten Brinke, A.; Bossuyt, P.M.; Bel, E.H. Biomarkers to identify sputum eosinophilia in different adult asthma phenotypes. *Eur. Respir. J.* **2015**, *46*, 688–696. [CrossRef]
28. Brusselle, G.G.; Maes, T.; Bracke, K.R. Eosinophils in the spotlight: Eosinophilic airway inflammation in nonallergic asthma. *Nat. Med.* **2013**, *19*, 977. [CrossRef]
29. Rosenberg, H.F.; Phipps, S.; Foster, P.S. Eosinophil trafficking in allergy and asthma. *J. Allergy Clin. Immunol.* **2007**, *119*, 1303–1310. [CrossRef]
30. Koenderman, L. Priming: A Critical Step in the Control of Eosinophil Activation. In *Eosinophils in Health and Disease*; Lee, J., Rosenberg, H., Eds.; Elsevier: Boston, MA, USA, 2013; pp. 170–178.

31. Gosens, R.; Stelmack, G.L.; Dueck, G.; McNeill, K.D.; Yamasaki, A.; Gerthoffer, W.T.; Unruh, H.; Gounni, A.S.; Zaagsma, J.; Halayko, A.J. Role of caveolin-1 in p42/p44 MAP kinase activation and proliferation of human airway smooth muscle. *Am. J. Physiol. Lung Cell Mol. Physiol.* **2006**, *291*, L523–L534. [CrossRef]
32. White, S.R.; Kulp, G.V.; Spaethe, S.M.; Van Alstyne, E.; Leff, A.R. A kinetic assay for eosinophil peroxidase activity in eosinophils and eosinophil conditioned media. *J. Immunol. Methods* **1991**, *144*, 257–263. [CrossRef]
33. Krug, N.; Napp, U.; Enander, I.; Eklund, E.; Rieger, C.; Schauer, U. Intracellular expression and serum levels of eosinophil peroxidase (EPO) and eosinophil cationic protein in asthmatic children. *Clin. Exp. Allergy* **1999**, *29*, 1507–1515. [CrossRef] [PubMed]
34. Busse, W.W.; Ring, J.; Huss-Marp, J.; Kahn, J.E. A review of treatment with mepolizumab, an anti-IL-5 mAb, in hypereosinophilic syndromes and asthma. *J. Allergy Clin. Immunol.* **2010**, *125*, 803–813. [CrossRef] [PubMed]
35. Pavord, I.D.; Korn, S.; Howarth, P.; Bleecker, E.R.; Buhl, R.; Keene, O.N.; Ortega, H.; Chanez, P. Mepolizumab for severe eosinophilic asthma (DREAM): A multicentre, double-blind, placebo-controlled trial. *Lancet* **2012**, *380*, 651–659. [CrossRef]
36. Negewo, N.A.; McDonald, V.M.; Baines, K.J.; Wark, P.A.; Simpson, J.L.; Jones, P.W.; Gibson, P.G. Peripheral blood eosinophils: A surrogate marker for airway eosinophilia in stable COPD. *Int. J. Chronic Obstr. Pulm. Dis.* **2016**, *11*, 1495. [CrossRef] [PubMed]
37. Johansson, M.W.; Mosher, D.F. Integrin activation states and eosinophil recruitment in asthma. *Front. Pharmacol.* **2013**, *4*, 33. [CrossRef] [PubMed]
38. Johansson, M.W.; Han, S.T.; Gunderson, K.A.; Busse, W.W.; Jarjour, N.N.; Mosher, D.F. Platelet activation, P-selectin, and eosinophil β1-integrin activation in asthma. *Am. J. Respir. Crit. Care Med.* **2012**, *185*, 498–507. [CrossRef] [PubMed]
39. Johansson, M.W.; Kelly, E.A.; Busse, W.W.; Jarjour, N.N.; Mosher, D.F. Up-regulation and activation of eosinophil integrins in blood and airway after segmental lung antigen challenge. *J. Immunol.* **2008**, *180*, 7622–7635. [CrossRef] [PubMed]
40. Luo, B.H.; Springer, T.A. Integrin structures and conformational signaling. *Curr. Opin. Cell Biol.* **2006**, *18*, 579–586. [CrossRef] [PubMed]
41. Askari, J.A.; Buckley, P.A.; Mould, A.P.; Humphries, M.J. Linking integrin conformation to function. *J. Cell Sci.* **2009**, *122*, 165–170. [CrossRef] [PubMed]
42. Asquith, K.L.; Ramshaw, H.S.; Hansbro, P.M.; Beagley, K.W.; Lopez, A.F.; Foster, P.S. The IL-3/IL-5/GM-CSF common β receptor plays a pivotal role in the regulation of Th2 immunity and allergic airway inflammation. *J. Immunol.* **2008**, *180*, 1199–1206. [CrossRef] [PubMed]
43. Byron, A.; Morgan, M.R.; Humphries, M.J. Adhesion signalling complexes. *Curr. Biol.* **2010**, *20*, R1063–R1067. [CrossRef] [PubMed]
44. Bergeron, C.; Boulet, L.P. Structural changes in airway diseases: Characteristics, mechanisms, consequences and pharmacologic modulation. *Chest* **2006**, *129*, 1068–1087. [CrossRef] [PubMed]
45. Duronio, R.J.; Xiong, Y. Signaling pathways that control cell proliferation. *Cold Spring Harb. Perspect. Biol.* **2013**, *5*, a008904. [CrossRef] [PubMed]
46. Rothenberg, M.E.; Hogan, S.P. The eosinophil. *Annu. Rev. Immunol.* **2006**, *24*, 147–174. [CrossRef] [PubMed]
47. Aderele, W.; Ette, S.; Oduwole, O.; Ikpeme, S. Plasma vitamin C (ascorbic acid) levels in asthmatic children. *Afr. J. Med. Med. Sci.* **1985**, *14*, 115–120. [PubMed]
48. Checkley, W.; Deza, M.P.; Klawitter, J.; Romero, K.M.; Klawitter, J.; Pollard, S.L.; Wise, R.A.; Christians, U.; Hansel, N.N. Identifying biomarkers for asthma diagnosis using targeted metabolomics approaches. *Respir. Med.* **2016**, *121*, 59–66. [CrossRef]
49. HATA, R.I.; Sunada, H.; Arai, K.; Sato, T.; Ninomiya, Y.; Nagai, Y.; Senoo, H. Regulation of collagen metabolism and cell growth by epidermal growth factor and ascorbate in cultured human skin fibroblasts. *Eur. J. Biochem.* **1988**, *173*, 261–267. [CrossRef] [PubMed]
50. Chan, D.; Lamande, S.R.; Cole, W.; Bateman, J.F. Regulation of procollagen synthesis and processing during ascorbate-induced extracellular matrix accumulation in vitro. *Biochem. J.* **1990**, *269*, 175–181. [CrossRef]
51. Mesnil, C.; Raulier, S.; Paulissen, G.; Xiao, X.; Birrell, M.A.; Pirottin, D.; Janss, T.; Starkl, P.; Ramery, E.; Henket, M. Lung-resident eosinophils represent a distinct regulatory eosinophil subset. *J. Clin. Investig.* **2016**, *126*, 3279–3295. [CrossRef]

52. Castillo, J.R.; Peters, S.P.; Busse, W.W. Asthma Exacerbations: Pathogenesis, Prevention, and Treatment. *J. Allergy Clin. Immunol. Pract.* **2017**, *5*, 918–927. [CrossRef] [PubMed]
53. Lambrecht, B.N.; Hammad, H. The immunology of asthma. *Nat. Immunol.* **2015**, *16*, 45. [CrossRef] [PubMed]
54. Lavinskiene, S.; Malakauskas, K.; Jeroch, J.; Hoppenot, D.; Sakalauskas, R. Functional activity of peripheral blood eosinophils in allergen-induced late-phase airway inflammation in asthma patients. *J. Inflamm.* **2015**, *12*, 25. [CrossRef] [PubMed]
55. Tang, W.; Smith, S.G.; Salter, B.; Oliveria, J.P.; Mitchell, P.; Nusca, G.M.; Howie, K.; Gauvreau, G.M.; O'Byrne, P.M.; Sehmi, R. Allergen-induced increases in interleukin-25 and interleukin-25 receptor expression in mature eosinophils from atopic asthmatics. *Int. Arch. Allergy Immunol.* **2016**, *170*, 234–242. [CrossRef] [PubMed]

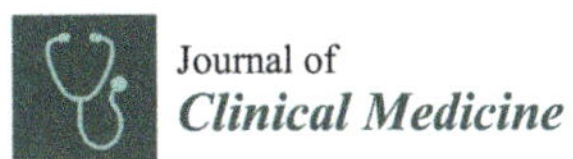
Journal of
Clinical Medicine

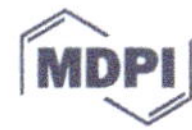

Review

Severe Eosinophilic Asthma

Agamemnon Bakakos, Stelios Loukides and Petros Bakakos *

Department of Respiratory Medicine, National and Kapodistrian University of Athens, 10561 Athens, Greece
* Correspondence: petros44@hotmail.com

Received: 25 July 2019; Accepted: 29 August 2019; Published: 2 September 2019

Abstract: Asthma is a heterogeneous disease with varying severity. Severe asthma is a subject of constant research because it greatly affects patients' quality of life, and patients with severe asthma experience symptoms, exacerbations, and medication side effects. Eosinophils, although at first considered insignificant, were later specifically associated with features of the ongoing inflammatory process in asthma, particularly in the severe case. In this review, we discuss new insights into the pathogenesis of severe asthma related to eosinophilic inflammation and the pivotal role of cytokines in a spectrum that is usually referred to as "T2-high inflammation" that accounts for almost half of patients with severe asthma. Recent literature is summarized as to the role of eosinophils in asthmatic inflammation, airway remodeling, and airway hypersensitivity. Major advances in the management of severe asthma occurred the past few years due to the new targeted biological therapies. Novel biologics that are already widely used in severe eosinophilic asthma are discussed, focusing on the choice of the right treatment for the right patient. These monoclonal antibodies primarily led to a significant reduction of asthma exacerbations, as well as improvement of lung function and patient quality of life.

Keywords: severe asthma; eosinophil; inflammation; interleukin-5 (IL-5); anti-IL-5; interleukin-4

---

1. Severe Asthma and Eosinophils

It is well established that asthma is a disease with a great spectrum of symptoms among patients and wide differences in treatment efficacy. In particular, severe asthma is noted to include various specific phenotypes and endotypes, which differ in their clinical presentation, their unique pathogenetic mechanisms, and their responsiveness to treatment [1]. In order to determine the severity of asthma, it is crucial to evaluate patients' responsiveness to the controller therapy, such as inhaled corticosteroids (ICS) and long-acting β2 agonists (LABA). In other words, clinicians need to evaluate how difficult it is to control asthma symptoms and exacerbations [2]. Therefore, severe asthma presents a challenge as it is defined as a disease which cannot be handled by conventional means of treatment—a medium–high dose of ICS combined with LABA or even oral corticosteroids [3]. A different approach has to be taken to improve asthma outcomes in these patients, and researchers began analyzing the cellular mechanisms that characterize severe asthma. The results were quite intriguing, as they yielded a number of different "types" of severe asthma which have to be recognized and treated accordingly. Eosinophils emerged as the hallmark of a prevalent type of severe asthma, which also involves T cells (T helper 2 (Th2) mainly, but also type 2 innate lymphoid cells) and was labeled the T2-high endotype [4].

Eosinophils were described almost 150 years ago by Paul Ehrlich as granulocytic leucocytes with a bilobed nucleus. Their primary location is within tissue and not in the bone marrow, residing mostly in the gastrointestinal tract in normal conditions [5]. They contain numerous cationic proteins, with four being the most notable: major basic protein (MBP), eosinophil cationic protein (ECP), eosinophil peroxidase (EPO), and eosinophil-derived neurotoxin (EDN); they are mostly associated with parasitic infections, since they have the ability to orchestrate the immune response against helminths in a Th2 cytokine cascade, very similar to that in asthmatic patients with the Th2 endotype [6]. This cascade commences when immunoglobulin E (IgE) reacts with an antigen; although, in helminthic infections, the antigen is indeed threatening for the host, in asthmatic patients, IgE targets are rather innocuous agents such as tree pollen or animal fur. Nevertheless, IgE activates mast cells, macrophages, and basophils, which in turn lead to the production of histamine and other inflammatory cytokines. The ongoing inflammatory process attracts cluster of differentiation 4 $(CD4)^+$ T cells and more eosinophils to the site of damage in this aberrant reaction, leading to the Th2-high endotype of severe asthma with high blood and sputum eosinophils [7].

2. Eosinophil Production and Development in the Bone Marrow

First of all, it is important to distinguish the two major types of eosinophils in the lungs. Even though the simplistic view we had in the past about eosinophils is still viable, recent studies showed that, except for eosinophils that emerge from the bone marrow and are directly recruited to sites of inflammation, a distinct type of eosinophil with different characteristics resides in tissues in homeostatic conditions. This eosinophil population is called "homeostatic eosinophils" (hEos) [8]. These hEos were mostly examined in mice, and they differ from the regular inflammatory eosinophils (iEos). Both of these populations are produced in the bone marrow from the $CD34^+$ progenitor stem cells and specialized $CD34^+$ interleukin-5 receptor $(IL\text{-}5R)^+$ hematopoietic progenitor cells via a complex activation of transcription factors, the most important being GATA-1, PU.1, and CAAT enhancer-binding proteins α and ε [9]. Notably, the actions of GATA-1 and PU.1 are antagonistic regarding the differentiation of other hematopoietic cells; nevertheless, they synergize when it comes to eosinophil production, as it was shown in studies where in vitro enhancement of PU.1 resulted in an amplified GATA-1 transcriptomic effect [10].

Several cytokines also take part in the development of eosinophils apart from the transcription factors previously mentioned, IL-5, IL-3, and GM-CSF(Granulocyte-macrophage colony-stimulating factor). IL-3 and GM-CSF are not selective, and they stimulate the development of other leucocytes such as neutrophils and macrophages more efficiently; however, IL-5 solely affects eosinophils and basophils [11]. The major difference in the production and recruitment of the two eosinophil populations is that hEos are differentiated in the bone marrow semi-independently from IL-5, while iEos need IL-5 in order to be produced from their precursor cells and trafficked to the lungs [12]. This was proven in IL-5 knock-out (KO) mice which could not produce a Th2-high response due to the lack of IL-5, but the number of hEos in the lung was only reduced by half, meaning that they could be recruited via different pathways. It also explains why, in patients treated with an anti-IL-5 agent, eosinophils can still be found in both their blood and lungs [13]. Moreover, stimulation of $CD34^+$ progenitor cells with IL-3, IL-5, and GM-CSF resulted in an upregulation of the IL-5R in these stem cells, thus prolonging eosinophil differentiation as long as they were stimulated by IL-5 [14]. However, mice that were lacking GM-CSF/IL-3/IL-5 functions were not observed to have a complete halt of eosinophil production. Instead, these mice had the ability to produce low numbers of eosinophils, indicating that there are more unidentified factors taking part in their development [15].

Even more interesting is the observation that hEos do not take active part in the allergic inflammation, as well as halting this aberrant response. They express several genes that cannot be found in the normal iEos that take part in the immunoregulation of lung and reduce the Th2 response after contact with allergens. Mice who were stripped of the prevalent eosinophil production gene (ΔdblGATA) showed a more severe allergic reaction after contact with dust mites, proving that hEos do not participate in the inflammatory process and they also downregulate the Th2 response, most probably by inhibiting the functionality of dendritic cells [12].

3. Eosinophil Migration to the Lung

Eosinophil trafficking from the bone marrow to the lungs is the first major step of the blooming inflammatory process. Even though various chemoattractants were discovered, most of them are not selective and can also draw other leucocytes. Activated Th2 cells and type 2 innate lymphoid cells (ILC2) synthesize IL-4, IL-5, and IL-13, while eotaxin-1 (CCL11) is produced by epithelial and endothelial cells after an allergen challenge. Specifically, IL-5 and eotaxin-1 play a pivotal role in eosinophil trafficking and synergize in promoting lung eosinophilia [16]. Although IL-4 is not a direct eosinophil mediator, it is crucial in the activation of the IgE cascade while also promoting the development of more Th2 lymphocytes, thus sustaining the migratory process [17]. The same applies to IL-13 as it induces eotaxin production [18].

IL-5 is the most crucial cytokine not only in recruiting eosinophils but also in prolonging their survival in tissues. This was observed in IL-5 KO mice which showed a greatly reduced number of eosinophils in the lungs when compared to IL-5 transgenic mice [19,20]. This is largely attributed to the IL-5 receptor that is also expressed in mature eosinophils apart from their progenitors, thus being able to respond to the stimulus of the cytokine via a Janus kinase signal transducer and prolong their half-life ($T_{1/2}$) by almost 50% [21]. IL-5 was also administered routinely to guinea pigs over a period of time, resulting in a reduction of eosinophils in the bone marrow and a concomitant increase of their number in circulation, indicating that it clearly mobilizes them and aids their trafficking into tissues [22]. It is synthesized mostly by activated Th2 lymphocytes and in smaller proportions by eosinophils and mast cells. IL-5 is already the primary target of monoclonal antibody treatment in asthmatic patients, highlighting even more its central role in the pathogenesis of the T2-high inflammatory response. Another source of IL-5 is innate lymphocytes termed ILC-2 cells that may initiate or amplify eosinophilic inflammation. These cells may also produce other Th2-related cytokines such as IL-4, IL-9, and IL-13. That is why the cytokine pattern above is usually termed as T2 instead of Th2 [23].

Eotaxin-1 was first described as a novel component in the bronchoalveolar lavage (BAL) of guinea pigs sensitized and challenged by ovalbumin and was later isolated from human tissue as well. It was the first eosinophil-specific chemoattractant discovered until two more CC chemokines named eotaxin-2 and eotaxin-3 were isolated later on [24]. Eotaxins are produced by epithelial cells of the lung but also in lower numbers by eosinophils, mast cells, macrophages of the alveoli, vascular endothelial cells, and smooth muscle cells of the airways after stimulation by IL-4 and IL-13 [25]. Eosinophils express receptors for the CC groups of chemokines, a classic G-protein transmembrane receptor, while eotaxins interact specifically with the CCR3 receptor and synergize with IL-5 and between themselves, in order to recruit eosinophils to the lungs [26]. It should be noted that the CCR3 receptor is constantly expressed on the eosinophil membrane, but its expression is further increased after an inflammatory stimulus [27]. Characteristically, it was demonstrated that the airways of asthmatic patients have a higher number of cells producing messenger RNA (mRNA) for CCR3 and its ligands, compared to healthy individuals [28]. Other cells expressing CCR3 receptors are basophils, mast cells, Th2 cells, and eosinophil progenitor cells. Activation of the CCR3 receptor by eotaxin results in the internalization of the ligand and induces chemotaxis via calcium mobilization and actin polymerization [29]. Studies showed that all three eotaxins are upregulated after an allergen challenge and have a pivotal role in different phases of the immune response.

Eotaxin-1 is needed in the first steps of the inflammatory response, whereas eotaxins 2 and 3 are needed to prolong eosinophil survival later on [30]. Their synergistic role is clearly demonstrated in studies between single eotaxin-1 or eotaxin-2 KO mice and both eotaxin 1 and 2 KO mice. The latter group had far fewer eosinophils in their lungs after an allergen challenge when compared to the single KO group [31]. Eotaxin-1 is also crucial in mobilizing eosinophils from the bone marrow, with its levels being correlated with the eosinophil number in blood and lungs in pig specimens. However, inhibition of IL-5 in those pigs showed that eotaxin-1 alone cannot mobilize eosinophils from the bone marrow, thus highlighting the importance of the cooperation between those two chemokines [32]. The same applies to their mobilization from circulation to tissues, since administration of eotaxin-1 without abolishing IL-5 effects increases blood eosinophilia but fails to increase their number in tissue. On the contrary, administration of IL-5 without abolishing eotaxin-1 demonstrated a notably higher number of tissue eosinophils, further underlining the important role of IL-5 in the tissue infiltration process [33]. Eotaxin-2 synergizes with IL-5 and drives the production of IL-13, with which it later synergizes to promote lung eosinophilia [34]. Eotaxin-3 levels start to rise at a later time, and it is thought to prolong the eosinophil recruitment in lungs [35]. The CCR3 receptor was targeted for the development of new targeted treatment of asthma, since it is expressed in all the cells taking part in the inflammatory process, making it evident that blocking the eotaxin/CCR3 axis might prove greatly important in future trials.

Eosinophils, which are found in circulation after being mobilized mostly by IL-5 and eotaxin-1 as previously mentioned, still need to migrate from the vasculature to the lung tissue. In this phase, several eosinophil-specific adhesion molecules with the most important being the β1 integrin very late antigen (VLA-4), the vascular cell adhesion molecule (VCAM-1), and the P-selectin glycoprotein ligand (PSGL-1) play an important role [36]. VLA-4 is an integrin which is expressed on the membrane of eosinophils after a stimulus from eotaxin-1. It ligands with the VCAM-1 integrin expressed at the vasculature membrane, resulting in the activation and firm adhesion of eosinophils to it, aiding their transit from the endothelium to tissues [36]. Usage of inhibitors of the VLA-4 and VCAM-1 interaction in mice studies showed a greatly reduced inflammatory response and eosinophil number in lungs, compared to normal mice [37]. Apparently, this ligand is a selective eosinophil adhesion chemokine, since it does not cause the adhesion of other leucocytes to the endothelium; therefore, more research is needed as to whether a VLA-4/VCAM-1 inhibitor could be used in the treatment of severe eosinophilic asthma. PSGL-1 on the other hand binds to P-selectin and modulates the first steps of the interaction between eosinophils and the endothelium, more specifically the rolling and adhesion stages. It is also solely expressed by eosinophils, which means that tampering with the PSGL-1/P-selectin ligand can reduce the transit of eosinophils to tissue. Trials were conducted in mice with ablation of the P-selectin gene and, indeed, those mice had fewer eosinophils in their lungs [38]. Inhibitors targeting this selectin ligand are currently being investigated in clinical trials; however, they are yet to yield promising results.

Recent studies highlighted the fact that eosinophilopoiesis can also occur in situ in the airways of severe asthmatics, since the number of $CD34^+$ and $CD34^+$ IL-5Rα^+ hematopoietic progenitor cells was much higher in this population's sputum when compared to mild asthmatics. Even more interesting was the fact that eosinophil progenitor cells did not vanish after anti-IL-5 treatment in these patients, which means that in situ eosinophilopoiesis is an important mechanism of persistent eosinophilia in the airways [39]. This could be attributed to the action of bronchial epithelial cells which, after being triggered by an extraneous stimulus, produce several cytokines, such as IL-25 and IL-33, along with thymic stromal lymphoid proteins (TSLPs) known as alarmins. Their expression was found to be higher in the airways of asthmatic patients, while they also correlate with disease severity [40]. The T2 cascade is sustained by the production of these alarmins, since they can promote eosinophil progenitor cell recruitment and trigger T2 cells, especially ILC2 cells, in producing IL-4, IL-5, and IL-13 [41]. This persistent production of cytokines by ILC2 cells facilitates the eosinophil progenitor cell homing to the lungs and provides fertile soil for their in situ maturation, causing persistent eosinophilia in these patients [42].

4. Eosinophilic Inflammation in the Lung

Eosinophils are the predominant cells of the inflammatory response in the lungs, contributing greatly to two major events: the remodeling and the hyperresponsiveness of the airways (AHR). Persistent inflammation caused by eosinophils leads to constant damage of the airways. The regeneration process is not flawless and results in hypertrophy of the smooth muscles, hyperplasia of goblet cells, and deposition of extracellular matrix proteins, causing membrane thickening and fibrosis [43].

The damage caused at the bronchial level is attributed to the degranulation of eosinophils and the release of their toxic proteins. Degranulation can occur in three different ways: (i) exocytosis, (ii) piecemeal degranulation, and (iii) cytolysis. In exocytosis, most specifically the subtype compound exocytosis, multiple granules inside the cell fuse and are then secreted to the extracellular space. This is the classic way that eosinophils act against helminths [44]. Piecemeal degranulation was demonstrated to be the most prevalent mechanism of eosinophil degranulation in asthmatic patients. In this highly regulated mechanism, the cytoplasmic proteins are "packaged" selectively in small vesicles, and then transported to the membrane through a tubulovesicular system until they are finally released by exocytosis. Various chemokines carefully regulate this process, such as Interferon-gamma (IFN-γ) and eotaxin-1, with studies showing that stimulating human eosinophils with a cytokine leads to the selective release of an eosinophilic protein [45,46]. In cytolysis, the cell dies; however, unlike apoptosis, its granules are released in the microenvironment, fully potent and active. Eosinophils which do not undergo piecemeal degranulation release their content through cytolysis [47]. Even if these mechanisms normally exist to protect tissues from damage, in this inflammatory process, the released proteins damage the epithelium, increase vascular permeability, and activate mast cells [48].

The release of eosinophilic granules and other mediators was proven to damage the airways in multiple ways. The smooth muscles of the airways contract via the M3 receptor after being triggered by acetylcholine. The M2 receptor limits its release and acts as a regulatory mechanism [49]. Eosinophils release MBP which is an allosteric antagonist of the M2 receptor, leading to an uncontrollable stimulation of the M3 receptor by acetylcholine and, thus, to bronchoconstriction [50]. MBP and other eosinophilic proteins were also shown to damage epithelial cells in vitro in similar concentrations to those found in the lungs of asthmatic patients, further proving their toxic effects [51]. However, MBP-abolished mice were not protected from AHR, meaning that other factors also contribute to this process [52]. Leukotrienes are abundant inside eosinophils, and their release causes bronchoconstriction and activates mast cells and basophils, which also excrete prostaglandins, histamine, and more leukotrienes to support the ongoing inflammation [53]. Eosinophils may induce AHR in a more indirect way, since eosinophil-ablated mice could still develop AHR when injected with T cells producing IL-13, which was demonstrated to cause AHR despite the absence of eosinophils [54]. More studies highlighted this indirect effect on AHR, since mast cells were proven to be more important in developing AHR in patients with eosinophilic asthma [55]. Blocking both CCR3 and IL-5 experimentally could not distinguish the effects of eosinophils and mast cells in AHR, since CCR3 is expressed in both types of cells. Nevertheless, use of CCR3 antagonists showed a significant reduction of both AHR and airway remodeling in animal studies, demonstrating the importance of the CCR3/eotaxin-1 axis [56]. Genetic ablation of eosinophils in mice via the *GATA-1* gene showed no protection from AHR when compared to normal mice in asthmatic models [57]. Therefore, while AHR is definitely one of the hallmarks of asthma, its correlation with eosinophils is debatable and seems to be more of a secondary effect of the generalized inflammatory process.

Nevertheless, eosinophils were proven to be one of the main factors behind airway remodeling. In a study designed with the same concept as the previous one mentioned, Δdbl-GATA mice were challenged by allergens and compared with wild-type mice. The latter group was found to exhibit all the features of airway remodeling, whereas the eosinophil-naïve mice were protected from it [58]. Similar results were demonstrated in both IL-5 KO mice and patients treated with anti-IL-5 agents, proving that reducing the number of eosinophils indeed reduces the deposition of extracellular matrix proteins (ECMs) such as collagen I in the airway lumen [59–61]. Eosinophils are activated by the effect of tumor necrosis factor-alpha (TNF-α) and, as recent studies showed, by IL-1beta; they secrete matrix metalloproteinase-9 which is one of the main enzymes found in asthmatic patients, highly correlated with the remodeling process and the persistent recruitment of eosinophils [62,63]. They also are a potent resource of transforming growth factor-β (TGF-β) which acts as a chemoattractant for fibroblasts and activates local fibroblasts to differentiate into myofibroblasts and even into smooth muscle cells, inducing ECM production in the meantime [64]. Mice treated with an anti TGF-β agent did not show evidence of airway remodeling, even if the inflammatory process was not altered, highlighting the pivotal role of TGF-β—mostly its correlation with the thickening of the basement membranes [65]. TGF-β is not only an eosinophil product; its mRNA was found increased in all the inflammation stages, with reports suggesting that eosinophils are its primary source in the first stages of the disease [61]. Nitric oxide (NO) is another toxic molecule secreted from eosinophils, and its levels correlate with the biomarker FeNO which is discussed later on [66]. Reactive oxygen species (ROS) are yet another product of eosinophils with clear potential to damage the airway and induce a fibrotic process [67]. Summarizing, eosinophils clearly contribute to airway remodeling, and the inhibition of eosinophil adhesion and activation may also reduce the inflammatory process and airway remodeling.

5. Biomarkers in Severe Eosinophilic Asthma and Endotyping

There was always a notion that the heterogeneity of asthma is due to the different phenotypes and endotypes of the disease. Nevertheless, endotyping became a necessity throughout the years; therefore, the need for specific biomarkers of every distinct type increased. These biomarkers include serum IgE, blood eosinophil levels, sputum eosinophils, and levels of exhaled nitric oxide in breath (widely known as FeNO) [68].

Sputum eosinophils are the most interesting biomarker in severe eosinophilic asthma due to the insight they provide into airway eosinophilia, despite the difficulty of collecting and analyzing them in every patient routinely. Treatment of patients based on sputum eosinophils showed a reduction of the rate of exacerbations, especially in those with severe asthma. [69] Both European Respiratory Society/American Thoracic Society (ERS/ATS) and Global Initiative for Asthma (GINA) guidelines support the use of sputum eosinophils for severe asthma management [1]. Sputum eosinophils ≥ 3% are correlated with airway eosinophilia [70]. Sputum mRNA can also be used in order to determine whether patients belong in the T2-high or the T2-low group, according to the expression of cytokines found in their sputum. Although this is a more costly method, it can "mark" candidates for biological treatments [71].

Blood eosinophils were used in the past few years as a marker for severe eosinophilic asthma requiring biological treatment with an anti-IL-5 agent, since they are correlated with sputum eosinophils. The threshold was put in several counts during trials, with the most often picked numbers being 150 cells/μL or 300 cells/μL; however, the most important from a clinical point of view is that blood eosinophil count—an easy and inexpensive biomarker—was chosen over sputum eosinophil number for eligibility for anti-IL-5 therapy [72]. During the anti-IL-5 trials, many biomarkers were evaluated, but none were deemed superior to blood eosinophils. The use of blood eosinophil counts as a biomarker for airway eosinophilia is based upon the relationship between blood and sputum eosinophil counts [73]. However, it should be noted that, although airway eosinophils are considered to better reflect eosinophil involvement in airway inflammation, peripheral blood eosinophils do not necessarily parallel airway eosinophils. High blood eosinophil numbers present good specificity for airway eosinophilia [74,75]. On the other hand, low blood eosinophil numbers might not accurately reflect the absence of airway eosinophilia [76,77]. This was demonstrated in a study including children with severe asthma, in which, despite 86% of them having blood eosinophil counts within normal levels, 84% still presented airway eosinophilia [78]. It should also be taken under consideration that blood eosinophil counts are influenced by high-dose ICS and mainly oral corticosteroids (OCS) [79]. A single measurement of blood eosinophil count of at least 150 cells/μL was shown to predict subsequent measurements on average of at least 150 cells/μL in 85% of patients [80].

FeNO is another marker that is used commonly and can inform us about the ICS response we should expect from a patient [81]. Nevertheless, there are several protruding factors that can confuse the results, the most important being smoking, allergic rhinitis, and female gender [82,83]. FeNO >50 ppb in adults suggests the presence of Th2-high inflammation, whereas FeNO < 25ppb suggests a Th2-low process. In another study, it was shown that, in patients with severe asthma refractory to treatment, an FeNO level >19ppb was indicative of sputum eosinophilia [84]. However, current guidelines from ATS/ERS do not recommend FeNO-guided management for patients with severe asthma [1]. This could be attributed to the fact that FeNO is correlated with the NO produced in asthmatic airways by other cells apart from eosinophils, such as epithelial cells and macrophages.

Thus, NO cannot be solely linked to eosinophils and the need for biological treatment, and it is more likely correlated with other aspects of the Th2 inflammation [85].

Volatile organic compounds (known as VOCs) are a modern biomarker also found in exhaled breath, like FeNO, and they are bound to predict with great accuracy both eosinophil and neutrophil counts in blood, while they are also correlated with eosinophil number in BAL [86]. They are processed by a meticulous algorithm called eNOSE (electronic nose), and early research suggested that they could be superior in estimating the risk of exacerbations and insensitivity to corticosteroids [87]. A recent study demonstrated that particular VOCs (hexane and 2-hexanone) had a high classification performance for eosinophilic asthma in a large asthmatic population classified according to their sputum cell count. Moreover, the combination of FeNO, blood eosinophils, and VOCs gave a very satisfactory prediction of eosinophilic asthma with an area under the curve (AUC) of 0.9 [88]. However, more data are needed if this method is to be applied on a daily basis. Last but not least, serum periostin, which derives from epithelial cells of the lung after stimulation by IL-13, was used as a biomarker of the T2-high endotype [89]. It was used in various studies as a predictor of Th2 inflammation and, even though the BOBCAT study showed that it was superior to regular biomarkers, the follow-up studies could not support these findings [75].

A combination of biomarkers may be better than using one alone, and this trend was followed in many studies. In the U-BIOPRED cohort study, a specific endotype of severe asthma involving eosinophils was described as "late-onset asthma with past or current smoking and chronic airflow obstruction with a high blood eosinophil count" [90]. A similar endotype was discovered by both the SARP and the Leicester cohorts using blood eosinophilia as an inflammatory marker, describing "late onset asthma associated with nasal polyps and resistance to corticosteroid therapy" and "a late-onset disease along with rhinosinusitis and numerous exacerbations", respectively [91]. The majority of these patients needed oral corticosteroids to achieve control of the disease and minimize exacerbations [92]. Although endotyping may not seem simple, it reveals individual therapeutic targets by means of specific treatable traits and mechanisms, leading to precision medicine, with the aid of biomarkers. For instance, Th2-high patients with severe asthma under ICS and LABA had higher FeNO, as well as blood and sputum eosinophil counts, compared to those with Th2-low inflammation in research using the *IL-13* genes in epithelial cells of the bronchial tree.

Concluding, it is clear that biomarkers have a role to play in guiding therapy of severe asthma. However, a combination of biomarkers may be used in order to achieve a greater predictive value. Also, new biomarkers with better correlation to specific endotypes and their respective molecular pathways need to be discovered in order to achieve optimal therapy.

6. Anti-IL-5 Therapy in Severe Eosinophilic Asthma

6.1. Mepolizumab

The story of anti-IL-5 treatment in asthma is definitely a fascinating one. Given the central role of eosinophils both in the allergic and non-allergic cascade of asthmatic inflammation, along with the fact that IL-5 is the cytokine mainly responsible for the differentiation, maturation, airway trafficking, and survival of eosinophils, the development of monoclonal antibodies against IL-5 raised high expectations for new treatment approaches, primarily in severe asthma.

However, the first studies were somewhat disappointing. In one study, mepolizumab prevented the rise in eosinophil numbers both in blood and sputum after inhaled allergen challenge, but it did not ameliorate allergen-induced asthmatic responses [93]. In another study including a small number of patients with difficult-to-treat asthma who were receiving high-dose ICS and/or oral CS, anti-IL-5 was able to reduce blood eosinophils but did not have an effect on other clinical outcomes apart from a small improvement in lung function— forced expiratory volume in the 1st second (FEV1) [94]. A few years later, in another study, mepolizumab was administered in a large group of not well-controlled patients with moderate to severe asthma, despite being treated with ICS and receiving four puffs of beta2-agonist daily as recue medication. Again, anti-IL-5 diminished blood eosinophils but did not manage to improve any clinically important outcome [70]. In the high-dose group, there was a trend toward reducing severe exacerbations, but the study was not powered to show such an effect. In spite of the consistent effect of anti-IL-5 in the reduction of blood eosinophils, the lack of a favorable effect in clinical asthma outcomes was obvious. These findings supported the dismal statement of the "final nail in the coffin for anti-IL-5 treatment in asthma".

However, in 2009, two small but well-designed randomized controlled trials were contracted that meant to change the road of anti-IL-5 treatment in asthma. In the first study, 20 asthmatics received either mepolizumab or placebo at five monthly intravenous infusions. These patients had corticosteroid-resistant eosinophilic asthma, and it is important to note that, although they were receiving a median dose of 10 mg of prednisone for a mean time of nine years and a high ICS dose, they still had >10% sputum eosinophils [95]. In the second study, 61 asthmatics received 12 infusions of either mepolizumab or placebo monthly [85]. Both studies revealed a significant reduction of exacerbations, accompanying a significant reduction in blood and sputum eosinophils. In the first study, the reduction of exacerbations occurred along with a reduction in prednisone dose. Still, there was no other clinically meaningful improvement in symptoms or lung function (FEV1) in both studies. These studies highlighted the importance of eosinophils in the pathogenesis of asthma exacerbations, but more clearly paved the way for the future of anti-IL-5 treatment by focusing—in contrast to previous studies—on two main determinants. Firstly, the primary outcome benefit from anti-IL-5 treatment relies mainly on the reduction of exacerbations; secondly, this benefit is obvious when selecting asthmatics with persistent eosinophilic inflammation despite regular corticosteroid (inhaled and/or oral) treatment.

Apart from a clear link with exacerbations, eosinophils are also important in airway remodeling in asthma. TGF-beta derived from eosinophils is involved in this process. In a study including 24 atopic asthmatics, anti-IL-5 treatment with mepolizumab reduced airway eosinophil numbers and significantly decreased the expression of three extracellular matrix proteins (tenascin, lumican, procollagen III) in the reticular basement membrane. It also reduced the percentage and the number of eosinophils expressing TGF-beta 1. These findings are extremely important, especially taking into consideration that the asthmatics included in this study were mild and received only short acting beta agonists (SABA) and not ICS. Firstly, these findings indicate that remodeling is present even in mild asthma, and it is driven to some degree by eosinophil-derived TGF-beta 1; secondly, anti-IL-5 can prevent this process by regulating the TGF-beta-enhanced deposition of matrix proteins through the reduction of eosinophils [60].

One of the largest studies in severe asthma, the DREAM study, including 621 patients was undertaken in order to examine the effect of mepolizumab in reducing the rate of clinically significant exacerbations. As such were defined the exacerbations that required oral corticosteroids or visit to an emergency department or hospitalization. All asthmatics had a history of at least two exacerbations requiring systemic corticosteroids in the previous year and signs of eosinophilic inflammation despite treatment. These signs were either sputum eosinophils >3%, peripheral blood eosinophils > 300×10^6/L, FeNO > 50 ppb, or loss of asthma control after a ≤ 25% reduction in regular corticosteroid dose (inhaled or oral). The study had a duration of 52 weeks, and patients received 13 infusions of one of three doses of IV mepolizumab (75, 250, and 750 mg). All three doses equally and significantly reduced the rate of asthma exacerbations. Moreover, they reduced the number of blood and sputum eosinophils and they were well tolerated. No improvements in FEV1 and AQLQ (asthma quality of life questionnaire) were observed, and this, in accordance with previous studies, indicated the dissociation of measures of control and exacerbations. This study also provided clinically valuable information regarding predictors of efficacy of mepolizumab treatment. The two main determinants were the baseline peripheral blood eosinophil number and the number of exacerbations in the previous year. Higher numbers indicated a more likely response to treatment. Other factors such as baseline FEV1, acute response to bronchodilators, IgE level, and atopic status were not associated with probability of response to mepolizumab [73].

In a following study (MENSA), 576 asthmatics treated with high-dose ICS with or without oral corticosteroids were randomized to receive either 75 mg of mepolizumab IV, 100 mg of mepolizumab subcutaneously (SC), or placebo every four weeks for 52 weeks. These asthmatics had at least two exacerbations requiring systemic corticosteroids the previous year and evidence of eosinophilic inflammation reflected by an eosinophil count of 150 cells/μL at screening or above 300 cells/μL at some time point in the previous year. The primary outcome was the annualized rate of exacerbations, and they were significantly reduced by both IV and SC mepolizumab by 47% and 53%, respectively. This was the first study to show that mepolizumab was associated with a significant improvement in lung function (FEV1), quality of life (AQLQ), and asthma control (ACQ-5) [96].

Another study (SIRIUS) explored the systemic corticosteroid-sparing effect of mepolizumab. In total, 135 asthmatics with severe eosinophilic asthma were randomized to receive either mepolizumab (100 mg SC) or placebo every four weeks for 20 weeks, and the primary outcome was the percentage reduction of the oral corticosteroid dose. The evidence of eosinophilic asthma was determined—similar to MENSA—by an eosinophil count of 150 cells/μL at screening or above 300 cells/μL at some time point in the previous year. In contrast to the MENSA study where 25% of asthmatics received oral steroids, in SIRIUS, all of the included patients received a mean dose of 10 mg of prednisone. This study involved a so-called optimization phase, in which a reduction of the dose of oral steroids was attempted before the start of mepolizumab, so as to establish that the patients genuinely needed this dose for their asthma control. The study showed that mepolizumab permitted the reduction of oral corticosteroid dose; moreover, despite this reduction, it also significantly reduced the rate of exacerbations and improved asthma control and quality of life (secondary outcomes in this study) [97].

In a 12-month open-label extension study of MENSA after the cessation of mepolizumab treatment, it was found that eosinophils increased both in blood and sputum, returning to pre-treatment levels within three months of cessation. As for asthma control, 12 months after the stop of medication, the exacerbation rates were similar to the pretreatment levels [98]. This study showed deterioration in exacerbation frequency after the cessation of mepolizumab that was preceded by a rebound worsening of eosinophilic inflammation.

In a post hoc analysis of the DREAM and MENSA studies, patients were stratified according to baseline blood eosinophil count in order to evaluate whether this biomarker could be used to predict response to mepolizumab. It was shown that using a threshold of 150 cells/μL could predict a favorable outcome in reducing exacerbations. Most importantly, this reduction was higher with increasing baseline blood eosinophil count (52% versus placebo for those with baseline blood eosinophils >150 and 70% for those with baseline blood eosinophils >500 cells/μL) [99]. In a subgroup analysis of the studies DREAM, MENSA, SIRIUS, and MUSCA, it was demonstrated that asthmatics with baseline eosinophils 150–300 cells/μL showed benefits in terms of reducing exacerbations and reducing the need for systemic corticosteroids that were clinically meaningful and comparable to patients with baseline >300 eosinophils/μL [100].

In patients with severe eosinophilic asthma previously treated with omalizumab, a post hoc analysis from MENSA and SIRIUS demonstrated that the response to mepolizumab was the same regardless of previous use of omalizumab [101]. This is clinically important because a subgroup of patients eligible for mepolizumab is also eligible for omalizumab treatment. Accordingly, a lack of response to omalizumab does not preclude a favorable response to mepolizumab in such asthmatics.

Another 32-week study (OSMO) included 145 patients who were eligible for both omalizumab and mepolizumab and were not controlled with omalizumab (median time of omalizumab treatment was 29.6 months). These asthmatics were switched immediately after the last dose of omalizumab to mepolizumab and achieved significant improvement, reflected by a 64% reduction in exacerbations compared to the previous year, better asthma control (measured by ACQ-5), and better quality of life (measured by Saint George's respiratory questionnaire—SGRQ). These outcomes were achieved early within 8–12 weeks and were kept or even improved during the study, indicating no evidence of possible additional action of the two antibodies until the wash-out of omalizumab. This study provided support to clinical practice in terms of switching from one biologic agent to another [102].

A study (MUSCA) assessed the effect of mepolizumab in the quality of life of patients with severe eosinophilic asthma and found a significant improvement in SGRQ of 7.7 (surpassing the minimal clinically important difference of four units), with a safety profile comparable to placebo [103].

Regarding safety, in a 52-week, open-label extension study of MENSA and SIRIUS (COSMOS study), mepolizumab had a favorable long-term safety profile, without any increase in the rate of adverse events [104]. Similarly, in the COLOMBUS study, an extension of the DREAM study lasting 3.5 years with a maximum exposure of 4.5 years, mepolizumab was safe and maintained its efficacy in the reduction of exacerbations [105].

Using data from five phase III studies with mepolizumab, it was shown that few patients developed anti-drug antibodies that had no impact on safety or efficacy of mepolizumab. Only one patient (from the SIRIUS study) was positive for neutralizing antibodies, but pharmacokinetic samples were not quantifiable during follow-up. These data show the low immunogenic response of mepolizumab [106].

6.2. Reslizumab

Reslizumab is a humanized anti-IL-5 IgG4 monoclonal antibody that binds with high affinity to the alpha subunit of the cytokine IL-5, thus preventing the interaction with its receptor [107].

Initially, a pilot safety study including 32 asthmatics showed that reslizumab at a dose of 1 mg/kg given intravenously reduced blood and sputum eosinophils but had no effect in lung function and airway hyperresponsiveness [94]. In the following phase IIb randomized, double-blind, placebo-controlled study, 106 patients with asthma and sputum eosinophils ≥3% were administered reslizumab at a dose 3 mg/kg IV every four weeks. Reslizumab managed to decrease sputum eosinophils significantly and improve FEV1, as well as improve asthma control (ACQ) in those patients with nasal polyps [108].

The two main phase III studies included 953 asthmatics that were randomized to receive either reslizumab (3 mg/kg IV) or placebo. All included patients had a baseline peripheral blood eosinophil count of > 400 cells/μL, ACQ-7 >1.5, at least 12% FEV1 reversibility, and at least one exacerbation requiring OCS in the last year; they were also on regular treatment with high-dose ICS plus additional controller with or without OCS (up to 10 mg of prednisone). The duration of the studies was 52 weeks, and the primary outcome was the rate of exacerbations defined either as need for OCS or doubling the ICS dose. Reslizumab was effective in reducing exacerbations significantly, improving FEV1, ACQ-7, and AQLQ, as well as reducing rescue medication and blood eosinophils [109]. In a post hoc analysis of these two studies, it was demonstrated that late-onset asthma (defined as onset after the age of 40) showed a better response to reslizumab compared to early-onset asthma [110].

In conclusion, these studies showed that reslizumab at a dose of 3 mg/kg IV is safe and more effective in patients with severe eosinophilic asthma and a peripheral blood eosinophil count > 400 cells/μL.

In another study including 10 patients with oral corticosteroid-dependent asthma, weight-adjusted intravenous reslizumab was more effective in reducing sputum eosinophilia compared to fixed-dose SC mepolizumab that was administered for at least one year with inadequate response. This was associated with a greater improvement in asthma control measured by ACQ-5 [111].

6.3. Benralizumab

Benralizumab is a humanized, afucosylated, monoclonal antibody targeting the IL-5α receptor. In comparison to anti-IL-5 monoclonal antibodies, benralizumab induces a direct, fast, and nearly complete depletion of blood eosinophils through enhanced antibody-dependent cell-mediated cytotoxicity, via natural killer cells [112]. As IL-5 receptors are expressed not only on eosinophils, but also on eosinophil progenitors and basophils, it is expected to affect all these populations. A study evaluating the effect of benralizumab on eosinophils in different compartments such as bone marrow, peripheral blood, sputum, and airways showed that bone marrow and peripheral blood eosinophils were completely suppressed while airway eosinophils (tissue and sputum) were also extensively depleted [113]. Two phase III trials, SIROCCO and CALIMA demonstrated that benralizumab significantly reduced the rate of asthma exacerbations in patients with severe, uncontrolled asthma and blood eosinophil counts ≥300 cells/μL [114,115]. In the SIROCCO study, benralizumab administered either every four weeks or every eight weeks (after the first three doses given every four weeks) reduced the rate of exacerbations by up to 51% after 48 weeks of treatment. It also improved lung function (expressed as an increase in pre-bronchodilator FEV1) and asthma control [114]. The effect compared to placebo was greater for the eight-weekly dosage, with the potential to lower the burden of asthma and reduce costs in comparison to other biologics that need to be given on a monthly basis. In CALIMA, a study of similar design to SIROCCO with a duration of 56 weeks, it was confirmed that benralizumab reduced asthma exacerbations up to 36% in patients with severe eosinophilic asthma and blood eosinophil counts ≥ 300 cells/μL. Again, as found in SIROCCO, a substantial improvement in lung function and asthma symptoms was observed [115]. Although there were no direct comparisons between biologics, it seems that the increases in lung function were greater with benralizumab than with other biologics.

In both studies, benralizumab produced a direct, rapid, and nearly complete depletion of eosinophils as early as four weeks, providing support for its mechanism of action directly on the IL-5α receptor, causing eosinophil apoptosis. Benralizumab depletes eosinophils directly, whereas mepolizumab and reslizumab reduce eosinophil number rather than deplete them entirely. This way, benralizumab is likely to overtake potential issues such as the induction of increased cytokine production due to cytokine-directed antibodies. A pooled analysis from the SIROCCO and CALIMA studies demonstrated that benralizumab was safe and effective in patients with severe eosinophilic asthma and blood eosinophils > 150 cells/μL [116].

A subsequent pooled analysis of the SIROCCO and CALIMA studies stratified patients according to baseline blood eosinophil count and by number of exacerbations (two and three or more). In this analysis, the rates of asthma exacerbations were increasingly reduced with increasing blood eosinophil thresholds and with greater exacerbation history. These reductions were even greater with a combination of high blood eosinophils and a history of more frequent exacerbations [117].

Another phase III study, ZONDA, showed that benralizumab significantly reduced the dose of oral prednisone in OCS-dependent patients, while also reducing the rate of exacerbations. All patients received oral corticosteroids for at least six months prior entering the study. The study included a run-in phase where the dose of prednisone was reduced to the minimum while maintaining asthma control, and this preceded the first administration of benralizumab. After 28 weeks, 50% of the patients managed to stop oral corticosteroids, while the likelihood of reducing the dose was four times higher in benralizumab-treated than in placebo-treated asthmatics [118].

A phase III extension study, BORA, included patients who completed the SIROCCO and CALIMA studies and evaluated the safety and tolerability of benralizumab. Interestingly, patients that received placebo in SIROCCO and CALIMA were randomized to receive benralizumab either every four weeks or every eight weeks (after administration of the first three doses every four weeks). The study confirmed the two-year safety of benralizumab as the percentage of patients experiencing adverse events was not different between BORA and the SIROCCO and CALIMA studies. No increased risk of infection was observed in patients receiving benralizumab for two years despite the long-term depletion of eosinophils. Moreover, asthmatics who were treated with benralizumab in BORA but received placebo in SIROCCO and CALIMA showed a comparable reduction in exacerbation rate with those receiving the active drug from the first year [119].

It is of high clinical importance to assess baseline characteristics in patients with severe eosinophilic asthma that may predict the response to treatment with benralizumab. In a study including patients from the SIROCCO and CALIMA phase III studies, it was shown that OCS use, nasal polyps, forced vital capacity (FVC) < 65% pred adult onset of asthma (>18 years), and three or more exacerbations in the previous year were associated with a greater response to benrlizumab, measured either as annual exacerbation rate or change in pre-bronchodilator FEV1 for those with > 300 eosinophils/μL.

Interestingly, OCS use, nasal polyps, and FVC < 65% pred could predict a better response to benralizumab in decreasing the rate of exacerbations, even in patients with < 300 eosinophils/μL [120]. This study highlights the importance of assessing these clinical features when evaluating an asthmatic patient eligible for benralizumab, and adds to the already known baseline blood eosinophil count predictive information for responsiveness to treatment.

Another study assessed the effect of benralizumab treatment by stratifying patients according to atopic status (atopic or non-atopic) and IgE level (high > 150 kU/L or low < 150 kU/L). The study again included patients from the phase III SIROCCO and CALIMA studies and demonstrated that the efficacy of benralizumab in reducing the exacerbation rate and improving lung function was not affected by atopic status and serum IgE level [121]. This is clinically important because it indicates that benralizumab is effective in patients with severe eosinophilic asthma that might be eligible for omalizumab treatment as well.

There are no head-to-head trials for direct comparison between the different anti-IL-5 biologics. In a matching-adjusted indirect comparison, benralizumab and mepolizumab similarly reduced exacerbation rate and improved lung function. No comparison could be made between benralizumab and reslizumab due to differences in study populations [122]. Another indirect comparison demonstrated that, in patients with similar blood eosinophil counts, mepolizumab was more effective in reducing exacerbations than benralizumab and reslizumab. As for lung function, benralizumab was associated with a greater improvement in FEV1 compared to reslizumab for patients with a blood eosinophil count > 400 cells/μL [123]. However, all these findings of the indirect comparison trials should be viewed with caution because of the differences in study populations and in the number of exacerbations in the previous year of the included patients. Moreover, there were differences in the treatment the patients received before starting the biologic (either the ICS dose and/or OCS dose). The studies for reslizumab enrolled asthmatics with baseline blood eosinophils > 400 cells/μL, a higher number compared to those enrolled in studies for mepolizumab and benralizumab. Accordingly, a greater effect might have been expected.

There are no studies evaluating possible co-administration of biologics with different mechanisms such as anti-IgE and anti-IL-5 for those who present a mixed phenotype (severe allergic and eosinophilic asthma). In these patients, it is logical to assess the predominant characteristics and decide which biologic to start [124].

It is suggested that anti-IL-5 antibodies be administered for at least 16 weeks in order to assess efficacy. However, this time may be extended up to 12 months as there are some late-responders, and 16 weeks is possibly too short a length of time to evaluate reduction in exacerbations [125].

There are still some unanswered questions with major clinical importance. How long should an anti-IL-5 be prescribed in a patient with severe eosinophilic asthma? It seems that, after stopping it, there is a relapse of exacerbations following an increase in blood and sputum eosinophils, and this was shown with mepolizumab and benralizumab. This relapse of eosinophilic inflammation is compatible with a lack of long-term bone marrow suppression after discontinuation of medication [98,119]. Is there a rationale for moving from an anti-IL-5 antibody to an anti-IL-5 receptor antibody or vice versa? The mechanism of action is different, and benralizumab is associated with almost a depletion of blood eosinophils while mepolizumab reduces them significantly but does not deplete them. However, no difference in efficacy in any outcome (exacerbation rate, lung function) was observed. One possible explanation is that these antibodies exert their effect by reducing the eosinophil pool in the bone marrow, thus reducing exacerbations through the reduction of eosinophils that are available for mobilization and trafficking in the airways.

7. Anti-IL-4 therapy in Severe Asthma

Dupilumab

Dupilumab is a fully human anti-interleukin-4α receptor monoclonal antibody, recently approved for moderate-to-severe eosinophilic asthma or oral steroid-dependent asthma. It blocks interleukin-4 and interleukin-13, which are key mediators in type-2-mediated inflammation.

The first study on dupilumab included 52 asthmatics with severe eosinophilic asthma and a baseline blood eosinophil count of > 300 cells/μL or sputum eosinophils > 3% who were treated with medium-to-high-dose ICS plus LABA. The patients received dupilumab (300 mg SC) or placebo weekly for 12 weeks or until an exacerbation occurred. The design of the study was provocative since asthmatics discontinued LABA by week four and gradually tapered and discontinued ICS at weeks 6–9. Dupilumab was associated with an 87% reduction in exacerbations compared to placebo and also improved lung function and reduced markers of Th2 inflammation [126].

The following phase IIb study included 769 patients with severe asthma on medium-to-high ICS plus LABA, irrespective of baseline blood eosinophil count. They received 200 mg or 300 mg of dupilumab or placebo every two or every four weeks for a total duration of 24 weeks. Dupilumab improved FEV1 and reduced the exacerbation rate significantly in the total population and also in the subgroups of patients with less than or more than 300 eosinophils/μL [127]. In a post hoc analysis of this study, the favorable effects of dupilumab were demonstrated regardless of the exacerbation frequency in the previous year, although treatment effects tended to be greater with higher number of exacerbations in the year prior to study entry. In another post hoc analysis of the above study, dupilumab (200 mg SC) every two or every four weeks was associated with clinically meaningful improvements in asthma control (as assessed by ACQ-5) and quality of life (assessed by AQLQ), while it also improved asthma symptoms and reduced productivity loss [128]. In another study of similar design, 1902 patients with severe uncontrolled asthma were assigned to receive dupilumab (200 or 300 mg SC) or matched placebo every two weeks for 52 weeks. The study again confirmed the favorable effect of both doses in reducing annual exacerbation rate and improving lung function. These effects, although observed irrespective of baseline blood eosinophils, were greater in those with > 300 cells/μL [129].

As with anti-IL-5 antibodies, dupilumab was assessed regarding its efficacy in reducing OCS in asthmatics with oral steroid-dependent asthma. Accordingly, 210 patients received dupilumab (300 mg) or placebo every two weeks for 24 weeks. Oral steroid doses were reduced from week four to week 20 and then remained at a stable dose for another four weeks. Dupilumab reduced oral corticosteroid dose by 70% compared to 42% reduction of placebo, and simultaneously decreased the rate of exacerbation by 59% compared to placebo; this effect was observed despite the reduction in the OCS dose. It also significantly improved lung function [130]. In the studies by Castro et al. and Rabe et al., transient eosinophilia was observed in few patients who received dupilumab.

A meta-analysis involving 3369 asthmatics from five studies concluded that treatment with dupilumab was effective in reducing exacerbations and improving lung function, asthma symptoms, asthma control and quality of life. Dupilumab was safe and well tolerated, and the most frequent adverse event was injection-site reaction [131].

Chronic rhinosinusitis with nasal polyps (CRSwNP) is often a comorbidity of severe eosinophilic asthma. In a subgroup analysis of a study involving patients with CRSwNP who received dupilumab as add-on therapy to mometasone fuorate nasal spray, those patients with comorbid asthma showed improvements not only in nasal polyp burden but also in asthma control, quality of life, and lung function [132].

8. Anti-IgE Therapy in Severe Asthma

Omalizumab

Omalizumab is a humanized monoclonal antibody that binds free IgE and prevents it from binding to the high-affinity IgE receptor on basophils and mast cells [133]. Omalizumab is now approved for the treatment of moderate-to-severe allergic asthma in patients > 6 years of age. Omalizumab was the first biologic approved for use in asthma 15 years ago. To be eligible for omalizumab, the asthmatic should demonstrate sensitization to one of the perennial allergens on skin prick testing. Levels of total IgE combined with body weight are used to calculate the dose and the frequency of dosing. Omalizumab is administered subcutaneously either once a month or every two weeks. It was extensively studied in both clinical trials and real-world observational studies and was found to reduce the annual relative risk of asthma exacerbation by 38% and the risk of emergency visits by 47% compared with controls, according to pooled data from seven randomized studies [134]. The benefit of omalizumab in reducing exacerbations in relation to the presence of biomarkers reflective of T2 inflammation was evaluated in a study, showing that asthmatics with peripheral blood eosinophils ≥ 260 cells/μL and FeNO ≥19.5 ppb had a greater reduction of exacerbations compared to those with biomarker values below the above cut-off levels [135]. Accordingly, these biomarkers could be beneficial in selecting patients who are more likely to respond to omalizumab treatment. However, more recent data from real-world studies suggest that blood eosinophil levels are not predictors of reduction in exacerbations [136,137].

9. Other Therapies

Thymic stromal lymphopoietin (TSLP) is produced by airway epithelial cells in response to inhaled allergens and proinflammatory stressors [138,139].

Tezepelumab is a human monoclonal antibody that binds to TSLP, inhibiting its stimulatory action on dendritic cells and innate lymphoid cells, thus preventing the induction of type 2 cytokines (e.g., IL-5, IL-4, and IL-13). One phase II, randomized, double-blind, placebo-controlled trial evaluated the efficacy and safety of tezepelumab in patients with uncontrolled asthma, despite treatment with long-acting beta-agonists and medium-to-high doses of inhaled corticosteroids. Three dose levels of subcutaneous tezepelumab were compared to placebo over 52 weeks. The primary end point was the annualized rate of asthma exacerbations. Exacerbation rates were significantly reduced in tezepelumab groups—regardless of the baseline blood eosinophil count—compared to placebo by 61% in the low-dose group, 71% in the medium-dose group, and 66% in the high-dose group. Lung function was improved irrespective of the dose, while health-related quality of life improved only in the high-dose group [140].

Prostaglandin D2 (PGD2) is mainly released from mast cells, but platelets, alveolar macrophages, Th2 cells, and dendritic cells can also produce smaller amounts of PGD2. Prostaglandin D2 contributes to T2 inflammation through binding of the G-protein-coupled receptor chemoattractant receptor-homologous molecule expressed on Th2 cells (CRTH2) [141]. Fevipiprant is an oral competitive antagonist of CRTH2.

In a phase II study, including 170 patients with mild-to-moderate persistent, allergic asthma, fevipiprant produced a significant improvement in FEV1 AUC_{0-24} only in patients with high serum IgE and blood eosinophils > 300/μL [142].

In another phase II study, including 61 patients with moderate-to-severe, persistent asthma and sputum eosinophilia (≥ 2%), fevipiprant produced a significant, 3.5-fold greater decrease in sputum eosinophilia than placebo during the 12-week treatment period. In addition, fevipiprant reduced bronchial submucosal eosinophil numbers in bronchial biopsies compared to placebo. However, no change in blood eosinophil count was observed [143].

Finally, in another phase IIb study, including 1058 patients with allergic asthma uncontrolled with inhaled corticosteroids, fevipiprant—as well as montelukast—improved pre-dose FEV1 compared to placebo. However, no evidence of a higher efficacy in any predefined subgroup, including blood eosinophil count was observed [144].

10. Summary

In order to consider a biologic therapy for severe asthma, it is fundamental to firstly confirm asthma diagnosis and then solve possible problems related to non-adherence to medication, improper inhaler technique, and treatment of comorbid conditions.

For severe eosinophilic asthma, targeted therapies directed against IL-5 and IL-4 are available up to date (Table 1). These agents proved effective mainly in reducing asthma exacerbations but also in improving lung function and asthma control. It is clinically desirable that these antibodies seem to work specifically for uncontrolled asthma despite the use of daily oral corticosteroids. This led to the option of systemic steroids as the last alternative for GINA step 5, which will likely be entirely erased as a treatment option in the years to come.

Another major benefit from the use of biologics in severe asthma is the opportunity for a better insight into asthma pathophysiology mechanisms. An important but still unanswered question is whether biologics have an effect on moderate asthma or produce a disease-modifying effect. Until then, and while expecting more biologics to come (e.g., tezepelumab), we hope to gain experience and understand more from the longer use of the current anti-T2 biologics.

Table 1. Studies on biologic therapies for severe eosinophilic asthma.

Study	Medication	Patients	Duration	Outcome
Pavord et al. [73] (DREAM study) Phase III	Mepolizumab	621	52 weeks	Reduced number of exacerbations
Ortega et al. [96] (MENSA study) Phase III	Mepolizumab	576	52 weeks	Reduced number of exacerbations and improved lung function (FEV1), asthma control (ACQ-5), and quality of life (AQLQ)
Bel et al. [97] (SIRIUS study) Phase III	Mepolizumab	135	20 weeks	Reduced oral corticosteroid dose and number of exacerbations
Chapman et al. [102] (OSMO study) Phase III	Mepolizumab	145	32 weeks	Reduced number of exacerbations and improvement in asthma control (ACQ-5) and quality of life (SGRQ)
Chupp et al. [103] (MUSCA study) Phase III	Mepolizumab	551	24 weeks	Improvement in the SGRQ total score
Castro et al. [109] Phase III	Reslizumab	953	52 weeks	Reduced number of exacerbations and improvement in lung function (FEV1), asthma control (ACQ-7), and quality of life (AQLQ)
Bleecker et al. [114] (SIROCCO study) Phase III	Benralizumab	1205	48 weeks	Reduced number of exacerbations, improved lung function (FEV1), and asthma control
FitzGerald et al. [115] (CALIMA study) Phase III	Benralizumab	1306	56 weeks	Reduced number of exacerbations and improved lung function (FEV1)
Nair et al. [118] (ZONDA study) Phase III	Benralizumab	220	28 weeks	Reduced oral corticosteroid dose and number of exacerbations
Busse et al. [119] (BORA study) Phase III	Benralizumab	1576	56 weeks	Validated 2-year safety of benralizumab use
Wenzel et al. [127] Phase IIb	Dupilumab	769	24 weeks	Reduced number of exacerbations and improved lung function (FEV1)

Table 1. *Cont.*

Study	Medication	Patients	Duration	Outcome
Castro et al. [129] Phase IIb	Dupilumab	1902	52 weeks	Reduced number of exacerbations and improved lung function (FEV1)
Rabe et al. [130] Phase III	Dupilumab	210	24 weeks	Reduced oral corticosteroid dose, number of exacerbations, and improved lung function (FEV1)
Corren et al. [140] Phase II	Tezepelumab	550	52 weeks	Improved lung function (FEV1) and reduced number of exacerbations
Erpenbeck et al. [142] Phase II	Fevipiprant	170	28 days	Improved lung function (FEV1) in patients with high blood eosinophil number or high serum immunoglobulin E (IgE)
Gonem et al. [143] Phase II	Fevipiprant	61	12 weeks	Reduced sputum eosinophilia
Bateman et al. [144] Phase IIb	Fevipiprant	1058	12 weeks	Improved lung function (FEV1)

Abbreviations: FEV1—forced expiratory volume in the first second; ACQ—asthma control questionnaire; AQLQ—asthma quality of life questionnaire; SGRQ—Saint George's respiratory questionnaire.

Author Contributions: A.B., S.L. and P.B. have substantially contributed to the conception of the work, drafted and revised the manuscript and made the final approval of the version to be published.

Conflicts of Interest: The authors declare no conflict of interest.

References

1. Chung, K.F.; Wenzel, S.E.; Brozek, J.L.; Bush, A.; Castro, M.; Sterk, P.J.; Adcock, I.M.; Bateman, E.D.; Bel, E.H.; Bleecker, E.R.; et al. International ERS/ATS guidelines on definition, evaluation and treatment of severe asthma. *Eur. Respir. J.* **2014**, *43*, 343–373. [CrossRef]
2. Reddel, H.K.; Taylor, D.R.; Bateman, E.D.; Boulet, L.-P.; Boushey, H.A.; Busse, W.W.; Casale, T.B.; Chanez, P.; Enright, P.L.; Gibson, P.G.; et al. An official American Thoracic Society/European Respiratory Society statement: Asthma control and exacerbations: Standardizing endpoints for clinical asthma trials and clinical practice. *Am. J. Respir. Crit. Care Med.* **2009**, *180*, 59–99. [CrossRef]
3. Bateman, E.D.; Boushey, H.A.; Bousquet, J.; Busse, W.W.; Clark, T.J.H.; Pauwels, R.A.; Pedersen, S.E. Can guideline-defined asthma control be achieved? The Gaining Optimal Asthma ControL study. *Am. J. Respir. Crit. Care Med.* **2004**, *170*, 836–844. [CrossRef]
4. Pavlidis, S.; Takahashi, K.; Kwong, F.N.K.; Xie, J.; Hoda, U.; Sun, K.; Elyasigomari, V.; Agapow, P.; Loza, M.; Baribaud, F.; et al. "T2-high" in severe asthma related to blood eosinophil, exhaled nitric oxide and serum periostin. *Eur. Respir. J.* **2019**. [CrossRef]
5. Rothenberg, M.E.; Hogan, S. The eosinophil. *Annu. Rev. Immunol.* **2006**, *24*, 147–174. [CrossRef]
6. Klion, A.D.; Nutman, T.B. The role of eosinophils in host defense against helminth parasites. *J. Allergy Clin. Immunol.* **2004**, *113*, 30–37. [CrossRef]
7. Bousquet, J.; Jeffery, P.K.; Busse, W.W.; Johnson, M.; Vignola, A.M. Asthma. From bronchoconstriction to airways inflammation and remodeling. *Am. J. Respir. Crit. Care Med.* **2000**, *161*, 1720–1745. [CrossRef]
8. Marichal, T.; Mesnil, C.; Bureau, F. Homeostatic Eosinophils: Characteristics and Functions. *Front. Med.* **2017**, *4*, 101. [CrossRef]
9. Du, J.; Stankiewicz, M.J.; Liu, Y.; Xi, Q.; Schmitz, J.E.; Lekstrom-Himes, J.A.; Ackerman, S.J. Novel combinatorial interactions of GATA-1, PU.1, and C/EBPepsilon isoforms regulate transcription of the gene encoding eosinophil granule major basic protein. *J. Biol. Chem.* **2002**, *277*, 43481–43494.
10. Trivedi, S.G.; Lloyd, C.M. Eosinophils in the pathogenesis of allergic airways disease. *Cell. Mol. Life Sci.* **2007**, *64*, 1269–1289. [CrossRef]
11. Sanderson, C.J. Interleukin-5, eosinophils, and disease. *Blood* **1992**, *79*, 3101–3109.
12. Mesnil, C.; Raulier, S.; Paulissen, G.; Xiao, X.; Birrell, M.A.; Pirottin, D.; Janss, T.; Starkl, P.; Ramery, E.; Henket, M.; et al. Lung-resident eosinophils represent a distinct regulatory eosinophil subset. *J. Clin. Investig.* **2016**, *126*, 3279–3295. [CrossRef]

13. Flood-Page, P.T.; Menzies-Gow, A.N.; Kay, A.B.; Robinson, D.S. Eosinophil's role remains uncertain as anti-interleukin-5 only partially depletes numbers in asthmatic airway. *Am. J. Respir. Crit. Care Med.* **2003**, *167*, 199–204. [CrossRef]
14. Tavernier, J.; Van der Heyden, J.; Verhee, A.; Brusselle, G.; Van Ostade, X.; Vandekerckhove, J.; North, J.; Rankin, S.M.; Kay, A.B.; Robinson, D.S. Interleukin 5 regulates the isoform expression of its own receptor alpha-subunit. *Blood* **2000**, *95*, 1600–1607.
15. Nishinakamura, R.; Miyajima, A.; Mee, P.J.; Tybulewicz, V.L.; Murray, R. Hematopoiesis in mice lacking the entire granulocyte-macrophage colony-stimulating factor/interleukin-3/interleukin-5 functions. *Blood* **1996**, *88*, 2458–2464.
16. Pease, J.E. Asthma, allergy and chemokines. *Curr. Drug Targets* **2006**, *7*, 3–12. [CrossRef]
17. Kelly-Welch, A.; Hanson, E.M.; Keegan, D. Interleukin-4 (IL-4) pathway. *Sci. STKE* **2005**, *2005*, cm9. [CrossRef]
18. Kelly-Welch, A.; Hanson, E.M.; Keegan, A.D. Interleukin-13 (IL-13) pathway. *Sci. STKE* **2005**, *2005*, cm8. [CrossRef]
19. Dent, L.A.; Strath, M.; Mellor, A.L.; Sanderson, C.J. Eosinophilia in transgenic mice expressing interleukin 5. *J. Exp. Med.* **1990**, *172*, 1425–1431. [CrossRef]
20. Foster, P.S.; Hogan, S.P.; Ramsay, A.J.; Matthaei, K.I.; Young, I.G. Interleukin 5 deficiency abolishes eosinophilia, airways hyperreactivity, and lung damage in a mouse asthma model. *J. Exp. Med.* **1996**, *183*, 195–201. [CrossRef]
21. Martinez-Moczygemba, M.; Huston, D. Biology of common beta receptor-signaling cytokines: IL-3, IL-5, and GM-CSF. *J. Allergy Clin. Immunol.* **2003**, *112*, 653–665.
22. Collins, P.D.; Marleau, S.; Griffiths-Johnson, D.A.; Jose, P.J.; Williams, T.J. Cooperation between interleukin-5 and the chemokine eotaxin to induce eosinophil accumulation in vivo. *J. Exp. Med.* **1995**, *182*, 1169–1174. [CrossRef]
23. Robinson, D.; Humbert, M.; Buhl, R.; Cruz, A.A.; Inoue, H.; Korom, S.; Hanania, N.A.; Nair, P. Revisiting Type 2-high and Type 2-low airway inflammation in asthma: Current knowledge and therapeutic implications. *Clin. Exp. Allergy* **2017**, *47*, 161–175. [CrossRef]
24. Griffiths-Johnson, D.A.; Collins, P.D.; Rossi, A.G.; Jose, P.J.; Williams, T.J. The chemokine, eotaxin, activates guinea-pig eosinophils in vitro and causes their accumulation into the lung in vivo. *Biochem. Biophys. Res. Commun.* **1993**, *197*, 1167–1172. [CrossRef]
25. Gutierrez-Ramos, J.C.; Lloyd, C.; Gonzalo, J.A. Eotaxin: From an eosinophilic chemokine to a major regulator of allergic reactions. *Immunol. Today* **1999**, *20*, 500–504. [CrossRef]
26. Simson, L.; Foster, P.S. Chemokine and cytokine cooperativity: Eosinophil migration in the asthmatic response. *Immunol. Cell Biol.* **2000**, *78*, 415–422. [CrossRef]
27. Sehmi, R.; Dorman, S.; Baatjes, A.; Watson, R.; Foley, R.; Ying, S.; Robinson, D.S.; Kay, A.B.; O'Byrne, P.M.; Denburg, J.A. Allergen-induced fluctuation in CC chemokine receptor 3 expression on bone marrow CD34+ cells from asthmatic subjects: Significance for mobilization of haemopoietic progenitor cells in allergic inflammation. *Immunology* **2003**, *109*, 536–546. [CrossRef]
28. Ying, S.; Meng, Q.; Zeibecoglou, K.; Robinson, D.S.; Macfarlane, A.; Humbert, M.; Kay, A.B. Eosinophil chemotactic chemokines (eotaxin, eotaxin-2, RANTES, monocyte chemoattractant protein-3 (MCP-3), and MCP-4), and C-C chemokine receptor 3 expression in bronchial biopsies from atopic and nonatopic (Intrinsic) asthmatics. *J. Immunol.* **1999**, *163*, 6321–6329.
29. Zimmermann, N.; Conkright, J.J.; Rothenberg, M.E. CC chemokine receptor-3 undergoes prolonged ligand-induced internalization. *J. Biol. Chem.* **1999**, *274*, 12611–12618. [CrossRef]
30. Ravensberg, A.J.; Ricciardolo, F.L.M.; van Schadewijk, A.; Rabe, K.F.; Sterk, P.J.; Hiemstra, P.S.; Mauad, T. Eotaxin-2 and eotaxin-3 expression is associated with persistent eosinophilic bronchial inflammation in patients with asthma after allergen challenge. *J. Allergy Clin. Immunol.* **2005**, *115*, 779–785. [CrossRef]
31. Pope, S.M.; Zimmermann, N.; Stringer, K.F.; Karow, M.L.; Rothenberg, M.E. The eotaxin chemokines and CCR3 are fundamental regulators of allergen-induced pulmonary eosinophilia. *J. Immunol.* **2005**, *175*, 5341–5350. [CrossRef]

32. Humbles, A.A.; Conroy, D.M.; Marleau, S.; Rankin, S.M.; Palframan, R.T.; Proudfoot, A.E.I.; Wells, T.N.C.; Li, D.; Jeffery, P.K.; Griffiths-Johnson, D.A.; et al. Kinetics of eotaxin generation and its relationship to eosinophil accumulation in allergic airways disease: Analysis in a guinea pig model in vivo. *J. Exp. Med.* **1997**, *186*, 601–612. [CrossRef]
33. Mould, A.W.; Matthaei, K.I.; Young, I.G.; Foster, P.S. Relationship between interleukin-5 and eotaxin in regulating blood and tissue eosinophilia in mice. *J. Clin. Investig.* **1997**, *99*, 1064–1071. [CrossRef]
34. Mattes, J.; Foster, P.S. Regulation of eosinophil migration and Th2 cell function by IL-5 and eotaxin. *Curr. Drug Targets Inflamm. Allergy* **2003**, *2*, 169–174. [CrossRef]
35. Kalomenidis, I.; Stathopoulos, G.T.; Barnette, R.; Guo, Y.; Peebles, R.S.; Blackwell, T.S.; Light, R.W. Eotaxin-3 and interleukin-5 pleural fluid levels are associated with pleural fluid eosinophilia in post-coronary artery bypass grafting pleural effusions. *Chest* **2005**, *127*, 2094–2100. [CrossRef]
36. Jia, G.-Q.; Gonzalo, J.-A.; Hidalgo, A.; Wagner, D.; Cybulsky, M.; Gutierrez-Ramos, J.C. Selective eosinophil transendothelial migration triggered by eotaxin via modulation of Mac-1/ICAM-1 and VLA-4/VCAM-1 interactions. *Int. Immunol.* **1999**, *11*, 1–10. [CrossRef]
37. Koo, G.C.; Shah, K.; Ding, G.J.F.; Xiao, J.Y.; Wnek, R.; Doherty, G.; Tong, X.C.; Pepinsky, R.B.; Lin, K.-C.; Hagmann, W.K. A small molecule very late antigen-4 antagonist can inhibit ovalbumin-induced lung inflammation. *Am. J. Respir. Crit. Care Med.* **2003**, *167*, 1400–1409. [CrossRef]
38. Broide, D.H.; Sullivan, S.; Gifford, T.; Sriramarao, P. Inhibition of pulmonary eosinophilia in P-selectin- and ICAM-1-deficient mice. *Am. J. Respir. Cell Mol. Biol.* **1998**, *18*, 218–225. [CrossRef]
39. Sehmi, R.; Smith, S.G.; Kjarsgaard, M.; Radford, K.; Boulet, L.P.; Lemiere, C.; Prazma, C.M.; Ortega, H.; Martin, J.G.; Nair, P. Role of local eosinophilopoietic processes in the development of airway eosinophilia in prednisone-dependent severe asthma. *Clin. Exp. Allergy* **2016**, *46*, 793–802. [CrossRef]
40. Mitchell, P.D.; O'Byrne, P.M. Biologics and the lung: TSLP and other epithelial cell-derived cytokines in asthma. *Pharmacol. Ther.* **2017**, *169*, 104–112. [CrossRef]
41. Fallon, P.G.; Ballantyne, S.J.; Mangan, N.E.; Barlow, J.L.; Dasvarma, A.; Hewett, D.R.; McIlgorm, A.; Jolin, H.E.; McKenzie, A.N. Identification of an interleukin (IL)-25-dependent cell population that provides IL-4, IL-5, and IL-13 at the onset of helminth expulsion. *J. Exp. Med.* **2006**, *203*, 1105–1116. [CrossRef]
42. Smith, S.G.; Chen, R.; Kjarsgaard, M.; Huang, C.; Oliveria, J.P.; O'Byrne, P.M.; Gauvreau, G.M.; Boulet, L.P.; Lemiere, C.; Martin, J.; et al. Increased numbers of activated group 2 innate lymphoid cells in the airways of patients with severe asthma and persistent airway eosinophilia. *J. Allergy Clin. Immunol.* **2016**, *137*, 75–86 e8. [CrossRef]
43. Chakir, J.; Shannon, J.; Molet, S.; Fukakusa, M.; Elias, J.; Laviolette, M.; Boulet, L.P.; Hamid, Q. Airway remodeling-associated mediators in moderate to severe asthma: Effect of steroids on TGF-beta, IL-11, IL-17, and type I and type III collagen expression. *J. Allergy Clin. Immunol.* **2003**, *111*, 1293–1298. [CrossRef]
44. Hafez, I.; Stolpe, A.; Lindau, M. Compound exocytosis and cumulative fusion in eosinophils. *J. Biol. Chem.* **2003**, *278*, 44921–44928. [CrossRef]
45. Lacy, P.; Mahmudi-Azer, S.; Bablitz, B.; Hagen, S.C.; Velazquez, J.R.; Man, S.F.; Moqbel, R. Rapid mobilization of intracellularly stored RANTES in response to interferon-gamma in human eosinophils. *Blood* **1999**, *94*, 23–32.
46. Carmo, L.A.; Bonjour, K.; Ueki, S.; Neves, J.S.; Liu, L.; Spencer, L.A.; Dvorak, A.M.; Weller, P.F.; Melo, R.C. CD63 is tightly associated with intracellular, secretory events chaperoning piecemeal degranulation and compound exocytosis in human eosinophils. *J. Leukoc. Biol.* **2016**, *100*, 391–401. [CrossRef]
47. Saffari, H.; Hoffman, L.H.; Peterson, K.A.; Fang, J.C.; Leiferman, K.M.; Pease, L.F., 3rd; Gleich, G.J. Electron microscopy elucidates eosinophil degranulation patterns in patients with eosinophilic esophagitis. *J. Allergy Clin. Immunol.* **2014**, *133*, 1728–1734. [CrossRef]
48. Piliponsky, A.M.; Gleich, G.J.; Bar, I.; Levi-Schaffer, F. Effects of eosinophils on mast cells: A new pathway for the perpetuation of allergic inflammation. *Mol. Immunol.* **2002**, *38*, 1369. [CrossRef]
49. Fryer, A.D.; Maclagan, J. Muscarinic inhibitory receptors in pulmonary parasympathetic nerves in the guinea-pig. *Br. J. Pharmacol.* **1984**, *83*, 973–978. [CrossRef]
50. Jacoby, D.B.; Gleich, G.J.; Fryer, A.D. Human eosinophil major basic protein is an endogenous allosteric antagonist at the inhibitory muscarinic M2 receptor. *J. Clin. Investig.* **1993**, *91*, 1314–1318. [CrossRef]

51. Gleich, G.J.; Flavahan, N.A.; Fujisawa, T.; Vanhoutte, P.M. The eosinophil as a mediator of damage to respiratory epithelium: A model for bronchial hyperreactivity. *J. Allergy Clin. Immunol.* **1988**, *81*, 776–781. [CrossRef]
52. Denzler, K.L.; Farmer, S.C.; Crosby, J.R.; Borchers, M.; Cieslewicz, G.; Larson, K.A.; Cormier-Regard, S.; Lee, N.A.; Lee, J.J. Eosinophil major basic protein-1 does not contribute to allergen-induced airway pathologies in mouse models of asthma. *J. Immunol.* **2000**, *165*, 5509–5517. [CrossRef]
53. Kay, A.B. Mediators of hypersensitivity and inflammatory cells in the pathogenesis of bronchial asthma. *Eur. J. Respir. Dis. Suppl.* **1983**, *129*, 1–44.
54. Mattes, J.; Yang, M.; Mahalingam, S.; Kuehr, J.; Webb, D.C.; Simson, L.; Hogan, S.P.; Koskinen, A.; McKenzie, A.N.; Dent, L.A.; et al. Intrinsic defect in T cell production of interleukin (IL)-13 in the absence of both IL-5 and eotaxin precludes the development of eosinophilia and airways hyperreactivity in experimental asthma. *J. Exp. Med.* **2002**, *195*, 1433–1444. [CrossRef]
55. Bradding, O.; Brightling, C. Mast cell infiltration of airway smooth muscle in asthma. *Respir. Med.* **2007**, *101*, 1045–1047. [CrossRef]
56. Wegmann, M.; Goggel, R.; Sel, S.; Sel, S.; Erb, K.J.; Kalkbrenner, F.; Renz, H.; Garn, H. Effects of a low-molecular-weight CCR-3 antagonist on chronic experimental asthma. *Am. J. Respir. Cell Mol. Biol.* **2007**, *36*, 61–67. [CrossRef]
57. Siegle, J.S.; Hansbro, N.; Herbert, C.; Yang, M.; Foster, P.S.; Kumar, R.K. Airway hyperreactivity in exacerbation of chronic asthma is independent of eosinophilic inflammation. *Am. J. Respir. Cell Mol. Biol.* **2006**, *35*, 565–570. [CrossRef]
58. Humbles, A.A.; Lloyd, C.M.; McMillan, S.J.; Friend, D.S.; Xanthou, G.; McKenna, E.E.; Ghiran, S.; Gerard, N.P.; Yu, C.; Orkin, S.H.; et al. A critical role for eosinophils in allergic airways remodeling. *Science* **2004**, *305*, 1776–1779. [CrossRef]
59. Kay, A.B.; Phipps, S.; Robinson, D.S. A role for eosinophils in airway remodelling in asthma. *Trends Immunol.* **2004**, *25*, 477–482. [CrossRef]
60. Flood-Page, P.; Menzies-Gow, A.; Phipps, S.; Ying, S.; Wangoo, A.; Ludwig, M.S.; Barnes, N.; Robinson, D.; Kay, A.B. Anti-IL-5 treatment reduces deposition of ECM proteins in the bronchial subepithelial basement membrane of mild atopic asthmatics. *J. Clin. Investig.* **2003**, *112*, 1029–1036. [CrossRef]
61. Tanaka, H.; Komai, M.; Nagao, K.; Ishizaki, M.; Kajiwara, D.; Takatsu, K.; Delespesse, G.; Nagai, H. Role of interleukin-5 and eosinophils in allergen-induced airway remodeling in mice. *Am. J. Respir. Cell Mol. Biol.* **2004**, *31*, 62–68. [CrossRef]
62. Esnault, S.; Kelly, E.A.; Johnson, S.H.; DeLain, L.P.; Haedt, M.J.; Noll, A.L.; Sandbo, N.; Jarjour, N.N. Matrix Metalloproteinase-9-Dependent Release of IL-1beta by Human Eosinophils. *Mediat. Inflamm.* **2019**, *2019*, 7479107. [CrossRef]
63. Schwingshackl, A.; Duszyk, M.; Brown, N.; Moqbel, R. Human eosinophils release matrix metalloproteinase-9 on stimulation with TNF-alpha. *J. Allergy Clin. Immunol.* **1999**, *104*, 983–989. [CrossRef]
64. Wicks, J.; Haitchi, H.M.; Holgate, S.T.; Davies, D.E.; Powell, R.M. Enhanced upregulation of smooth muscle related transcripts by TGF beta2 in asthmatic (myo) fibroblasts. *Thorax* **2006**, *61*, 313–319. [CrossRef]
65. McMillan, S.J.; Xanthou, G.; Lloyd, C.M. Manipulation of allergen-induced airway remodeling by treatment with anti-TGF-beta antibody: Effect on the Smad signaling pathway. *J. Immunol.* **2005**, *174*, 5774–5780. [CrossRef]
66. Roos, A.B.; Mori, M.; Gronneberg, R.; Osterlund, C.; Claesson, H.E.; Wahlstrom, J.; Grunewald, J.; Eklund, A.; Erjefalt, J.S.; Lundberg, J.O.; et al. Elevated exhaled nitric oxide in allergen-provoked asthma is associated with airway epithelial iNOS. *PLoS ONE* **2014**, *9*, e90018. [CrossRef]
67. MacPherson, J.C.; Comhair, S.A.; Erzurum, S.C.; Klein, D.F.; Lipscomb, M.F.; Kavuru, M.S.; Samoszuk, M.K.; Hazen, S.L. Eosinophils are a major source of nitric oxide-derived oxidants in severe asthma: Characterization of pathways available to eosinophils for generating reactive nitrogen species. *J. Immunol.* **2001**, *166*, 5763–5772. [CrossRef]
68. Chung, K.F. Asthma phenotyping: A necessity for improved therapeutic precision and new targeted therapies. *J. Intern. Med.* **2016**, *279*, 192–204. [CrossRef]
69. Petsky, H.L.; Cates, C.J.; Kew, K.M.; Chang, A.B. Tailoring asthma treatment on eosinophilic markers (exhaled nitric oxide or sputum eosinophils): A systematic review and meta-analysis. *Thorax* **2018**, *73*, 1110–1119. [CrossRef]

70. Flood-Page, P.; Swenson, C.; Faiferman, I.; Matthews, J.; Williams, M.; Brannick, L.; Robinson, D.; Wenzel, S.; Busse, W.; Hansel, T.T.; et al. A study to evaluate safety and efficacy of mepolizumab in patients with moderate persistent asthma. *Am. J. Respir. Crit. Care Med.* **2007**, *176*, 1062–1071. [CrossRef]
71. Seys, S.F.; Grabowski, M.; Adriaensen, W.; Decraene, A.; Dilissen, E.; Vanoirbeek, J.A.; Dupont, L.J.; Ceuppens, J.L.; Bullens, D.M. Sputum cytokine mapping reveals an 'IL-5, IL-17A, IL-25-high' pattern associated with poorly controlled asthma. *Clin. Exp. Allergy* **2013**, *43*, 1009–1017. [CrossRef]
72. Pouliquen, I.J.; Kornmann, O.; Barton, S.V.; Price, J.A.; Ortega, H.G. Characterization of the relationship between dose and blood eosinophil response following subcutaneous administration of mepolizumab. *Int. J. Clin. Pharmacol. Ther.* **2015**, *53*, 1015–1027. [CrossRef]
73. Pavord, I.D.; Korn, S.; Howarth, P.; Bleecker, E.R.; Buhl, R.; Keene, O.N.; Ortega, H.; Chanez, P. Mepolizumab for severe eosinophilic asthma (DREAM): A multicentre, double-blind, placebo-controlled trial. *Lancet* **2012**, *380*, 651–659. [CrossRef]
74. Fowler, S.J.; Tavernier, G.; Niven, R. High blood eosinophil counts predict sputum eosinophilia in patients with severe asthma. *J. Allergy Clin. Immunol.* **2015**, *135*, 822–824. [CrossRef]
75. Wagener, A.H.; de Nijs, S.B.; Lutter, R.; Sousa, A.R.; Weersink, E.J.; Bel, E.H.; Sterk, P.J. External validation of blood eosinophils, FE(NO) and serum periostin as surrogates for sputum eosinophils in asthma. *Thorax* **2015**, *70*, 115–120. [CrossRef]
76. Hastie, A.T.; Moore, W.C.; Li, H.; Rector, B.M.; Ortega, V.E.; Pascual, R.M.; Peters, S.P.; Meyers, D.A.; Bleecker, E.R.; National Heart, L.; et al. Biomarker surrogates do not accurately predict sputum eosinophil and neutrophil percentages in asthmatic subjects. *J. Allergy Clin. Immunol.* **2013**, *132*, 72–80. [CrossRef]
77. Korevaar, D.A.; Westerhof, G.A.; Wang, J.; Cohen, J.F.; Spijker, R.; Sterk, P.J.; Bel, E.H.; Bossuyt, P.M. Diagnostic accuracy of minimally invasive markers for detection of airway eosinophilia in asthma: A systematic review and meta-analysis. *Lancet Respir. Med.* **2015**, *3*, 290–300. [CrossRef]
78. Ullmann, N.; Bossley, C.J.; Fleming, L.; Silvestri, M.; Bush, A.; Saglani, S. Blood eosinophil counts rarely reflect airway eosinophilia in children with severe asthma. *Allergy* **2013**, *68*, 402–406. [CrossRef]
79. Yancey, S.W.; Keene, O.N.; Albers, F.C.; Ortega, H.; Bates, S.; Bleecker, E.R.; Pavord, I. Biomarkers for severe eosinophilic asthma. *J. Allergy Clin. Immunol.* **2017**, *140*, 1509–1518. [CrossRef]
80. Katz, L.E.; Gleich, G.J.; Hartley, B.F.; Yancey, S.W.; Ortega, H.G. Blood eosinophil count is a useful biomarker to identify patients with severe eosinophilic asthma. *Ann. Am. Thorac. Soc.* **2014**, *11*, 531–536. [CrossRef]
81. Dweik, R.A.; Boggs, P.B.; Erzurum, S.C.; Irvin, C.G.; Leigh, M.W.; Lundberg, J.O.; Olin, A.C.; Plummer, A.L.; Taylor, D.R.; American Thoracic Society Committee on Interpretation of Exhaled Nitric Oxide Levels (FENO) for Clinical Applications. An official ATS clinical practice guideline: Interpretation of exhaled nitric oxide levels (FENO) for clinical applications. *Am. J. Respir. Crit. Care Med.* **2011**, *184*, 602–615. [CrossRef]
82. Kostikas, K.; Minas, M.; Papaioannou, A.I.; Papiris, S.; Dweik, R.A. Exhaled nitric oxide in asthma in adults: The end is the beginning? *Curr. Med. Chem.* **2011**, *18*, 1423–1431. [CrossRef]
83. Zuiker, R.G.; Boot, J.D.; Calderon, C.; Piantone, A.; Petty, K.; de Kam, M.; Diamant, Z. Sputum induction with hypertonic saline reduces fractional exhaled nitric oxide in chronic smokers and non-smokers. *Respir. Med.* **2010**, *104*, 917–920. [CrossRef]
84. Tseliou, E.; Bessa, V.; Hillas, G.; Delimpoura, V.; Papadaki, G.; Roussos, C.; Papiris, S.; Bakakos, P.; Loukides, S. Exhaled nitric oxide and exhaled breath condensate pH in severe refractory asthma. *Chest* **2010**, *138*, 107–113. [CrossRef]
85. Haldar, P.; Brightling, C.E.; Hargadon, B.; Gupta, S.; Monteiro, W.; Sousa, A.; Marshall, R.P.; Bradding, P.; Green, R.H.; Wardlaw, A.J.; et al. Mepolizumab and exacerbations of refractory eosinophilic asthma. *N. Engl. J. Med.* **2009**, *360*, 973–984. [CrossRef]
86. Diamant, Z.; Vijverberg, S.; Alving, K.; Bakirtas, A.; Bjermer, L.; Custovic, A.; Dahlen, S.E.; Gaga, M.; Gerth van Wijk, R.; Del Giacco, S.; et al. Towards clinically applicable biomarkers for asthma—An EAACI position paper. *Allergy* **2019**. [CrossRef]
87. Brinkman, P.; van de Pol, M.A.; Gerritsen, M.G.; Bos, L.D.; Dekker, T.; Smids, B.S.; Sinha, A.; Majoor, C.J.; Sneeboer, M.M.; Knobel, H.H.; et al. Exhaled breath profiles in the monitoring of loss of control and clinical recovery in asthma. *Clin. Exp. Allergy* **2017**, *47*, 1159–1169. [CrossRef]
88. Schleich, F.N.; Zanella, D.; Stefanuto, P.H.; Bessonov, K.; Smolinska, A.; Dallinga, J.W.; Henket, M.; Paulus, V.; Guissard, F.; Graff, S.; et al. Exhaled Volatile Organic Compounds are Able to Discriminate between Neutrophilic and Eosinophilic Asthma. *Am. J. Respir. Crit. Care Med.* **2019**. [CrossRef]

89. Simpson, J.L.; Yang, I.A.; Upham, J.W.; Reynolds, P.N.; Hodge, S.; James, A.L.; Jenkins, C.; Peters, M.J.; Jia, G.; Holweg, C.T.; et al. Periostin levels and eosinophilic inflammation in poorly-controlled asthma. *BMC Pulm. Med.* **2016**, *16*, 67. [CrossRef]
90. Lefaudeux, D.; De Meulder, B.; Loza, M.J.; Peffer, N.; Rowe, A.; Baribaud, F.; Bansal, A.T.; Lutter, R.; Sousa, A.R.; Corfield, J.; et al. U-BIOPRED clinical adult asthma clusters linked to a subset of sputum omics. *J. Allergy Clin. Immunol.* **2017**, *139*, 1797–1807. [CrossRef]
91. Wu, W.; Bleecker, E.; Moore, W.; Busse, W.W.; Castro, M.; Chung, K.F.; Calhoun, W.J.; Erzurum, S.; Gaston, B.; Israel, E.; et al. Unsupervised phenotyping of Severe Asthma Research Program participants using expanded lung data. *J. Allergy Clin. Immunol.* **2014**, *133*, 1280–1288. [CrossRef]
92. Buhl, R.; Humbert, M.; Bjermer, L.; Chanez, P.; Heaney, L.G.; Pavord, I.; Quirce, S.; Virchow, J.C.; Holgate, S.; expert group of the European Consensus Meeting for Severe Eosinophilic Asthma. Severe eosinophilic asthma: A roadmap to consensus. *Eur. Respir. J.* **2017**. [CrossRef]
93. Leckie, M.J.; ten Brinke, A.; Khan, J.; Diamant, Z.; O'Connor, B.J.; Walls, C.M.; Mathur, A.K.; Cowley, H.C.; Chung, K.F.; Djukanovic, R.; et al. Effects of an interleukin-5 blocking monoclonal antibody on eosinophils, airway hyper-responsiveness, and the late asthmatic response. *Lancet* **2000**, *356*, 2144–2148. [CrossRef]
94. Kips, J.C.; O'Connor, B.J.; Langley, S.J.; Woodcock, A.; Kerstjens, H.A.; Postma, D.S.; Danzig, M.; Cuss, F.; Pauwels, R.A. Effect of SCH55700, a humanized anti-human interleukin-5 antibody, in severe persistent asthma: A pilot study. *Am. J. Respir. Crit. Care Med.* **2003**, *167*, 1655–1659. [CrossRef]
95. Nair, P.; Pizzichini, M.M.; Kjarsgaard, M.; Inman, M.D.; Efthimiadis, A.; Pizzichini, E.; Hargreave, F.E.; O'Byrne, P.M. Mepolizumab for prednisone-dependent asthma with sputum eosinophilia. *N. Engl. J. Med.* **2009**, *360*, 985–993. [CrossRef]
96. Ortega, H.G.; Liu, M.C.; Pavord, I.D.; Brusselle, G.G.; FitzGerald, J.M.; Chetta, A.; Humbert, M.; Katz, L.E.; Keene, O.N.; Yancey, S.W.; et al. Mepolizumab treatment in patients with severe eosinophilic asthma. *N. Engl. J. Med.* **2014**, *371*, 1198–1207. [CrossRef]
97. Bel, E.H.; Wenzel, S.E.; Thompson, P.J.; Prazma, C.M.; Keene, O.N.; Yancey, S.W.; Ortega, H.G.; Pavord, I.D.; SIRIUS Investigators. Oral glucocorticoid-sparing effect of mepolizumab in eosinophilic asthma. *N. Engl. J. Med.* **2014**, *371*, 1189–1197. [CrossRef]
98. Haldar, P.; Brightling, C.E.; Singapuri, A.; Hargadon, B.; Gupta, S.; Monteiro, W.; Bradding, P.; Green, R.H.; Wardlaw, A.J.; Ortega, H.; et al. Outcomes after cessation of mepolizumab therapy in severe eosinophilic asthma: A 12-month follow-up analysis. *J. Allergy Clin. Immunol.* **2014**, *133*, 921–923. [CrossRef]
99. Ortega, H.G.; Yancey, S.W.; Mayer, B.; Gunsoy, N.B.; Keene, O.N.; Bleecker, E.R.; Brightling, C.E.; Pavord, I.D. Severe eosinophilic asthma treated with mepolizumab stratified by baseline eosinophil thresholds: A secondary analysis of the DREAM and MENSA studies. *Lancet Respir. Med.* **2016**, *4*, 549–556. [CrossRef]
100. Yancey, S.W.; Bradford, E.S.; Keene, O.N. Disease burden and efficacy of mepolizumab in patients with severe asthma and blood eosinophil counts of >/=150-300cells/muL. *Respir. Med.* **2019**, *151*, 139–141. [CrossRef]
101. Magnan, A.; Bourdin, A.; Prazma, C.M.; Albers, F.C.; Price, R.G.; Yancey, S.W.; Ortega, H. Treatment response with mepolizumab in severe eosinophilic asthma patients with previous omalizumab treatment. *Allergy* **2016**, *71*, 1335–1344. [CrossRef]
102. Chapman, K.R.; Albers, F.C.; Chipps, B.; Munoz, X.; Devouassoux, G.; Bergna, M.; Galkin, D.; Azmi, J.; Mouneimne, D.; Price, R.G.; et al. The clinical benefit of mepolizumab replacing omalizumab in uncontrolled severe eosinophilic asthma. *Allergy* **2019**. [CrossRef]
103. Chupp, G.L.; Bradford, E.S.; Albers, F.C.; Bratton, D.J.; Wang-Jairaj, J.; Nelsen, L.M.; Trevor, J.L.; Magnan, A.; Ten Brinke, A. Efficacy of mepolizumab add-on therapy on health-related quality of life and markers of asthma control in severe eosinophilic asthma (MUSCA): A randomised, double-blind, placebo-controlled, parallel-group, multicentre, phase 3b trial. *Lancet Respir. Med.* **2017**, *5*, 390–400. [CrossRef]
104. Lugogo, N.; Domingo, C.; Chanez, P.; Leigh, R.; Gilson, M.J.; Price, R.G.; Yancey, S.W.; Ortega, H.G. Long-term Efficacy and Safety of Mepolizumab in Patients with Severe Eosinophilic Asthma: A Multi-center, Open-label, Phase IIIb Study. *Clin. Ther.* **2016**, *38*, 2058–2070. [CrossRef]
105. Khatri, S.; Moore, W.; Gibson, P.G.; Leigh, R.; Bourdin, A.; Maspero, J.; Barros, M.; Buhl, R.; Howarth, P.; Albers, F.C.; et al. Assessment of the long-term safety of mepolizumab and durability of clinical response in patients with severe eosinophilic asthma. *J. Allergy Clin. Immunol.* **2019**, *143*, 1742–1751. [CrossRef]

106. Ortega, H.G.; Meyer, E.; Brusselle, G.; Asano, K.; Prazma, C.M.; Albers, F.C.; Mallett, S.A.; Yancey, S.W.; Gleich, G.J. Update on immunogenicity in severe asthma: Experience with mepolizumab. *J. Allergy Clin. Immunol. Pract.* **2019**. [CrossRef]
107. Egan, R.W.; Athwal, D.; Bodmer, M.W.; Carter, J.M.; Chapman, R.W.; Chou, C.C.; Cox, M.A.; Emtage, J.S.; Fernandez, X.; Genatt, N.; et al. Effect of Sch 55700, a humanized monoclonal antibody to human interleukin-5, on eosinophilic responses and bronchial hyperreactivity. *Arzneimittelforschung* **1999**, *49*, 779–790. [CrossRef]
108. Castro, M.; Mathur, S.; Hargreave, F.; Boulet, L.P.; Xie, F.; Young, J.; Wilkins, H.J.; Henkel, T.; Nair, P.; Res-5-Study, G. Reslizumab for poorly controlled, eosinophilic asthma: A randomized, placebo-controlled study. *Am. J. Respir. Crit. Care Med.* **2011**, *184*, 1125–1132. [CrossRef]
109. Castro, M.; Zangrilli, J.; Wechsler, M.E.; Bateman, E.D.; Brusselle, G.G.; Bardin, P.; Murphy, K.; Maspero, J.F.; O'Brien, C.; Korn, S. Reslizumab for inadequately controlled asthma with elevated blood eosinophil counts: Results from two multicentre, parallel, double-blind, randomised, placebo-controlled, phase 3 trials. *Lancet Respir. Med.* **2015**, *3*, 355–366. [CrossRef]
110. Brusselle, G.; Germinaro, M.; Weiss, S.; Zangrilli, J. Reslizumab in patients with inadequately controlled late-onset asthma and elevated blood eosinophils. *Pulm. Pharmacol. Ther.* **2017**, *43*, 39–45. [CrossRef]
111. Mukherjee, M.; Aleman Paramo, F.; Kjarsgaard, M.; Salter, B.; Nair, G.; LaVigne, N.; Radford, K.; Sehmi, R.; Nair, P. Weight-adjusted Intravenous Reslizumab in Severe Asthma with Inadequate Response to Fixed-Dose Subcutaneous Mepolizumab. *Am. J. Respir. Crit. Care Med.* **2018**, *197*, 38–46. [CrossRef]
112. Kolbeck, R.; Kozhich, A.; Koike, M.; Peng, L.; Andersson, C.K.; Damschroder, M.M.; Reed, J.L.; Woods, R.; Dall'acqua, W.W.; Stephens, G.L.; et al. MEDI-563, a humanized anti-IL-5 receptor alpha mAb with enhanced antibody-dependent cell-mediated cytotoxicity function. *J. Allergy Clin. Immunol.* **2010**, *125*, 1344–1353 e2. [CrossRef]
113. Laviolette, M.; Gossage, D.L.; Gauvreau, G.; Leigh, R.; Olivenstein, R.; Katial, R.; Busse, W.W.; Wenzel, S.; Wu, Y.; Datta, V.; et al. Effects of benralizumab on airway eosinophils in asthmatic patients with sputum eosinophilia. *J. Allergy Clin. Immunol.* **2013**, *132*, 1086–1096 e5. [CrossRef]
114. Bleecker, E.R.; FitzGerald, J.M.; Chanez, P.; Papi, A.; Weinstein, S.F.; Barker, P.; Sproule, S.; Gilmartin, G.; Aurivillius, M.; Werkstrom, V.; et al. Efficacy and safety of benralizumab for patients with severe asthma uncontrolled with high-dosage inhaled corticosteroids and long-acting beta2-agonists (SIROCCO): A randomised, multicentre, placebo-controlled phase 3 trial. *Lancet* **2016**, *388*, 2115–2127. [CrossRef]
115. FitzGerald, J.M.; Bleecker, E.R.; Nair, P.; Korn, S.; Ohta, K.; Lommatzsch, M.; Ferguson, G.T.; Busse, W.W.; Barker, P.; Sproule, S.; et al. Benralizumab, an anti-interleukin-5 receptor alpha monoclonal antibody, as add-on treatment for patients with severe, uncontrolled, eosinophilic asthma (CALIMA): A randomised, double-blind, placebo-controlled phase 3 trial. *Lancet* **2016**, *388*, 2128–2141. [CrossRef]
116. Goldman, M.; Hirsch, I.; Zangrilli, J.G.; Newbold, P.; Xu, X. The association between blood eosinophil count and benralizumab efficacy for patients with severe, uncontrolled asthma: Subanalyses of the Phase III SIROCCO and CALIMA studies. *Curr. Med. Res. Opin.* **2017**, *33*, 1605–1613. [CrossRef]
117. FitzGerald, J.M.; Bleecker, E.R.; Menzies-Gow, A.; Zangrilli, J.G.; Hirsch, I.; Metcalfe, P.; Newbold, P.; Goldman, M. Predictors of enhanced response with benralizumab for patients with severe asthma: Pooled analysis of the SIROCCO and CALIMA studies. *Lancet Respir. Med.* **2018**, *6*, 51–64. [CrossRef]
118. Nair, P.; Wenzel, S.; Rabe, K.F.; Bourdin, A.; Lugogo, N.L.; Kuna, P.; Barker, P.; Sproule, S.; Ponnarambil, S.; Goldman, M.; et al. Oral Glucocorticoid-Sparing Effect of Benralizumab in Severe Asthma. *N. Engl. J. Med.* **2017**, *376*, 2448–2458. [CrossRef]
119. Busse, W.W.; Bleecker, E.R.; FitzGerald, J.M.; Ferguson, G.T.; Barker, P.; Sproule, S.; Olsson, R.F.; Martin, U.J.; Goldman, M.; BORA Study Investigators. Long-term safety and efficacy of benralizumab in patients with severe, uncontrolled asthma: 1-year results from the BORA phase 3 extension trial. *Lancet Respir. Med.* **2019**, *7*, 46–59. [CrossRef]
120. Bleecker, E.R.; Wechsler, M.E.; FitzGerald, J.M.; Menzies-Gow, A.; Wu, Y.; Hirsch, I.; Goldman, M.; Newbold, P.; Zangrilli, J.G. Baseline patient factors impact on the clinical efficacy of benralizumab for severe asthma. *Eur. Respir. J.* **2018**, *52*. [CrossRef]
121. Chipps, B.E.; Newbold, P.; Hirsch, I.; Trudo, F.; Goldman, M. Benralizumab efficacy by atopy status and serum immunoglobulin E for patients with severe, uncontrolled asthma. *Ann. Allergy Asthma Immunol.* **2018**, *120*, 504–511. [CrossRef]

122. Bourdin, A.; Husereau, D.; Molinari, N.; Golam, S.; Siddiqui, M.K.; Lindner, L.; Xu, X. Matching-adjusted indirect comparison of benralizumab versus interleukin-5 inhibitors for the treatment of severe asthma: A systematic review. *Eur. Respir. J.* **2018**, *52*. [CrossRef]
123. Busse, W.; Chupp, G.; Nagase, H.; Albers, F.C.; Doyle, S.; Shen, Q.; Bratton, D.J.; Gunsoy, N.B. Anti-IL-5 treatments in patients with severe asthma by blood eosinophil thresholds: Indirect treatment comparison. *J. Allergy Clin. Immunol.* **2019**, *143*, 190–200. [CrossRef]
124. Zervas, E.; Samitas, K.; Papaioannou, A.I.; Bakakos, P.; Loukides, S.; Gaga, M. An algorithmic approach for the treatment of severe uncontrolled asthma. *ERJ Open Res.* **2018**, *4*. [CrossRef]
125. Difficult-to-Treat and Severe Asthma in Adolescent and Adult Patients Diagnosis and Management. 2019, A GINA Pocket Guide for Health Professionals. Available online: www.ginasthma.org (accessed on 30 April 2019.).
126. Wenzel, S.; Ford, L.; Pearlman, D.; Spector, S.; Sher, L.; Skobieranda, F.; Wang, L.; Kirkesseli, S.; Rocklin, R.; Bock, B.; et al. Dupilumab in persistent asthma with elevated eosinophil levels. *N. Engl. J. Med.* **2013**, *368*, 2455–2466. [CrossRef]
127. Wenzel, S.; Castro, M.; Corren, J.; Maspero, J.; Wang, L.; Zhang, B.; Pirozzi, G.; Sutherland, E.R.; Evans, R.R.; Joish, V.N.; et al. Dupilumab efficacy and safety in adults with uncontrolled persistent asthma despite use of medium-to-high-dose inhaled corticosteroids plus a long-acting beta2 agonist: A randomised double-blind placebo-controlled pivotal phase 2b dose-ranging trial. *Lancet* **2016**, *388*, 31–44. [CrossRef]
128. Corren, J.; Castro, M.; Chanez, P.; Fabbri, L.; Joish, V.N.; Amin, N.; Graham, N.M.H.; Mastey, V.; Abbe, A.; Taniou, C.; et al. Dupilumab improves symptoms, quality of life, and productivity in uncontrolled persistent asthma. *Ann. Allergy Asthma Immunol.* **2019**, *122*, 41–49. [CrossRef]
129. Castro, M.; Corren, J.; Pavord, I.D.; Maspero, J.; Wenzel, S.; Rabe, K.F.; Busse, W.W.; Ford, L.; Sher, L.; FitzGerald, J.M.; et al. Dupilumab Efficacy and Safety in Moderate-to-Severe Uncontrolled Asthma. *N. Engl. J. Med.* **2018**, *378*, 2486–2496. [CrossRef]
130. Rabe, K.F.; Nair, P.; Brusselle, G.; Maspero, J.F.; Castro, M.; Sher, L.; Zhu, H.; Hamilton, J.D.; Swanson, B.N.; Khan, A.; et al. Efficacy and Safety of Dupilumab in Glucocorticoid-Dependent Severe Asthma. *N. Engl. J. Med.* **2018**, *378*, 2475–2485. [CrossRef]
131. Xiong, X.F.; Zhu, M.; Wu, H.X.; Fan, L.L.; Cheng, D.Y. Efficacy and safety of dupilumab for the treatment of uncontrolled asthma: A meta-analysis of randomized clinical trials. *Respir. Res.* **2019**, *20*, 108. [CrossRef]
132. Bachert, C.; Nan, Z. Medical Algorithm: Diagnosis and Treatment of Chronic Rhinosinusitis. *Allergy* **2019**. [CrossRef]
133. Schulman, E.S. Development of a monoclonal anti-immunoglobulin E antibody (omalizumab) for the treatment of allergic respiratory disorders. *Am. J. Respir. Crit. Care Med.* **2001**, *164*, S6–S11. [CrossRef]
134. Humbert, M.; Busse, W.; Hanania, N.A.; Lowe, P.J.; Canvin, J.; Erpenbeck, V.J.; Holgate, S. Omalizumab in asthma: An update on recent developments. *J. Allergy Clin. Immunol. Pract.* **2014**, *2*, 525–536. [CrossRef]
135. Hanania, N.A.; Wenzel, S.; Rosen, K.; Hsieh, H.J.; Mosesova, S.; Choy, D.F.; Lal, P.; Arron, J.R.; Harris, J.M.; Busse, W. Exploring the effects of omalizumab in allergic asthma: An analysis of biomarkers in the EXTRA study. *Am. J. Respir. Crit. Care Med.* **2013**, *187*, 804–811. [CrossRef]
136. Casale, T.B.; Luskin, A.T.; Busse, W.; Zeiger, R.S.; Trzaskoma, B.; Yang, M.; Griffin, N.M.; Chipps, B.E. Omalizumab Effectiveness by Biomarker Status in Patients with Asthma: Evidence From PROSPERO, A Prospective Real-World Study. *J. Allergy Clin. Immunol. Pract.* **2019**, *7*, 156–164. [CrossRef]
137. Humbert, M.; Taille, C.; Mala, L.; Le Gros, V.; Just, J.; Molimard, M.; STELLAIR Investigators. Omalizumab effectiveness in patients with severe allergic asthma according to blood eosinophil count: The STELLAIR study. *Eur. Respir. J.* **2018**, *51*. [CrossRef]
138. Lambrecht, B.N.; Hammad, H. The role of dendritic and epithelial cells as master regulators of allergic airway inflammation. *Lancet* **2010**, *376*, 835–843. [CrossRef]
139. Licona-Limon, P.; Kim, L.K.; Palm, N.W.; Flavell, R.A. TH2, allergy and group 2 innate lymphoid cells. *Nat. Immunol.* **2013**, *14*, 536–542. [CrossRef]
140. Corren, J.; Parnes, J.R.; Wang, L.; Mo, M.; Roseti, S.L.; Griffiths, J.M.; van der Merwe, R. Tezepelumab in Adults with Uncontrolled Asthma. *N. Engl. J. Med.* **2017**, *377*, 936–946. [CrossRef]
141. Kostenis, E.; Ulven, T. Emerging roles of DP and CRTH2 in allergic inflammation. *Trends Mol. Med.* **2006**, *12*, 148–158. [CrossRef]

142. Erpenbeck, V.J.; Popov, T.A.; Miller, D.; Weinstein, S.F.; Spector, S.; Magnusson, B.; Osuntokun, W.; Goldsmith, P.; Weiss, M.; Beier, J. The oral CRTh2 antagonist QAW039 (fevipiprant): A phase II study in uncontrolled allergic asthma. *Pulm. Pharmacol. Ther.* **2016**, *39*, 54–63. [CrossRef]
143. Gonem, S.; Berair, R.; Singapuri, A.; Hartley, R.; Laurencin, M.F.M.; Bacher, G.; Holzhauer, B.; Bourne, M.; Mistry, V.; Pavord, I.D.; et al. Fevipiprant, a prostaglandin D2 receptor 2 antagonist, in patients with persistent eosinophilic asthma: A single-centre, randomised, double-blind, parallel-group, placebo-controlled trial. *Lancet Respir. Med.* **2016**, *4*, 699–707. [CrossRef]
144. Bateman, E.D.; Guerreros, A.G.; Brockhaus, F.; Holzhauer, B.; Pethe, A.; Kay, R.A.; Townley, R.G. Fevipiprant, an oral prostaglandin DP2 receptor (CRTh2) antagonist, in allergic asthma uncontrolled on low-dose inhaled corticosteroids. *Eur. Respir. J.* **2017**, *50*. [CrossRef]

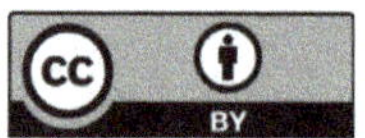

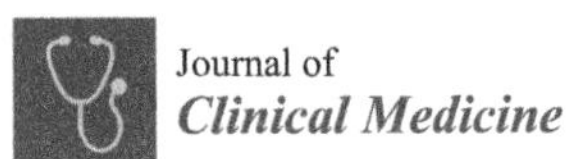
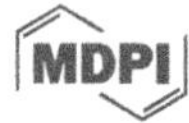

Review

The Co-Existence of Obstructive Sleep Apnea and Bronchial Asthma: Revelation of a New Asthma Phenotype?

Angeliki Damianaki [1,2], Emmanouil Vagiakis [3], Ioanna Sigala [3], Athanasia Pataka [4], Nikoletta Rovina [5], Athina Vlachou [2], Vasiliki Krietsepi [1], Spyros Zakynthinos [2,3] and Paraskevi Katsaounou [2,3,*]

1 Pulmonary Department "Saint George" General Hospital of Chania, 73300 Crete, Greece; angeldam@hotmail.com (A.D.); vikkikrietsepi@yahoo.gr (V.K.)
2 First ICU Clinic, National and Kapodistrian University of Athens, 10561 Athens, Greece; athvlachou@yahoo.com (A.V.); szakynthinos@yahoo.com (S.Z.)
3 Sleep Lab, First ICU Clinic Evangelismos Hospital, 10676 Athens, Greece; sleeplabathens@yahoo.gr (E.V.); giannasig@yahoo.com (I.S.)
4 Respiratory Failure Unit, G. Papanikolaou Hospital, Exohi, Aristotle University of Thessaloniki, 57010 Thessaloniki, Greece; patakath@yahoo.gr
5 ICU, First Department of Pulmonary Medicine, Sotiria Hospital, 115 27 Athens, Greece; nikrovina@med.uoa.gr
* Correspondence: paraskevikatsaounou@gmail.com; Tel.: +30-213-204-3384

Received: 31 July 2019; Accepted: 5 September 2019; Published: 16 September 2019

Abstract: Bronchial asthma (BA) and obstructive sleep apnea (OSA) are common respiratory obstructive diseases that may coexist. It would be interesting to study the possible influence of that coexistence on both diseases. Until now, reviews focused mainly on epidemiology. The aim of this study was to review the literature in relation to epidemiology, pathophysiology, consequences, screening of patients, and treatment of the coexistence of OSA and BA. We pooled studies from the PubMed database from 1986 to 2019. OSA prevalence in asthmatics was found to be high, ranging from19% to 60% in non-severe BA, reaching up to 95% in severe asthma. Prevalence was correlated with the duration and severity of BA, and increased dosage of steroids taken orally or by inhalation. This high prevalence of the coexistence of OSA and BA diseases could not be a result of just chance. It seems that this coexistence is based on the pathophysiology of the diseases. In most studies, OSA seems to deteriorate asthma outcomes, and mainly exacerbates them. CPAP (continuous positive airway pressure) treatment is likely to improve symptoms, the control of the disease, and the quality of life in asthmatics with OSA. However, almost all studies are observational, involving a small number of patients with a short period of follow up. Although treatment guidelines cannot be released, we could recommend periodic screening of asthmatics for OSA for the optimal treatment of both the diseases.

Keywords: obstructive sleep apnea; bronchial asthma; alternative overlap syndrome

1. Introduction

Bronchial asthma is a common inflammatory respiratory disease affecting up to 1–18% of the population in different countries. It is characterized by bronchial hyper-responsiveness (BHR) and presents with variable symptoms including wheezing, shortness of breath, chest tightness, and cough that vary according to disease severity [1]. The gold standard for the diagnosis is the improvement of forced expiratory volume in the first second (FEV_1) >12% and 200 mL, 10–20 min after the inhalation of 100–200 mg of salbutamol [1].Almost 5–10% of asthmatics have severe, refractory asthma despite optimal therapy, and experience frequent exacerbations, hospital admissions, and healthcare utilization. They often use high doses of inhaled or oral steroids. A significant percentage of asthmatic patients, up to 70%, experience symptoms during sleep, and therefore have nocturnal asthma [2]. Both nocturnal symptoms in asthma and uncontrolled asthma have a profound effect on sleep quality [3]. The aim of asthma treatment is to achieve asthma control, which means having very few symptoms. Asthma control is assessed using validated questionnaires such as the asthma control questionnaire (ACQ) and the asthma control test (ACT) [1].

Obstructive sleep apnea (OSA) is the most frequent sleep-related breathing disorder. OSA with excessive daytime sleepiness ranged in frequency between 3% and 18% in men and 1–17% in women [4]. OSA is an under-diagnosed disorder [5] that is characterized by recurrent collapses of the upper airway during sleep, leading to a remarkable reduction or complete cessation of airflow despite ongoing breathing efforts. That airflow obstruction leads to repetitive hypoxia and fragmented sleep, and is therefore associated with hypertension, cardiovascular disease, diabetes, and stroke [6–8]. The gold standard diagnostic test is the overnight attended polysomnography (PSG), which is rather expensive and time-consuming. As a result, researchers often use validated questionnaires, such as the Berlin questionnaire (BQ), stop bang questionnaire (SBQ), and the sleep apnea scale of the sleep disorders questionnaire (SA–SDQ), to estimate the risk of having OSA [9–11]. The severity of OSA is determined using the apnea hypopnea index (AHI), which is defined as the number of apneas and hypopneas per hour of total sleep time (TST). Continuous positive airway pressure (CPAP) is the treatment of choice as it decreases long-term mortality [12].

OSA and BA share some common characteristics. First, they are both obstructive respiratory diseases, but with different mechanisms and anatomy of obstruction. A patient with BA and OSA has both upper and lower airway obstruction during sleep. Second, both diseases share common co–morbidities like obesity, allergic rhinitis, and gastro-esophageal reflux (GER). Patients with OSA and BA also have poor quality of sleep and may have increased morbidity and mortality. When they coexist, a bidirectional relationship may additionally affect each other. Since 2013, the coexistence of OSA and BA was defined as alternative overlap syndrome (AOS) to distinguish it from the overlap syndrome that is referred to as chronic obstructive pulmonary disease (COPD) and OSA [13]. While there are reviews in the literature, they mainly focused on the epidemiology. In order to determine the current state-of-the-art knowledge, we conducted a literature review, targeting epidemiology, pathophysiology, clinical consequences, screening, and treatment of AOS. We additionally aim to point out possible gaps for future research.

2. Methods

A review of the literature was performed pooling studies in English from the PUBMED database from 1986 to 2019. The following search terms were used: obstructive sleep apnea, bronchial asthma, and alternative overlap syndrome. We decided to focus on studies addressing the prevalence, diagnosis, pathophysiology, clinical outcomes, treatment, and screening of patients with obstructive sleep apnea and bronchial asthma (alternative overlap syndrome). During the search process, 673 articles emerged. Studies were excluded if not written in the English language or were carried out on a pediatric population (<18 years of age). Additionally, studies that were not relevant to our review were excluded. Finally, 92 articles were selected for this review.

3. Epidemiology

The vast majority of studies mainly referred to the prevalence of OSA in asthmatic populations. The prevalence was increased, ranging from 19% to 60% [14–16], and reaches up to 95% in severe BA in two studies [17,18], which suggests that the two diseases did not accidentally coexist. The great variability of this prevalence was the result of:

1. The diagnostic method used for OSA diagnosis. Early studies used questionnaires regarding OSA symptoms like habitual snoring, witnessed apneas, and daytime sleepiness [19–22]. Later, studies

used validated questionnaires estimating the risk of having OSA [23–25]. Some used cardio-respiratory polygraphy [18,26], while a few used attended overnight polysomnography [14,27–29]. Other studies used a combination of the above-referred sleep studies [30–32].

2. The cut-offs used for the determination of OSA diagnosis. Some studies used AHI ≥5 [14,33], others AHI ≥15 [18,34], while others used the RDI (respiratory disturbances index includes apneas, hypopneas, and respiratory effort related arousals) [17].

3. The diagnostic method used for BA diagnosis. Few studies used spirometry or provocation tests [28,33,35]. The majority used questionnaires, where patients were asked to answer if they had asthma symptoms, receive asthma medications, or they have been informed about having asthma by their physicians [14,27,29,31].

4. The heterogeneity of the populations in relation to age, smoking status, and weight.

Early questionnaire-based, cross-sectional studies depicted a statistically significant higher prevalence of OSA symptoms, such as habitual snoring and witnessed apneas, in patients with BA as compared to the general population, independently of the body mass index (BMI), gender, age, or smoking status [19–22]. BA has been confirmed as an independent risk factor for habitual snoring, which is the mild end of the spectrum of sleep disordered breathing (SDB) [36].

In 2015, a large retrospective cohort study using data from the National Health Insurance of Taiwan, collected 38.840 newly diagnosed asthmatics between 2000 and 2010. Each patient matched to four people without asthma according to gender, age, and the date of the diagnosis. The occurrence of OSA was followed until the end of 2011. The overall incidence of OSA was 2.51-fold greater in the asthma cohort than in the comparison group (12.1 vs. 4.84 per person-years). Among asthmatics, the adjusted hazard ratio (HR) for OSA increased to 1.78 for asthma patients with one or less annual emergency room (ER) visits, and 23.8 for those who visited the ER more than once per year. Additionally, the adjusted HR in patients with inhaled steroids compared to those without receiving steroids was 1.33. The authors concluded that asthmatics had a greater risk for OSA, which was much greater when the asthma was more severe [33].

The same year, in another large study, this time a prospective population-based study, 547 selected subjects free of OSA at baseline (AHI < 5) on two consecutive overnight-attended PSG studies were followed every four years for OSA incidence. The BA diagnosis was based on questionnaires. Patients with asthma had a 39% increase in the risk of developing incident OSA as compared with controls, independently of the baseline covariates such as BMI, AHI, and BMI change over time. The risk was duration-dependent: for each 5-year increment in asthma duration, the risk for incident OSA increased by 7%. An asthma duration >10 years increased the risk by 65% [14].

In a recent meta–analysis of 26 studies (7675 patients), the prevalence/relative risk of OSA and the OSA risk (OSA diagnosis based on questionnaires) was 49.5%/2.64 and 27.5%/3.73, respectively, in asthmatics. Patients with BA and OSA had significantly greater BMI (average difference 2.15 kg/m^2 $p < 0.004$), and sleepiness (average difference on the Epworth sleepiness scale, ESS = 3.98, $p = 0.004$) compared to asthmatics without OSA, while no difference was observed in FEV$_1$ [16].

There is evidence in the literature that the prevalence of OSA in asthmatics is positively correlated with the severity of BA, ranging from 50 to 95% in severe asthma [17,18], and with the dosage of the received oral or inhalational steroids in a dose-dependent manner [17,37]. The possible association between the severity of BA and the severity of OSA remain controversial [18,28].

While the vast majority of studies address asthmatic populations, Alhabri et al. studied the relation between OSA and BA in the opposite direction. They found that patients with OSA diagnosed with PSG had a 35% increased prevalence of BA and these patients had a greater BMI, AHI, and the lowest oxygen saturation during sleep compared with OSA patients without BA. It seems like BA deteriorated OSA. Obesity (BMI > 35 kg/m^2) was the only independent factor that could predict BA in OSA patients [27]. Increased prevalence of BA was also reported in OSA patients in some studies where the prevalence was not the primary endpoint. Kauppi et al., in a sample of 1586 patients with

OSA, reported 13% having BA based on a questionnaire [31], while Wang et al. studying a sample of 466 patients in a sleep laboratory found that 16.5% had BA [35].

4. Pathophysiology

The exact mechanisms through which these diseases interact with each other are unknown, although much work has been done regarding this issue. The role of inflammation is a key contributor. Common co–morbidities like allergic rhinitis, obesity and GER also play an important role. Some of the proposed mechanisms are discussed below.

5. How BA Could Affect or Lead to OSA?

5.1. Mechanical Effects

Asthmatics with nocturnal asthma symptoms demonstrate hyperinflation during the day, meaning their functional residual capacity (FRC) is increased compared to healthy controls. However, the normal drop in FRC during sleep is exaggerated in asthmatics and specifically during Rapid Eye Movement (REM) sleep. This results in an increased airway resistance as an inverse relationship between lung volume and airway resistance is known to exist [38]. Moreover, Irvin et al. demonstrated that in asthmatics with nocturnal symptoms, there is an airway–parenchyma uncoupling, probably due to neural mechanisms, meaning that during the night, airway resistance is increased independently of lung volume [39]. Airway resistance could attenuate the normal tracheal tug inducing upper airway collapse [40].

5.2. Alterations in the Upper Airway Anatomy

The inflammatory infiltration of the upper airway in asthma [41], the increased fat deposition in the pharyngeal walls due to steroids use [17], or the presence of comorbidities such as obesity [42], lead to a diminished cross-sectional diameter of the upper airway. Moreover, allergic rhinitis, nasal polyps, and adenoids hypertrophy, which frequently accompany asthma, increase airflow resistance and create high negative pressure during inspiration that increase the risk of upper airway collapse [43,44].

Additionally, bronchial asthma possibly influences pharyngeal muscle function, either directly affecting neural sensor pathways because of inflammation or indirectly due to muscle weakness caused from the steroids that is the cornerstone of BA treatment [1]. Pharyngeal muscle myopathy increases collapsibility of the upper airway, increasing the risk of OSA. Yigla et al. reported a high prevalence of OSA (95%) among asthmatics receiving long-term chronic or frequent bursts of oral steroid therapy and indentified a positive dose–response relationship between steroids and OSA [17]. Other studies reported similar results [33,37]. The possible mechanisms through which asthma affects OSA are summarized from the authors in the figure below, although the impact of steroidsuse still remains controversial (Table 1).

Table 1. The effect of asthma on Obstructive Sleep Apnea.

Attenuation of the Normal Tracheal Tug/Alteration in the Upper Airway Anatomy	
Diminished cross-sectional diameter of the upper airway due to Asthma inflammation	Nasal obstruction due to Nasal polyps
Increased fat deposition in the pharyngeal walls due to: • Sleep deprivation • Depression • Exercise limitation • Obesity • Steroids use	Adenoids hypertrophy
Upper airway muscle dysfunction • Steroid use • Disruption of sensory neural pathways due to inflammation	Allergic rhinitis

6. How Could OSA Affect or Lead to BA?

The key factor seems to be the inflammation induced by OSA, both through the airway and systemic. The repeated episodes of a collapsed upper airway lead to hypoxia and eventually oxidative stress, which then cascades to systemic inflammation with increased serum levels of cytokines such as C-reactive protein, interleukin-6 (IL-6), and tumor necrosis factor (TNF-α). The distal airway inflammation seen in BA increases the probability of asthma attacks [45,46].

Additionally, in OSA, a neutrophil-predominant inflammation seems to begin from the nose, expands to the distal airways infiltrating the airway walls [47,48], and is related to the disease severity. Studies in experimental animal models have showed that the increased inspiration effort against the closed upper airway combined with intermittent hypoxia is associated with inflammation of the lungs [49,50].

Teodorescu et al. studied a large and objectively diagnosed sample of 255 asthmatic patients and estimated the risk of having OSA using the SA-SDQ questionnaire. A higher SA-SDQ score was associated with increased asthma symptoms, β_2-agonist use, healthcare utilization, and worse asthma quality of life. They also conducted sputum induction and found higher percentages of neutrophils in asthmatics' sputum with a high OSA risk compared to those without a high OSA risk ($p = 0.001$), whereas sputum eosinophil percentages were similar ($p = 0.66$). There was a significant association of SA-SDQ with sputum neutrophils. Namely, each increase in SA-SDQ by its standard deviation (6.85 units) was associated with a rise in sputum neutrophils of 7.78% (95% CI 2.33–13.22, $p = 0.0006$), independently of obesity and other confounding factors [24]. Authors concluded that OSA may be an important contributor to neutrophilic asthma.

The same results were also confirmed in 55 patients with severe asthma and OSA diagnosed using cardiorespiratory polygraphy [26]. Furthermore, by receiving bronchial biopsies with bronchoscopy, researchers found that the thickness of the bronchial basement membrane was negatively associated with the AHI [26]. Although more studies are needed, we may suggest that the coexistence of OSA in asthma patients may divert asthma inflammation to being neutrophilic, may contribute to airway remodeling, and eventually may result in a difficult-to-treat asthma.

Moreover, additional factors seen in OSA like GER, cardiac dysfunction, obesity, and increased levels of vascular endothelial growth factor (VEGF) and leptin have been proposed to increase BHR and deteriorate asthma outcomes [51–54].

The overall pathophysiologic mechanisms involved in the BA–OSA interaction are depicted in Figure 1.

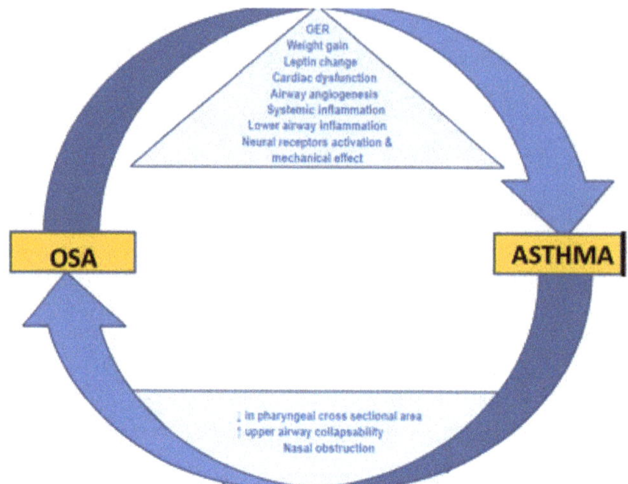

Figure 1. Pathophysiological mechanisms between Obstructive Sleep Apnea and Asthma. Adapted from Alkhalil et al. Sleep Medicine, 2009 [55].

7. Clinical Consequences of the Alternative Overlap Syndrome

There is strong clinical evidence to support the claim that OSA deteriorates BA outcomes.

Namely, the coexistence of OSA in asthmatics causes an increase in persistent nocturnal asthmatic symptoms compared with those without OSA [56–58]. Later, Teodorescu et al. investigated whether OSA was associated with daytime in addition to night-time asthma symptoms. Among 752 asthmatics, high OSA risk (using the SA-SDQ questionnaire) was associated with persistent daytime and night-time asthma symptoms ($p < 0.0001$ for each). A diagnosis of OSA was associated with both persistent daytime ($p < 0.0001$), in addition to night-time ($p = 0.0008$), asthma symptoms. The associations were retained in regression models where other known asthma aggravators, like obesity, were included. They concluded that unrecognized OSA may be the cause of persistent BA symptoms, both daytime and nocturnal [23].

OSA is the fifth independent risk factor (adjusted OR 3.4) among 13 clinical and environmental factors studied for recurrent exacerbations in difficult to treat asthma. The first four are psychological dysfunctioning, recurrent respiratory infections, GER, and severe chronic sinus disease [59]. Therefore, according to Global Initiative for Asthma (GINA) recommendations, chest physicians should investigate the possibility of underlying OSA in patients with difficult-to-treat asthma [1]. Moreover, in 2017, Wang et al. reported that the severity of OSA was independently correlated with the number of severe asthma exacerbations (OR = 1.32, $p < 0.001$) in a prospective cross–sectional cohort study [15].

Regarding asthma control, studies using ACT and ACQ questionnaires showed worse asthma control in asthmatics with OSA, although this was not statistically significant in all studies [25,60,61].

There is not much evidence addressing pulmonary function in asthmatic patients with OSA. The natural history of FEV_1 decline in asthmatic patients has been reported to be 38–40.9 mL/year [62]. Known factors contributing to FEV_1 decline in asthmatic patients are age, sex, smoking, acute exacerbations, obesity, and hypoxia [63–65]. In a recent retrospective study, using a sleep laboratory population with OSA patients, 77 asthmatic patients with OSA (diagnosed using PSG) were selected and followed for more than 5 years with spirometry. Asthmatic patients with OSA had substantially greater declines in FEV_1per year compared to those without OSA in an AHI–dependent manner. Asthma patients with severe OSA (AHI > 30) had a decline in $FEV_1$of 72.4 ± 61.7mL/year as compared to 41.9 ± 45.3 mL/year in those with mild to moderate OSA (5 < AHI ≤ 30) and 24.3 ± 27.5mL/year in those without OSA (AHI ≤ 5).The severity of OSA was the only independent factor for this decline after adjusting for other confounding factors like BMI, age, current smoking status, and number of emergency room visits/year. CPAP treatment significantly decreased the FEV_1decline in the patients with severe OSA [35]. However, in a meta-analysis, in asthmatic patients with and without OSA, no significant difference was seen in FEV_1 (mean difference = −2.28, $p = 0.32$) [16].

It is known that asthmatics have a low quality of sleep due to a variety of factors such as the increased frequency of nocturnal asthma, co-morbidities, bronchodilators, and corticosteroids [20,66]. As a result, they present excessive daytime sleepiness more frequently compared to controls [20]. For the first time in 2006 in a cross-sectional, clinic-based study investigating all these factors, Teodorescu et al. reported that sleepiness is common in asthmatics and may reflect occult OSA more often than the effects of asthma itself, other co-morbidities, or asthma medications [22]. Asthmatics with OSA have greater sleepiness than OSA-free asthmatics, scoring higher on the ESS [15,16].

The European Sleep Apnea Database (ESADA) cohort addressed the differences between asthmatics and non-asthmatics referred to sleep centers. An interesting finding was that asthmatic patients are under-referred for sleep studies, meaning that physicians are not aware or underestimate the coexistence of OSA and asthma in clinical practice. In that cohort, asthmatic women (with or without OSA) were more obese and reported more daytime sleepiness (according to ESS) than the non-asthmatic ones. This shows that obesity is the main factor for sleep referral in asthmatic women but may give implications about the existence of a specific phenotype as well [67].

There are very few reports investigating the objective parameters of sleep in subjects with AOS. In 2018, 384 adult women from the Sleep and Health Program in Sweden, an on-going community-based study, underwent overnight polysomnography. Women with both asthma and OSA had a longer sleep time in non-deep sleep stages $N_1$and N_2, and less time in the REM stage than the control group with no asthma or OSA. The group with BA and OSA had a lower mean oxygen saturation (93.4% vs. 94.7%, $p = 0.004$) than the group with OSA alone and spent more time with oxygen saturation below 90% than the patients with OSA only. The results remained after adjusting for age, BMI, and smoking status. BA was independently associated with lower oxygen saturation, while OSA was not. Authors concluded that coexisting OSA and BA is associated with poorer sleep quality and more profound nocturnal hypoxemia than either of the diseases alone [29]. Similar results concerning sleep architecture had already been reported in other studies [28,68].

While studies have highlighted OSA among asthma patients in outpatient settings, such data in the inpatient setting was sparse until 2015 when Becerra et al., using a 2009–2011 U.S. Nationwide Inpatient Sample, studied the impact of two common asthma co-morbidities—OSA and obesity—on the length and cost of hospitalization and on the need for invasive mechanical ventilation. They reported that OSA and obesity significantly increased the length of stay (OR = 1.07 in males and 1.14 in females, and 1.07 in males and 1.08 in females, respectively) and the total hospital charges in both genders (15% in males and 19% in females, and 8.6% in males and 9.6% in females, respectively). Furthermore, when they coexisted, this led to multiplied increases in the length of stay (OR = 1.19 in males and 1.24 in females) and hospital charges (24.9% in males and 28.5% in females).

OSA alone in asthmatics (OR = 2.56 in males and 3.22 in females) or in coexistence with obesity (OR = 2.85 in males and 3.60 in females) significantly increased the use of mechanical ventilation while obesity alone did not (OR = 0.97 in males and 1.01 in females) [69].

OSA and BA are associated with increased rates of systemic arterial hypertension [70,71], with inflammation being proposed as the basic pathophysiologic cause [72,73]. OSA in asthmatics lead to greater prevalence of arterial hypertension compared to asthmatics without OSA (adjusted OR = 2.20), as Ferguson et al. reported in a cross-sectional, questionnaire-based study. The authors concluded that the inflammation of the diseases act additionally [74].

The only study addressing the mortality in AOS is a retrospective study from South Korea. Kyu-Tae Han et al. used data from the National Health Insurance Service (NHIS) National Sample Cohort 2004–2013 in order to investigate the association between sleep disorders (International Classification of Diseases ICD-10: G.47) and mortality in patients with newly diagnosed BA (ICD-10: J.45) during outpatient care between 2004 and 2013. They excluded patients with sleep disorders diagnosed prior to the BA diagnosis. They studied asthmatic patients that were difficult to be controlled, had increased sleep disorders prevalence, and frequently used health services. The study sample consisted of 186.491 asthmatic patients newly diagnosed with asthma. A sleep disorders diagnosis that followed the asthma diagnosis and mortality was studied in these patients. A total of 5179 patients died during the study period (2.78%) because of lung cancer (10.5%), senility (6.1%), COPD (4.5%), myocardial infarction (4.4%), and stomach cancer (3.7%). Asthmatic patients with coexisting sleep disorders had an increased risk of death compared with asthmatics without sleep disorders after adjusting for confounding variables like age, sex, gender, income, and co-morbidities (hazard ratio [HR]: 1.451 (95% confidence interval [CI]: 1.253–1.681). The mean duration between the asthma diagnosis and death was shorter in asthmatics with sleep disorders (mean duration: 103.85 months), compared with asthmatics without sleep disorders (mean duration: 116.05 months, $p < 0.0001$). Authors concluded that the presence of sleep disorders in patients with asthma was associated with a high risk of mortality, as shown using Kaplan–Meier survival curves and a log rank test [75]. We summarize the findings concerning the impact of OSA on asthma in Table 2.

Table 2. Impact of Obstructive Sleep Apnea (OSA) on asthma.

Study	Study Design	Population	Asthma Diagnosis	OSA Diagnosis	Results
Teodorerscu, M et al. J Asthma 2012 [23]	Cross-sectional	$N = 828$ subjects with BA Allergy and pulmonary clinics	ATS guidelines	SA-SDQ and review of medical notes	High OSA risk associated with persistent daytime (OR = 1.96, 95% CI = 1.31–2.94) and night-time (OR = 1.97, 95% CI = 1.32–1.94) asthma symptoms.
Wang et al. Sleep Med 2016 [15]	Prospective cross-sectional cohort study	$N = 146$ asthmatics $N = 157$ controls Asthma follow-up in outpatient clinics	Physician diagnosis	PSG	Annual number of severe asthma exacerbations was significantly higher in the OSA group compared to the no-OSA group ($p < 0.001$). AHI significantly correlated with the number of exacerbations ($p < 0.001$).
Tay, T.R Respirology 2016 [60]	Cross-sectional	$N = 90$ asthmatics	Specialist physician diagnosis (76 had variable airflow obstruction)	Clinical symptoms and BQ or previous positive PSG	OSA or high OSA risk in 35/90 (38.9%). Univariate analysis showed asthmatics with OSA to have worse ACT ($p = 0.034$) and worse AQLQ ($p = 0.029$), but not in multivariate analysis.
Kim et al. Ann Allergy Asthma Immunol 2013 [25]	Cross-sectional	$N = 217$ asthmatics Controls = 0 Randomly recruited from tertiary care clinic	1. Airway reversibility with $FEV_1 > 12\%$ and 200 mL post SABA or positive metacholine provocation test 2. Persistent symptoms 3. Physician diagnosis of asthma (need all three)	BQ	A total of 89/217 (41%) were high risk for OSA. The high OSA risk group had a lower ACT score than the low OSA risk group but it was not statistically significant: 20.9 ± 3.6 vs. 21.5 ± 3.3 ($p = 0.091$).
Teodorescu et al. Chest 2010 [61]	Cross-sectional	$N = 472$ asthmatics from tertiary care clinic visits	Asthma or allergy specialist using ATS guidelines and ACQ for BA control	SA-SDQ	A total of 109/472 (23%) were high risk for OSA. High OSA risk associated with 2.87-fold higher odds for having poorly controlled asthma ($p = 0.0009$, 95% CI = 1.54–5.32).
Wang et al. BMC Pulm Med 2017 [35]	Retrospective	$N = 77$ asthmatics Sleep lab of a tertiary hospital	ATS criteria. Airway reversibility with $FEV_1 > 12\%$ and 200 mL post SABA or average daily diurnal peak flow variability was more than 10%. Regular follow up with pulmonary function tests at least every six months for more than 5 years.	PSG	The decline in FEV_1 among asthmatics with severe OSA (AHI > 30/h) was 72.4 ± 61.7 mL/year ($N = 34$), as compared to 41.9 ± 45.3 mL/year ($N = 33$, $p = 0.020$) in those with mild to moderate OSA (5 < AHI ≤ 30) and 24.3 ± 27.5 mL/year ($N = 10$, $p = 0.016$) in those without OSA (AHI ≤ 5).
Teodorescu et al. Sleep Med 2006 [22]	Cross-sectional	$N = 115$ asthmatics Routine asthma follow-up visits	Physician diagnosis	SA-SDQ	ESS associated with SA-SDQ ($p < 0.0001$) and asthma severity step ($p = 0.04$), but was not associated with asthma severity step in multiple regression analysis.
Sundbom et al. J Clin Sleep Med 2018 [29]	Cross-sectional	Women pooled from the Sleep and Health program in Sweden. $N = 36$ patients with BA $N = 15$ patientswith BA + OSA $N = 109$ patients with OSA	Positive answers to either of the following questions: 1. Have you an attack of asthma in the last 12 months? 2. Are you currently taking any medicine, including inhalers, aerosols, or tablets for asthma?	Full-night home PSG	Women with BA+OSA had a longer sleeping time in N1 and N2 sleep stages than the control group with no BA or OSA. They had also lower mean oxygen saturation (93.4% vs. 94.7%, $p = 0.04$) than the women with OSA alone. The results were consistent after multivariate analysis. BA was independently associated with lower oxygen saturation while OSA was not.

Table 2. *Cont.*

Study	Study Design	Population	Asthma Diagnosis	OSA Diagnosis	Results
Becerra et al. Respiratory Medicine 2016 [69]	Retrospective	2009–2011 U.S Nationwide Inpatient Sample International Classification of Diseases, 9th Revision, Clinical Modification (ICD–9–CM) 493.x to identify primary hospitalizations for asthma. N = 179.789 primary BA hospitalizations	Secondary diagnosis code for BA hospitalizations with comorbid conditions of obesity (ICD–9–CM 278.0x) and OSA (ICD–9–CM 327.23)	Secondary diagnose code for OSA (ICD–9–CM 327.23) objectively based OSA diagnosis	Increased hospital length of stay was associated with the presence of obesity (OR for males = 1.07, OR for females = 1.08), OSA (OR for males = 1.07, OR for females = 1.14), and both obesity and OSA (OR for males = 1.19, OR for females = 1.24). Increased total hospital charges was related to obesity (8.64% for males and 9.61% for females), OSA (15.39% for males and 19.13% for females), and both co-morbidities (24.94% for males and 28.50% for females). Presence of OSA alone increased the odds of needing mechanical ventilation for males (OR = 2.56) and females (OR = 3.22), as did presence of both co-morbidities (OR for males = 2.85, OR for females = 3.60).
Ferguson et al. Lung 2014 [74]	Cross-sectional, questionnaire-based	N = 812 asthmatics at routine follow-up at allergy and pulmonary clinics	ATS criteria, managed by an academic specialist	SA-SDQ	Hypertension was diagnosed in 191 asthmatics (24%), OSA in 65 (8%), and OSA or high OSA risk (combined OSA variable) in 239 (29%). With adjustment for covariates, associations with hypertension remained significant for some FEV_1% categories (70–79% odds ratio = 1.60 [95% CI: 0.90–2.87]; 60–69% OR = 2.73 [95% CI = 1.28–5.79]; < 60% OR = 0.96 [95% CI = 0.43–2.14]), and for OSA (OR = 2.20 [95% CI = 1.16–4.19]).
Han et al. BMC Pulmonary Medicine 2016 [75]	Retrospective	National Health Insurance Service (NHIS) National Sample Cohort 2004–2013 in South Korea. A total of 186.491 patients who were newly diagnosed with BA during the study period at outpatient care were followed for OSA development and mortality.	ICD–10: J.45	ICD–10:G.47 only when it followed a BA diagnosis	A total of 5179 (2.78%) patients died during the study period. Sleep disorders in patients previously diagnosed with asthma were associated with a higher risk of mortality (hazard ratio (HR): 1.451 (95% CI = 1.253–1.681). The mean duration between BA diagnosis and death was shorter in asthmatics with sleep disorders (mean duration = 103.85 months) compared to asthmatics without sleep disorders (mean duration = 116.05 months, $p < 0.0001$)

BA = Bronchial Asthma, OSA = Obstructive Sleep Apnea, ATS = American Thoracic Society, SA-SDQ = Sleep Apnea of Sleep Disorders Questionnaire, PSG = Polysomnography, AHI = Apnea Hypopnea Index, OR = Odds Ratio, CI = Confidence Interval, HR = Hazard Ratio, BQ = Berlin Questionnaire, ACT = Asthma Control Test, AQLQ = Asthma Quality of Life Questionnaire, SABA = Short Acting B Agonist, ACQ = Asthma Control Questionnaire, FEV_1 = Forced Expiratory Volume in the first second, ESS = Epworth Sleepiness Scale.

8. Treatment

Early CPAP application has shown a favorable effect on asthma parameters' main symptoms. Most of these studies were retrospective, included a small number of subjects (9to16), having a short period of follow up (maximum 9 months), adherence to treatment was not based on objectives criteria, and there was a broad heterogeneity regarding the assessment of the results [56–58].

The first study investigating the impact of the long-term use of CPAP on asthma symptoms and on the control of the disease in a large number of patients was a questionnaire-based one. A survey questionnaire was distributed to all OSA patients using CPAP therapy in 2013. They received 1586 answers and 13% of them had BA. The mean duration of CPAP-usage was 5.7 years and their CPAP daily use was 6.3 h. Self-reported asthma severity (measured using a visual analogue scale) decreased significantly and the ACT score increased significantly from 15.35 to 19.8 ($p < 0.001$) without a significant change in the BMI [31].

The first prospective, multicenter study recently conducted in Spain examined asthma outcomes 6 months after CPAP use in 99 adult asthmatics with OSA. ACQ and the mini–asthma quality of life questionnaire (mini–AQLQ) was used for asthma control and quality of life, respectively, and objective measures of BA (spirometry) and OSA (PSG) as well. Both the control of the disease and the quality of life were significantly improved in general, but when the diseases were categorized according to their severity, only patients with moderate and severe BA and severe OSA, and patients who used CPAP >4 h/day, were significantly improved. There was a significant decrease in the percentage of asthma exacerbations seen in the six months after the use of CPAP (from 35.4% to7.2%, $p = 0.015$), a significant improvement in bronchial reversibility, symptoms of GER, rhinitis, and exhaled nitric oxide levels (eNO) (all $p < 0.05$). However, no significant changes were observed in the asthma medication used, drugs, body weight, and other asthma co-morbidities [32].

The favorable impact of CPAP on AOS has been attributed to the decrease of the local and systemic inflammation [76,77], and the improvement of both the heterogeneity of alveolar ventilation [78] and GER [79].

There is one retrospective study that reported an improvement in FEV_1 after CPAP treatment [35]. This finding was not confirmed in other studies [32,58,80], but the follow-up period was too short (maximum 6 months).

The impact of CPAP on BHR in patients with AOS is still a matter of controversy. Although most studies reported a decrease in BHR [81,82], this was not a constant finding [80]. However, more research is needed using a longer follow-up period in order to draw conclusions regarding the effect of CPAP treatment on pulmonary function.

According to current OSA guidelines, there is clear evidence in treating patients with moderate or severe OSA, whereas treatment should be restricted in mild OSA patients that are symptomatic or have serious co-morbidities, but still, asthma is not one of them. Considering asthmatic patients with mild OSA, there is no clear evidence regarding the best practice for treating these patients.

We therefore conclude that the optimal treatment practice for AOS is the best treatment of each disease separately and the recognition and treatment of the co-morbidities like obesity, GER. and more importantly allergic rhinitis, which is probably the basic reason of the high prevalence of OSA among the asthmatics. In a recent population-based study, a history of allergic rhinitis was associated with an increased risk of sleep-disordered breathing in the elderly and it was an independent risk factor of OSA in asthmatics (adjusted OR = 1.90, $p = 0.046$), while neck circumference was not (adjusted OR = 1.02, $p = 0.654$), although this is traditionally the most significant factor that predicts OSA [34].Patients who received intranasal corticosteroids had a significant improvement in OSA [83]. Another issue that needs investigation is the heterogeneity of the severity of both diseases in the same patient. Perhaps all the possible combinations may co-exist. Therefore, patients may have severe moderate or mild BA with severe, moderate, or mild OSA in any combination, as it happens with chronic bronchitis and emphysema in COPD. Consequently, treatment should be personalized.

We summarize the main studies addressing the effects of CPAP treatment for OSA on asthma outcomes in Table 3.

The role of alternative treatment in OSA like uvulopalatopharyngoplasty, oral appliances, upper-airway stimulation, or surgical interventions on AOS has not been investigated yet. Bariatric surgery is known to improve asthma control, pulmonary function, BHR, and quality of life. Bariatric surgery also improves OSA parameters [84,85]. The effect of bariatric surgery on AOS has not been studied yet.

The effect of biological asthma treatments and leukotriene inhibitors have not been studied regarding AOS.

Table 3. Effects of C–PAP treatment for OSA on asthma outcomes.

Study Design	SAMPLE SIZE	Main Characteristics	C–Pap Treatment/Adherence	Method for OSA Diagnosis	Changes With C–Pap
Chan et al., single-center, control-CPAP, off-cCPAP Am Rev Resp Dis 1988 [56]	9 subjects	Severe asthma, AHI 21.1/h	2 weeks, no objective adherence	PSG	Improved symptoms, reduced bronchodilator use, improved AM and PM pre-/post-bronchodilator PEFR that paralleled the treatment period and returned to pretreatment levels during the CPAP-off period
Guilleminault et al., single-center Eur Resp J 1988 [57]	10 subjects	BA with moderate to severe obstruction (FEV_1 54% predicted), RDI = 51/h	6–9 months, no objective adherence	PSG	Improved symptoms
Ciftsi et al., single center Resp Med 2005 [58]	16 subjects	Nocturnal asthma, AHI 44/h	2 months, no objective adherence	PSG	Improved symptoms, no response in FEV_1
Lafond et al., single center Prospective Eur Resp J 2007 [80]	20 subjects	Stable asthma of various control levels, AHI = 48/h	6 weeks, objective adherence. CPAP use 6.7 h per night (subjects excluded if CPAP use <4 h per night).	PSG	Improved mini-AQLQ scores. No improvement in BHR (metacholine challenge) No changes in FEV_1
Kauppi et al., single center retrospective cross-sectional questionnaire study Sleep Breath 2006 [31]	152 subjects using CPAP in 2013	Self-reported physician-diagnosed BA, REI (respiratory event index) > 41.2/h	5.7 years, daily use 6.3 h, objective adherence	Home polygraphy	Decreased self-reported BA severity, improved ACT scores, reduced percentage of patients using rescue medication daily, no changes in BMI
Wang et al., single center, retrospective BMC Pulm Med 2017 [35]	Subset of 13 subjects	BA based on symptoms and spirometry Severe OSA AHI >30/h	2 years, objective adherence, CPAP use 6.4 h/night	PSG	Reduced annual decline in FEV_1 A trend toward reduced ER visits ($p = 0.058$)

Table 3. *Cont.*

Study Design	SAMPLE SIZE	Main Characteristics	C–Pap Treatment/Adherence	Method for OSA Diagnosis	Changes With C–Pap
Serrano Pariente et al., multicenter (15 centers), prospective Allergy 2017 [32]	99 subjects	BA: Intermittent: 11%, mild persistent:17%, moderate persistent:48%, severe persistent: 24%, RDI = 46.3/h	6 months, objective adherence recorded and non–compliant subjects were not excluded	PSG: 30% of patients or cardiorespiratory polygraphy: 70%	Improved symptoms; improved ACQ and mini-AQLQ scores in asthmatics with severe OSA (AHI > 30), as well in asthmatics with moderate to severe BA; improved ACQ and mini AQLQ scores in subjects who used CPAP > 4 h/night; reduced proportion of patients without a well-controlled asthma score; reduced bronchodilator use; reduced exacerbations; reduction in proportion of patients with positive bronchodilator response; improved symptoms of GER and rhinitis; improved exhaled nitric oxide values; no changes in FEV_1

OSA = Obstructive Sleep Apnea, C-pap = Continuous positive airway pressure, AHI = Apnea Hypopnea Index, h = hour, PSG = Polysomnography, AM = Morning, PM = Afternoon, PEFR = Peak Expiratory Flow Rate, BA = Bronchial Asthma, FEV_1 = Forced Expiratory Volume in the first second, RDI = Respiratory Disturbances Index, AQLQ = Asthma Quality of Life Questionnaire, BHR = Bronchial Hyper-responsiveness, REI = Respiratory Events Index, ACT = Asthma Control Test, BMI = Body Mass Index, ER = Emergency Room, ACQ = Asthma Control Questionnaire, GER = Gastro-Esophageal Reflux.

9. Screening

From the above-mentioned data it is obvious that BA is a risk factor for OSA occurrence and development, and OSA might aggravate BA reciprocally. OSA worsens asthma outcomes [25,59,69]. On the other hand, there is strong evidence that long-term use of CPAP in patients with BA and OSA improves symptoms, asthma control, and quality of life [31,32]. That is why the need for screening asthmatics for OSA is imperative. Apart from the overnight-attended PSG, which is an expensive and time-consuming method, and therefore, it is inconvenient for screening a large number of subjects, there is a gap in the literature regarding the use of OSA questionnaires in asthmatic populations. For the first time, Huan et al. compared the SBQ with BQ in 123 objectively diagnosed asthmatics undergoing overnight-attended PSG. Compared with BQ, SBQ had a higher diagnostic sensitivity (84.4% vs. 60%), lower specificity (79.5% vs. 91%), lower positive predictive value (70.4% vs. 79.4%), and higher negative predictive value (90% vs. 80%) to detect moderate-to-severe OSA at an AHI cut-off of 15/h. They concluded that SBQ is the preferable sleep questionnaire over BQ for detecting the risk of having moderate-to-severe OSA in asthmatics [86].

10. Summary

OSA has been found to have increased prevalence, ranging from 19 to 60%, in asthmatic patients, and even reaching 95% in severe asthma cases. The diagnosis of OSA has been made either using a questionnaire or an overnight-attended PSG. Home sleep apnea testing (HSAT) is likely to be much more accurate than questionnaires and better for identifying moderate to severe OSA, but it is not recommended in patients with severe cardiorespiratory disease and there are no special recommendations for asthmatic patients [87,88].Given that patients with AOS usually suffer from severe asthma, and therefore studies using HSAT would not have included them, we did not focus on HSAT in the current review. However, we included studies that have evaluated asthmatic patients using HSAT and PSG, as seen in Table 1 (Sundbom et al.) and Table 2 (Kauppi et al., Serrano Pariente et al.). It is difficult to accurately estimate the prevalence of AOS based on the fact that the prevalence of OSA depends on the definition used and the population studied, and ranges between 2% and 10% in women and between 4% and 31% in men [89–91]. More specifically, while the Wisconsin study found a prevalence of sleep-disordered breathing (SDB) defined as an AHI ≥5/hr to be 9% in women and 24% in men [89], in a more recent systematic review, the overall prevalence for AHI ≥5 events/h was found to range from 9% to 38% and was higher in males and in some elderly groups, and it increased reaching 90% in men and 78% in women. For AHI ≥15 events/h, the prevalence ranged from 6% to 17% in the general population, reaching 49% in the advanced ages. OSA prevalence increases with obesity and age [92].

The prevalence of OSA in asthmatics is positively correlated with the severity and duration of asthma and the dosage of oral or inhaled steroids. It seems that asthma is a risk factor for the OSA occurrence, but in order for a causal relationship to confirmed, large prospective studies are needed with objective pulmonary function and sleep measurements.

As the impact of OSA on asthma causes a neutrophilic inflammation, contributes to airway remodeling, increases nocturnal and diurnal persistent symptoms, worsens sleep quality and nocturnal hypoxemia increasing sleepiness the next day, deteriorates asthma outcomes, is an independent risk factor for asthma exacerbations, and increases the days of hospitalization and health resource utilization, OSA should not be seen as a simple co-morbidity. AOS is a new asthma phenotype that should be uncovered. Additionally, although it is clear that the co-existence of asthma and OSA increases asthma exacerbations, the association of the number of exacerbations with sleep parameters like AHI, ODI (oxygen desaturation index), and AI (arousal index) has not yet been defined.

Finally, since we lack data from double-blind studies, there are currently no available treatment guidelines for the combination of OSA and asthma, and the treatment of asthma and OSA is limited to each specific disease's guidelines. In Table 4, we outline the major take away points, as well as areas where further research is needed.

Table 4. Coexistence of Obstructive Sleep Apnea in asthmatics patients.

Section	Conclusions	Future Research Needed
Epidemiology	OSA is quite common among asthmatics, so a new asthma phenotype seems to emerge.	
Diagnosis	Clinicians should suspect OSA in asthmatic patients with the above characteristics: • obesity • sleepiness • allergic rhinitis • GER • severe uncontrolled asthma lasting over a decade requiring high doses of steroids	
Pathophysiology	• OSA and asthma interact in terms of pathophysiology • AOS inflammation is neutrophilic • AOS is a difficult-to-treat asthma phenotype • There is a possible causal relationship between asthma and OSA	• The exact pathophysiologic mechanisms remain unknown • More studies are needed to confirm neutrophilic inflammation in asthmatic patients with OSA • Large prospective studies with objective measures of pulmonary function and sleep are needed for a causal relationship to be confirmed
Clinical consequences	• Increased night-time and daytime symptoms • Increased asthma exacerbation (related to AHI) • Worse asthma control • Deterioration of sleep quality (increased sleep time of non-deep sleep stages (N1, N2), reduced sleep time in deeper stages (REM), excessive sleepiness the next day); it is associated with profound hypoxemia during sleep • Increased annual FEV_1 decline (related to OSA–severity) • Increased arterial hypertension • Increased hospitalization days and costs, especially when associated with obesity • Increased need of mechanical ventilation • Increased mortality (possible)	• The association between the number of asthma exacerbations and objective sleep parameters must be investigated • More studies are needed regarding sleep architecture and objective parameters like ODI, AI, and heart rate • Large prospective long-term studies are needed to show how pulmonary function is affected in asthmatics with OSA • More research is needed in order to study mortality, hypertension, hospital admissions, and hospitalization requirements

Table 4. *Cont.*

Section	Conclusions	Future Research Needed
Treatment	C-PAP treatment seems to have a favorable effect on asthma outcomes, where it: • Improves daytime and night–time symptoms • Reduces asthma exacerbations • Improves asthma control • Improves quality of life • Reduces BHR (still controversial) • Lessens annual FEV_1 decline • Improves GER and rhinitis symptoms • Reduces eNO levels	• Large prospective randomized controlled trials are needed to confirm the beneficial effects of C-PAP treatment on AOS • The effectiveness of alternative OSA treatments and asthma medications on AOS have to be explored • There is a gap in literature concerning the need of C-PAP treatment in asthmatics with mild OSA
Screening of patients with AOS	• The need for screening asthmatics presenting with the described phenotype is imperative • SBQ is recommended • If SBQ is indicative for OSA, patients must be referred to a sleep lab as well if the risk of having OSA remain high and SBQ is not indicative	More studies are needed in large asthmatic populations to confirm the diagnostic value of SBQ and investigate if other questionnaires have the potential to accurately estimate the risk of having OSA

OSA = Obstructive Sleep Apnea, GER = Gastro Esophageal Reflux, AOS = Alternative Overlap Syndrome, AHI = Apnea Hypopnea Index, REM = Rapid Eye Movement, FEV_1 = Forced Expiratory Volume in the first second, ODI = Oxygen Desaturation Index, AI = Arousal Index, C-PAP = Continuous positive airway pressure, BHR = Bronchial Hyper-responsiveness, eNO = exhaled Nitric Oxide, SBQ = Stop Bang Questionnaire.

GINA guidelines urge physicians to look for OSA in asthmatics [1]. However, there are limitations in diagnosing OSA in a primary care setting, which may lead to the under-diagnosis of OSA. This problem is worse when asthma coexists because of overlapping nocturnal symptoms. Although SBQ has not been validated in large asthmatic populations, there is an urgent need to use it periodically forasthmatics, especially in those with refractory asthma, obesity, allergic rhinitis, and GER. These patients will need to be tested for OSA at the sleep lab. Early diagnosis of OSA in asthmatic patients will lead to the appropriate treatment with CPAP and will stop the vicious circle of OSA worsening asthma control and escalating asthma pharmaceutical treatment.

We conclude that there is an urgent need for the early diagnosis of OSA in asthmatic patients in order to effectively treat both diseases and lessen the economic burden.

Author Contributions: This review is the result of A.D.'s thesis at her Master in Somnology, P.K. was her supervisor in her Thesis, revised it critically for important intellectual content, and funded the publication through her research grant, E.V. contributed in the conception and design of A.D.'s thesis, S.Z. is the Head of the First ICU Clinic, Academic Responsible for the Master of Somnology and member of A.D.'s Thesis Committee. All authors revised critically the text according to their expertise, agreed with the final version of the text to be submitted and to be accountable for the work.

Acknowledgments: We thank Eleni Loutrari for her help as a member of A.D.'s Thesis Committee

Conflicts of Interest: The authors declare no conflict of interest.

Abbreviations

AHI	Apnea Hypopnea Index
ACQ	Asthma Control Questionnaire
ACT	Asthma Control Test
AI	Arousal Index
AM	Morning
AOS	Alternative Overlap Syndrome
AQLQ	Asthma Quality of Life Questionnaire
BMI	Body Mass Index
BA	Bronchial Asthma
BHR	Bronchial Hyper-responsiveness
BQ	Berlin Questionnaire
CI	Confidence Interval
COPD	Chronic Obstructive Pulmonary Disease
CPAP	Continuous Positive Airway Pressure
CRP	C-Reactive Protein
e-NO	exhaled- Nitric Oxide
ER	Emergency Room
ESS	Epworth Sleepiness Scale
FEV1	Forced Expiratory Volume in One Second
FRC	Functional Residual Capacity
GER	Gastro-Esophageal Reflux
GINA	Global Initiative for Asthma
HSAT	Home Sleep Apnea Testing
HR	Hazard Ratio
ICD–10	International Classification of Diseases
IL–6	Interleukin–6
Mini–AQLQ	Mini Asthma Quality of Life Questionnaire
OSA	Obstructive Sleep Apnea
ODI	Oxygen Desaturation Index
OR	Odds Ratio
PEFR	Peak Expiratory Flow Rate

PM	Afternoon
PSG	Polysomnography
REI	Respiratory Events Index
REM	Rapid Eye Movement
RDI	Respiratory Disturbances Index
SABA	Short Acting B Agonist
SBQ	Stop Bang Questionnaire
SA-SDQ	Sleep Apnea of Sleep Disorders Questionnaire
SDB	Sleep Disordered Breathing
TNF	Tumor Necrosis Factor
TST	Total Sleep Time
VEGF	Vascular Endothelial Growth Factor

References

1. Global Initiative for Asthma. Global Strategy for Asthma Management and Prevention. 2017. Available online: http://www.ginasthma.org (accessed on 7 June 2019).
2. Dolan, C.M.; Fraher, K.E.; Bleecker, E.R.; Borish, L.; Chipps, B.; Hayden, M.L.; Weiss, S.; Zheng, B.; Johnson, C. Design and baseline characteristics of the epidemiology and natural history of asthma: Outcomes and treatment regimens (TENOR) study: A large cohort of patients with severe or difficult-to-treat asthma. *Ann. Allergy Asthma Immunol.* **2004**, *92*, 32–39. [CrossRef]
3. Luyster, F.S.; Teodorescu, M.; Bleecker, E.; Busse, W.; Calhoun, W.; Castro, M.; Fan Chung, K.; Erzurum, S.; Israel, E.; Strollo, P.J.; et al. Sleep quality and asthma control and quality of life in non-severe and severe asthma. *Sleep Breath.* **2012**, *16*, 1129–1137. [CrossRef] [PubMed]
4. Franklin, K.A.; Lindberg, E. Obstructive sleep apnea is a common disorder in the population—A review on the epidemiology of sleep apnea. *J. Thorac. Dis.* **2015**, *7*, 1311–1322. [PubMed]
5. Simpson, L.; Hillman, D.R.; Cooper, M.N.; Ward, K.L.; Hunter, M.; Cullen, S.; James, A.; Palmer, L.J.; Mukherjee, S.; Eastwood, P. High prevalence of undiagnosed sleep apnoea in the general population and methods for screening for representative controls. *Sleep Breath.* **2013**, *17*, 967–973. [CrossRef] [PubMed]
6. Kendzerska, T.; Gershon, A.S.; Hawker, G.; Tomlinson, G.; Leung, R.S. Obstructive sleep apnea and incident diabetes. A historical cohort study. *Am. J. Respir. Crit. Care Med.* **2014**, *190*, 218–225. [CrossRef] [PubMed]
7. Gottlieb, D.J.; Yenokyan, G.; Newman, A.B.; O'Connor, G.T.; Punjabi, N.M.; Quan, S.F.; Redline, S.; Resnick, H.E.; Tong, E.K.; Diener-West, M.; et al. Prospective study of obstructive sleep apnea and incident coronary heart disease and heart failure: The Sleep Heart Health Study. *Circulation* **2010**, *122*, 352–360. [CrossRef]
8. Redline, S.; Yenokyan, G.; Gottlieb, D.J.; Shahar, E.; O'Connor, G.T.; Resnick, H.E.; Diener-West, M.; Sanders, M.H.; Wolf, P.A.; Geraghty, E.M.; et al. Obstructive sleep apnea-hypopnea and incident stroke: The Sleep Heart Health Study. *Am. J. Respir. Crit. Care Med.* **2010**, *182*, 269–277. [CrossRef]
9. Douglass, A.B.; Bornstein, R.; Nino-Murcia, G.; Keenan, S.; Miles, L.; Zarcone, V.P.; Guilleminault, C.; Dement, W.C. The Sleep Disorders Questionnaire I: Creation and multivariate structure of SDQ. *Sleep* **1994**, *17*, 160–167. [CrossRef]
10. Netzer, N.C.; Stoohs, R.A.; Netzer, C.M.; Clark, K.; Strohl, K.P. Using the Berlin Questionnaire to identify patients at risk for the sleep apnea syndrome. *Ann. Intern. Med.* **1999**, *131*, 485–491. [CrossRef]
11. Chung, F.; Yegneswaran, B.; Liao, P.; Chung, S.A.; Vairavanathan, S.; Islam, S.; Khajehdehi, A.; Shapiro, C.M. STOP questionnaire—A tool to screen patients for obstructive sleep apnea. *Anesthesiology* **2008**, *108*, 812–821. [CrossRef]
12. Young, T.; Finn, L.; Peppard, P.E.; Szklo-Coxe, M.; Austin, D.; Nieto, F.J.; Stubbs, R.; Hla, K.M. Sleep disordered breathing and mortality: Eighteen-year follow-up of the Wisconsin sleep cohort. *Sleep* **2008**, *31*, 1071–1078. [PubMed]
13. Ioachimescu, O.C.; Teodorescu, M. Integrating the overlap of obstructive lung disease and obstructive sleep apnoea. OLDOSA syndrome. *Respirology* **2013**, *18*, 421–431. [CrossRef] [PubMed]
14. Teodorescu, M.; Barnet, J.H.; Hagen, W.; Palta, M.; Young, T.B.; Peppard, P.E. Association between Asthma and Risk of Developing Obstructive Sleep Apnea. *JAMA* **2015**, *313*, 156–164. [CrossRef] [PubMed]

15. Wang, Y.; Liu, K.; Hu, K.; Yang, J.; Li, Z.; Nie, M.; Dong, Y.; Huang, H.; Chen, J. Impact of obstructive sleep apnea on severe asthma exacerbations. *Sleep Med.* **2016**, *26*, 1–5. [CrossRef] [PubMed]
16. Kong, D.L.; Qin, Z.; Shen, H.; Jin, H.Y.; Wang, W.; Wang, Z.F. Association of Obstructive Sleep Apnea with Asthma: A Meta Analysis. *Sci. Rep.* **2017**, *7*, 4088. [CrossRef]
17. Yigla, M.; Tov, N.; Solomonov, A.; Rubin, A.H.; Harlev, D. Difficult-to-control asthma and obstructive sleep apnea. *J. Asthma* **2003**, *40*, 865–871. [CrossRef] [PubMed]
18. Julien, J.Y.; Martin, J.G.; Ernst, P.; Olivenstein, R.; Hamid, Q.; Lemiere, C.; Pepe, C.; Naor, N.; Olha, A.; Kimoff, R.J. Prevalence of obstructive sleep apnea-hypopnea in severe versus moderate asthma. *J. Allergy Clin. Immunol.* **2009**, *124*, 371–376. [CrossRef] [PubMed]
19. Fitzpatrick, M.; Martin, K.; Fossey, E.; Shapiro, C.M.; Elton, R.A.; Douglas, N.J. Snoring, asthma and sleep disturbance in Britain: A community-based survey. *Eur. Respir. J.* **1993**, *6*, 531–535. [PubMed]
20. Janson, C.; De Backer, W.; Gislason, T.; Plaschke, P.; Björnsson, E.; Hetta, J.; Kristbjarnarson, H.; Vermeire, P.; Boman, G. Increased prevalence of sleep disturbances and daytime sleepiness in subjects with bronchial asthma: A population study of young adults in three European countries. *Eur. Respir. J.* **1996**, *9*, 2132–2138. [CrossRef] [PubMed]
21. Larsson, L.G.; Lindberg, A.; Franklin, K.A.; Lundbäck, B. Obstructive Lung Disease in Northern Sweden Studies. Obstructive sleep apnea syndrome is common in subjects with chronic bronchitis. Report from the Obstructive Lung Disease in Northern Sweden studies. *Respiration* **2001**, *68*, 250–255. [CrossRef]
22. Teodorescu, M.; Consens, F.B.; Bria, W.F.; Coffey, M.J.; Mc Morris, M.S.; Weatherwax, K.; Durance, A.; Palmisano, J.; Senger, C.M.; Chervin, R.D. Correlates of daytime sleepiness in patients with asthma. *Sleep Med.* **2006**, *7*, 607–613. [CrossRef] [PubMed]
23. Teodorescu, M.; Polomis, D.A.; Teodorescu, M.C.; Gangnon, R.E.; Peterson, A.G.; Consens, F.B.; Chervin, R.D.; Jarjour, N.N. Association of obstructive sleep apnea risk or diagnosis with daytime asthma in adults. *J. Asthma* **2012**, *49*, 620–628. [CrossRef] [PubMed]
24. Teodorescu, M.; Broytman, O.; Curran-Everett, D.; Sorkness, R.L.; Crisafi, G.; Bleecker, E.R.; Erzurum, S.; Gaston, B.M.; Wenzel, S.E.; Jarjour, N.N. Obstructive Sleep Apnea Risk, Asthma Burden and Lower Airway Inflammation in Adults in the Severe Asthma Research Program (SARP) II. *J. Allergy Clin. Immunol. Pract.* **2015**, *3*, 566–575. [CrossRef] [PubMed]
25. Kim, M.Y.; Jo, E.J.; Kang, S.Y.; Chang, Y.S.; Yoon, I.Y.; Cho, S.H.; Min, K.U.; Kim, S.H. Obstructive sleep apnea is associated with reduced quality of life in adult patients with asthma. *Ann. Allergy Asthma Immunol.* **2013**, *110*, 253–2577. [CrossRef] [PubMed]
26. Taillé, C.; Rouve-Tallec, A.; Stoica, T.M.; Danel, C.; Dehoux, M.; Marin-Esteban, V.; Pretolani, M.; Aubier, M.; Ortho, M.P. Obstructive Sleep Apnoea Modulates Airway Inflammation and Remodelling in Severe Asthma. *PLoS ONE* **2016**, *11*, e0150042. [CrossRef]
27. Alharbi, M.; Almutairi, A.; Alotaibi, D.; Alotaibi, A.; Shaikh, S.; Bahammam, A.S. The prevalence of asthma in patients with obstructive sleep apnoea. *Prim. Care Respir. J.* **2009**, *18*, 328–330. [CrossRef] [PubMed]
28. Shaker, A. Study of obstructive sleep apnea (OSA) in asthmatics. *Egypt. J. Chest Dis. Tuberc.* **2017**, *66*, 293–298. [CrossRef]
29. Sundbom, F.; Janson, C.; Malinovschi, A.; Lindberg, E.; Lindberg, E. Effects of Co existing Asthma and Obstructive Sleep Apnea on Sleep Architecture, Oxygen Saturation, and Systemic Inflammation in Women. *J. Clin. Sleep Med.* **2018**, *14*, 253–259. [CrossRef]
30. Madama, D.; Silva, A.; Matos, M.J. Overlap syndrome—Asthma and obstructive sleep apnea. *Rev. Port. Pneumol.* **2016**, *22*, 6–10. [CrossRef]
31. Kauppi, P.; Bachour, P.; Maasilta, P.; Bachour, A. Long-term CPAP treatment improves asthma control in patients with asthma and obstructive sleep apnoea. *Sleep Breath.* **2016**, *20*, 1217–1224. [CrossRef]
32. Serrano-Pariente, J.; Plaza, V.; Soriano, J.B.; Mayos, M.; Lopez-Vina, A.; Picado, C.; Vigil, L.; on behalf of the CPASMA Trial Group. Asthma outcomes improve with continuous positive airway pressure for obstructive sleep apnea. *Allergy* **2017**, *72*, 802–812. [CrossRef]
33. Shen, T.C.; Lin, C.L.; Wei, C.C.; Chen, C.H.; Tu, C.Y.; Hsia, T.C.; Shih, C.M.; Hsu, W.H.; Sung, F.C.; Kao, C.H. Risk of obstructive sleep apnea in adult patients with asthma: A population-based cohort study in Taiwan. *PLoS ONE* **2015**, *10*, e0128461. [CrossRef] [PubMed]

34. Kim, S.H.; Won, H.K.; Moon, S.D.; Kim, B.K.; Chang, Y.S.; Kim, K.W.; Yoon, I.Y. Impact of self-reported symptoms of allergic rhinitis and asthma on sleep disordered breathing and sleep disturbances in the elderly with polysomnography study. *PLoS ONE* **2017**, *12*, e0173075. [CrossRef]
35. Wang, T.Y.; Lo, Y.L.; Lin, S.M.; Huang, C.D.; Chung, F.T.; Lin, H.C.; Wang, C.H.; Kuo, H.P. Obstructive sleep apnoea accelerates FEV_1 decline in asthmatic patients. *BMC Pulm. Med.* **2017**, *17*, 1–6. [CrossRef]
36. Knuiman, M.; James, A.; Divitini, M.; Bartholomew, H. Longitudinal study of risk factors for habitual snoring in a general adult population: The Busselton Health Study. *Chest* **2006**, *130*, 1779–1783. [CrossRef] [PubMed]
37. Teodorescu, M.; Consens, F.B.; Bria, W.F.; Coffey, M.G.; McMorris, M.S.; Weatherwax, K.; Palmisano, J.; Senger, C.M.; Ye, Y.; Kalbfleisch, J.D.; et al. Predictors of habitual snoring and obstructive sleep apnea risk in patients with asthma. *Chest* **2009**, *135*, 1125–1132. [CrossRef] [PubMed]
38. Ballard, R.D.; Irvin, C.G.; Martin, R.J.; Pak, J.; Pandey, R.; White, D.P. Influence of sleep on lung volume in asthmatic patients and normal subjects. *J. Appl. Physiol.* **1990**, *68*, 2034–2041. [CrossRef] [PubMed]
39. Irvin, C.G.; Pak, J.; Martin, R.J. Airway-parenchyma uncoupling in nocturnal asthma. *Am. J. Respir. Crit. Care Med.* **2000**, *161*, 50–56. [CrossRef] [PubMed]
40. Van de Graaff, W.B. Thoracic influence on upper airway patency. *J. Appl. Physiol.* **1988**, *65*, 2124–2131. [CrossRef] [PubMed]
41. Collett, P.W.; Brancatisano, A.P.; Engel, L.A. Upper airway dimensions and movements in bronchial asthma. *Am. Rev. Resp. Dis.* **1986**, *133*, 1143–1149.
42. Zielinski, T.A.; Brown, E.S.; Nejtek, V.A.; Khan, D.A.; Moore, J.J.; Rush, A.J. Depression in asthma: Prevalence and clinical implications. Prim Care Companion. *J. Clin. Psychiatry* **2000**, *2*, 153–158.
43. Togias, A. Rhinitis and asthma: Evidence for respiratory system integration. *J. Allergy Clin. Immunol.* **2003**, *111*, 1171–1183. [CrossRef] [PubMed]
44. Corey, J.P.; Houser, S.M.; Ng, B.A. Nasal congestion: A review of its etiology, evaluation, and treatment. *Ear Nose Throat J.* **2000**, *79*, 690–693. [CrossRef] [PubMed]
45. Salerno, F.G.; Carpagnano, E.; Guido, P.; Bonsignore, M.R.; Roberti, A.; Aliani, M.; Vignola, A.M.; Spanevello, A. Airway inflammation in patients affected by obstructive sleep apnea syndrome. *Respir. Med.* **2004**, *98*, 25–28. [CrossRef] [PubMed]
46. Yokoe, T.; Minoguchi, K.; Matsuo, H.; Oda, N.; Minoguchi, H.; Yoshino, G.; Hirano, T.; Adachi, M. Elevated levels of C-reactive protein and interleukin-6 in patients with obstructive sleep apnea syndrome are decreased by nasal continuous positive airway pressure. *Circulation* **2003**, *107*, 1129–1134. [CrossRef] [PubMed]
47. Bergeron, C.; Kimoff, J.; Hamid, Q. Obstructive sleep apnea syndrome and inflammation. *J. Allergy Clin. Immunol.* **2005**, *116*, 1393–1396. [CrossRef] [PubMed]
48. Li, A.M.; Hung, E.; Tsang, T.; Yin, J.; So, H.K.; Wong, E.; Fok, T.F.; Ng, P.C. Induced sputum inflammatory measures correlate with disease severity in children with obstructive sleep apnea. *Thorax* **2007**, *62*, 75–79. [CrossRef]
49. Calero, G.; Serrano-Mollar, A.; Farre, R.; Closa, D.; Navajas, D.; Montserrat, J.M. Lung inflammation in a rat model of obstructive sleep apnea. Role of strenuous breathing. *Am. J. Respir. Crit. Care Med.* **2004**, *169*, A432.
50. Yokoe, T.; Tanaka, A.; Yamamoto, Y.; Watanabe, Y.; Yamamoto, M.; Ohta, S.; Adachi, M.; Minoguchi, K. Intermittent hypoxia causes airway inflammation in C57BL/6J mice. *Am. J. Respir. Crit. Care Med.* **2009**, *179*, A5331.
51. Puthalapattu, S.; Ioachimescu, O.C. Asthma and obstructive sleep apnea: Clinical and pathogenic interactions. *J. Investig. Med. Off. Publ. Am. Fed. Clin. Res.* **2014**, *62*, 665–675. [CrossRef]
52. Beuther, D.A.; Sutherland, E.R. Overweight, obesity, and incident asthma. *Am. J. Respir. Crit. Care Med.* **2007**, *175*, 661–666. [CrossRef] [PubMed]
53. Simcock, D.E.; Kanabar, V.; Clarke, G.W.; O'Connor, B.J.; Lee, T.H.; Hirst, S.J. Proangiogenic activity in bronchoalveolar lavage fluid from patients with asthma. *Am. J. Respir. Crit. Care. Med.* **2007**, *176*, 146–153. [CrossRef] [PubMed]
54. Sideleva, O.; Suratt, B.T.; Black, K.E.; Tharp, W.G.; Pratley, R.E.; Forgione, P.; Dienz, O.; Irvin, C.G.; Dixon, A.E. Obesity and asthma: An inflammatory disease of adipose tissue not the airway. *Am. J. Respir. Crit. Care. Med* **2012**, *186*, 598–605. [CrossRef] [PubMed]

55. Alkhalil, M.; Schulman, E.; Getsy, J. Obstructive sleep apnea syndrome and asthma: What are the links? *J. Clin. Sleep Med.* **2009**, *15*, 71–78.
56. Chan, C.S.; Woolcock, A.J.; Sullivan, C.E. Nocturnal asthma: Role of snoring and obstructive sleep apnea. *Am. Rev. Respir. Dis.* **1988**, *137*, 1502–1504. [CrossRef]
57. Guilleminault, C.; Quera-Salva, M.A.; Powell, N.; Riley, R.; Romaker, A.; Partinen, M.; Baldwin, R.; Nino-Murcia, G. Nocturnal asthma: Snoring, small pharynx and nasal CPAP. *Eur. Respir. J.* **1988**, *1*, 902–907. [PubMed]
58. Ciftci, T.U.; Ciftci, B.; Guven, S.F.; Kokturk, O.; Turktas, H. Effect of nasal continuous positive airway pressure in uncontrolled nocturnal asthmatic patients with obstructive sleep apnea syndrome. *Respir. Med.* **2005**, *99*, 529–534. [CrossRef] [PubMed]
59. Ten Brinke, A.; Sterk, P.J.; Masclee, A.A.M.; Spinhoven, P.; Schmidt, J.T.; Zwindermane, A.H.; Rabe, K.F.; Bel, E.H. Risk factors of frequent exacerbations in difficult-to-treat asthma. *Eur. Respir. J.* **2005**, *26*, 812–818. [CrossRef]
60. Tay, T.R.; Radhakrishna, N.; Hore-Lacy, F.; Smith, C.; Hoy, R.; Dabscheck, E.; Hew, M. Comorbidities in difficult asthma are independent risk factors for frequent exacerbations, poor control and diminished quality of life. *Respirology* **2016**, *21*, 1384–1390. [CrossRef]
61. Teodorescu, M.; Polomis, D.A.; Hall, S.V.; Teodorescu, M.C.; Gangnon, R.E.; Peterson, A.G.; Xie, A.; Sorkness, C.A.; Jarjour, N.N. Association of obstructive sleep apnea risk with asthma control in adults. *Chest* **2010**, *138*, 543–550. [CrossRef]
62. Dijkstra, A.; Vonk, J.M.; Jongepier, H.; Koppelman, G.H.; Schouten, J.P.; Ten Hacken, N.H.; Timens, W.; Postma, D.S. Lung function decline in asthma: Association with inhaled corticosteroids, smoking and sex. *Thorax* **2006**, *61*, 105–110. [CrossRef] [PubMed]
63. Baek, K.J.; Cho, J.Y.; Rosenthal, P.; Alexander, L.E.; Nizet, V.; Broide, D.H. Hypoxia potentiates allergen induction of HIF-1alpha, chemokines, airway inflammation, TGF-beta1, and airway remodeling in a mouse model. *Clin. Immunol.* **2013**, *47*, 27–37. [CrossRef] [PubMed]
64. Matsunaga, K.; Akamatsu, K.; Miyatake, A.; Ichinose, M. Natural history and risk factors of obstructive changes over a 10-year period in severe asthma. *Respir. Med.* **2013**, *107*, 355–360. [CrossRef] [PubMed]
65. Lange, P.; Parner, J.; Vestbo, J.; Schnohr, P.; Jensen, G. A 15-year follow-up study of ventilatory function in adults with asthma. *N. Engl. J. Med.* **1998**, *339*, 1194–1200. [CrossRef] [PubMed]
66. Bixler, E.O.; Vgontzas, A.N.; Lin, H.M.; Calhoun, S.L.; Vela-Bueno, A.; Kales, A. Excessive daytime sleepiness in a general population sample: The role of sleep apnea, age, obesity, diabetes, and depression. *J. Clin. Endocrinol. Metab.* **2005**, *90*, 4510–4515. [CrossRef] [PubMed]
67. Bonsignore, M.R.; Pepin, J.L.; Anttalainen, U.; Schiza, S.E.; Basoglu, O.K.; Pataka, A.; Steiropoulos, P.; Dogas, Z.; Grote, L.; Hedner, J.; et al. ESADA Study Group. Clinical presentation of patients with suspected obstructive sleep apnea and self-reported physician-diagnosed asthma in the ESADA cohort. *J. Sleep Res.* **2018**, *27*, e12729. [CrossRef] [PubMed]
68. Guven, S.F.; Dursun, A.B.; Ciftci, B.; Erkekol, F.O.; Kurt, O.K. The prevalence of obstructive sleep apnea in patients with difficult-to-treat asthma. *Asian Pac. J. Allergy Immunol.* **2014**, *32*, 153–159. [CrossRef] [PubMed]
69. Becerra, M.B.; Becerra, B.J.; Teodorescu, M. Healthcare burden of obstructive sleep apnea and obesity among asthma hospitalizations: Results from the U.S.-based Nationwide Inpatient Sample. *Respir. Med.* **2016**, *117*, 230–236. [CrossRef] [PubMed]
70. Dogra, S.; Ardern, C.I.; Baker, J. The relationship between age of asthma onset and cardiovascular disease in Canadians. *J. Asthma Off. J. Assoc. Care Asthma* **2007**, *44*, 849–854. [CrossRef]
71. Chobanian, A.V.; Bakris, G.L.; Black, H.R.; Cushman, W.C.; Green, L.A.; Izzo, J.L.; Jones, D.W.; Materson, B.J.; Oparil, S.; Wright, J.T., Jr.; et al. NHLBI JNC on Prevention, Detection, Evaluation, and Treatment of High Blood Pressure; National High Blood Pressure Education Program Coordinating Committee. The Seventh Report of the Joint National Committee on Prevention, Detection, Evaluation, and Treatment of High Blood Pressure: The JNC 7 report. *JAMA* **2003**, *289*, 2560–2572.
72. Bjermer, L. Time for a paradigm shift in asthma treatment: From relieving bronchospasm to controlling systemic inflammation. *J. Allergy Clin. Immunol.* **2007**, *120*, 1269–1275. [CrossRef] [PubMed]

73. Ryan, S.; Taylor, C.T.; Mcnicholas, W.T. Systemic inflammation: A key factor in the pathogenesis of cardiovascular complications in obstructive sleep apnoea syndrome? *Thorax* **2009**, *64*, 631–636. [CrossRef] [PubMed]
74. Ferguson, S.; Teodorescu, M.C.; Gangnon, R.E.; Peterson, A.G.; Consens, F.B.; Chervin, R.D.; Teodorescu, M. Factors associated with systemic hypertension in asthma. *Lung* **2014**, *192*, 675–683. [CrossRef] [PubMed]
75. Han, K.T.; Bae, H.C.; Lee, S.G.; Kim, S.J.; Kim, W.; Lee, H.J.; Ju, Y.J.; Park, E.C. Are sleep disorders associated with increased mortality in asthma patients? *BMC Pulm. Med.* **2016**, *16*, 154. [CrossRef] [PubMed]
76. Alkhalil, M.; Schulman, E.S.; Getsy, J. Obstructive sleep apnea syndrome and asthma: The role of continuous positive airway pressure treatment. *Ann. Allergy Asthma Immunol.* **2008**, *101*, 350–357. [CrossRef]
77. Culla, B.; Guida, G.; Brussino, L.; Tribolo, A.; Cicolin, A.; Sciascia, S.; Badiu, I.; Mietta, S.; Bucca, C. Increased oral nitric oxide in obstructive sleep apnoea. *Respir. Med.* **2010**, *104*, 316–320. [CrossRef] [PubMed]
78. Hanon, S.; Schuermans, D.; Vincken, W.; Verbanck, S. Irreversible acinar airway abnormality in well controlled asthma. *Respir. Med.* **2014**, *108*, 1601–1607. [CrossRef]
79. Tawk, M.; Goodrich, S.; Kinasewitz, G.; Orr, W. The effect of 1week of continuous positive airway pressure treatment in obstructive sleep apnoea patients with concomitant gastro-esophageal reflux. *Chest* **2006**, *130*, 1003–1008. [CrossRef]
80. Lafond, C.; Sériès, F.; Lemière, C. Impact of CPAP on asthmatic patients with obstructive sleep apnoea. *Eur. Respir. J.* **2007**, *29*, 307–311. [CrossRef]
81. Busk, M.; Busk, N.; Puntenney, P.; Hurchins, J.; Yu, Z.; Gunst, S.J.; Tepper, R.S. Use of continuous positive airway pressure reduces airway reactivity in adults with asthma. *Eur. Respir. J.* **2013**, *41*, 317–322. [CrossRef]
82. Lin, H.C.; Wang, C.H.; Yang, C.T.; Huang, T.J.; Yu, C.T.; Shieh, W.B.; Kuo, H.P. Effect of nasal continuous positive airway pressure on methacholine-induced bronchoconstriction. *Respir. Med.* **1995**, *89*, 121–128. [CrossRef]
83. Liu, H.T.; Lin, Y.C.; Kuan, Y.; Huang, Y.H.; Hou, W.H.; Liou, T.H.; Chen, H.C. Intranasal corticosteroid therapy in the treatment of obstructive sleep apnea: A meta-analysis of randomized controlled trials. *Am. J. Rhinol. Allergy* **2016**, *30*, 215–221. [CrossRef] [PubMed]
84. Aguiar, I.C.; Freitas, W.R.; Santos, I.R.; Apostolico, N.; Nacif, S.R.; Urbano, J.J.; Fonsêca, N.T.; Thuler, F.R.; Ilias, E.J.; Kassab, P.; et al. Obstructive sleep apnea and pulmonary function in patients with severe obesity before and after bariatric surgery: A randomized clinical trial. *Multidiscip. Respir. Med.* **2014**, *9*, 43. [CrossRef] [PubMed]
85. Dixon, A.E.; Pratley, R.E.; Forgione, P.M.; Kaminsky, D.A.; Whittaker-Leclair, L.A.; Griffes, L.A.; Garudathri, J.; Raymond, D.; Poynter, M.E.; Bunn, J.Y.; et al. Effects of obesity and bariatric surgery on airway hyperresponsiveness, asthma control and inflammation. *J. Allergy Clin. Immunol.* **2011**, *128*, 508–515. [CrossRef] [PubMed]
86. Lu, H.; Fu, C.; Li, W.; Jiang, H.; Wu, X.; Li, S. Screening for obstructive sleep apnea syndrome in asthma patients: A prospective study based on Berlin and STOP-Bang questionnaires. *J. Thorac. Dis.* **2017**, *9*, 1945–1958. [CrossRef] [PubMed]
87. Kapur, V.K.; Auckley, D.H.; Chowdhuri, S.; Kuhlmann, D.C.; Mehra, R.; Ramar, K.; Harrod, C.G. Clinical practice guideline for diagnostic testing for adult obstructive sleep apnea: An American Academy of Sleep Medicine clinical practice guideline. *J. Clin. Sleep Med.* **2017**, *13*, 479–504. [CrossRef] [PubMed]
88. Rosen, I.M.; Kirsch, D.B.; Carden, K.A.; Malhotra, R.K.; Ramar, K.; Aurora, R.N.; Kristo, D.A.; Martin, J.L.; Olson, E.J.; Rosen, C.L.; et al. American Academy of Sleep Medicine Board of Directors. Clinical Use of a Home Sleep Apnea Test: An Updated American Academy of Sleep Medicine Position Statement. *J. Clin. Sleep Med.* **2018**, *14*, 2075–2077. [CrossRef]
89. Young, T.; Palta, M.; Dempsey, J.; Skatrud, J.; Weber, S.; Badr, S. The occurrence of sleep-disordered breathing among middle-aged adults. *N. Engl. J. Med.* **1993**, *328*, 1230–1235. [CrossRef]
90. Bixler, E.O.; Vgontzas, A.N.; Lin, H.M.; Ten Have, T.; Rein, J.; Vela-Bueno, A.; Kales, A. Prevalence of sleep-disordered breathing in women: Effects of gender. *Am. J. Respir. Crit. Care Med.* **2001**, *163*, 608–613. [CrossRef]

91. Heinzer, R.; Vat, S.; Marques-Vidal, P.; Marti-Soler, H.; Andries, D.; Tobback, N.; Mooser, V.; Preisig, M.; Malhotra, A.; Waeber, G.; et al. Prevalence of sleep-disordered breathing in the general population: The HypnoLaus study. *Lancet Respir. Med.* **2015**, *3*, 310–318. [CrossRef]
92. Senaratna, C.V.; Perret, J.L.; Lodge, C.J.; Lowe, A.J.; Campbell, B.E.; Matheson, M.C.; Hamilton, G.S.; Dharmage, S.C. Prevalence of obstructive sleep apnea in the general population: A systematic review. *Sleep Med. Rev.* **2017**, *34*, 70–81. [CrossRef] [PubMed]

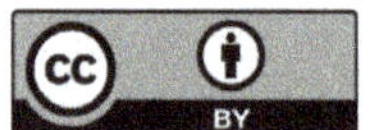

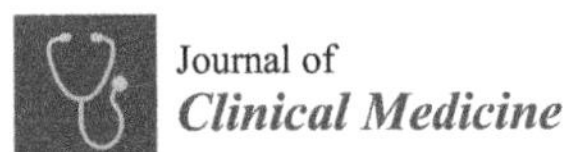
Journal of
Clinical Medicine

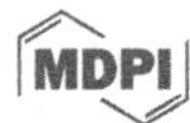

Article

Longitudinal Relationships between Asthma-Specific Quality of Life and Asthma Control in Children; The Influence of Chronic Rhinitis

Dillys van Vliet [1], Brigitte A. Essers [2], Bjorn Winkens [3], Jan W. Heynens [4], Jean W. Muris [5], Quirijn Jöbsis [1] and Edward Dompeling [1,*]

1 Department of Paediatric Pulmonology, School for Public Health and Primary Care (CAPHRI), Maastricht University Medical Centre (MUMC+), 6202 AZ Maastricht, The Netherlands; dillysv@hotmail.com (D.v.V.); r.jobsis@mumc.nl (Q.J.)
2 Department of Clinical Epidemiology and Medical Technology Assessment, MUMC+, 6229 HX Maastricht, The Netherlands; brigitte.essers@mumc.nl
3 Department of Methodology and Statistics, CAPHRI, MUMC+, 6229 HA Maastricht, The Netherlands; bjorn.winkens@maastrichtuniversity.nl
4 Department of Paediatrics, Zuyderland Medical Centre, 6162 BG Sittard-Geleen, The Netherlands; jan.heijnens@mumc.nl
5 Department of Primary Care Medicine, CAPHRI, MUMC+, 6229 HA Maastricht, The Netherlands; jean.muris@maastrichtuniversity.nl
* Correspondence: Edward.dompeling@mumc.nl; Tel.: +31-43-3877248; Fax: +31-43-3845246

Received: 10 January 2020; Accepted: 9 February 2020; Published: 18 February 2020

Abstract: Managing pediatric asthma includes optimizing both asthma control and asthma-specific quality of life (QoL). However, it is unclear to what extent asthma-specific QoL is related to asthma control or other clinical characteristics over time. The aims of this study were to assess in children longitudinally: (1) the association between asthma control and asthma-specific QoL and (2) the relationship between clinical characteristics and asthma-specific QoL. In a 12-month prospective study, asthma-specific QoL, asthma control, dynamic lung function indices, fractional exhaled nitric oxide, the occurrence of exacerbations, and the use of rescue medication were assessed every 2 months. Associations between the clinical characteristics and asthma-specific QoL were analyzed using linear mixed models. At baseline, the QoL symptom score was worse in children with asthma and concomitant chronic rhinitis compared to asthmatic children without chronic rhinitis. An improvement of asthma control was longitudinally associated with an increase in asthma-specific QoL (p-value < 0.01). An increased use of β_2-agonists, the occurrence of wheezing episodes in the year before the study, the occurrence of an asthma exacerbation in the 2 months prior to a clinical visit, and a deterioration of lung function correlated significantly with a decrease in the Pediatric Asthma Quality of Life Questionnaire (PAQLQ) total score (p-values ≤ 0.01). Chronic rhinitis did not correlate with changes in the PAQLQ score over 1 year. The conclusion was that asthma control and asthma-specific QoL were longitudinally associated, but were not mutually interchangeable. The presence of chronic rhinitis at baseline did influence QoL symptom scores. β_2-agonist use and exacerbations before and during the study were inversely related to the asthma-specific QoL over time.

Keywords: asthma; asthma-specific quality of life; chronic rhinitis; disease-specific quality of life; health-related quality of Life (HRQLQ); children; longitudinal study

1. Introduction

Respiratory symptoms have a significant influence on the daily life of children with asthma [1,2]. In the management of asthma, monitoring of both the asthma control and the quality of life (QoL) is important. International guidelines mention optimal QoL as an important objective in asthma management, but offer no guidance on how or when to base clinical decisions on asthma-specific QoL [3–5].

As guidelines recommend medication titration predominantly based on asthma control, additional knowledge about the longitudinal relationship between pediatric asthma control and asthma-specific QoL is important [3–5]. Studies focusing on asthma-specific QoL found a fair to good cross-sectional association between the QoL and the asthma level of disease control in children [1,6–12]. However, several important questions remain. First, as asthma is a chronic disease, it is relevant to know whether changes in the quality of life over the course of time are correlated with changes in the asthma control. To date, longitudinal data on this topic are lacking [1,6–13].

Second, there is no information available about the course and variation of asthma-specific QoL in children. This information may give insight into the frequency with which asthma-specific QoL should be monitored in clinical care. Third, as similar questions were used to assess the asthma control and the QoL in some studies, it is unclear to what extent this may have over-exaggerated the correlation between the asthma control and the QoL [9,12]. Fourth, very little is known about the longitudinal relationship between asthma-specific QoL and clinical characteristics, such as the presence of chronic rhinitis, the use of rescue medication, the daily dosage of inhaled corticosteroids, the exacerbation rate, lung function, atopy, airway inflammation (e.g., fractional exhaled nitric oxide (FeNO) levels), and bronchial hyperresponsiveness.

Although it is generally assumed that these clinical characteristics affect the QoL, there are little longitudinal data in children to confirm this.

Therefore, the objectives of this study are to determine the association over time:

1) between asthma control and asthma-specific QoL;
2) between clinical characteristics (e.g., the presence of chronic rhinitis, daily dosage of inhaled corticosteroids, lung function impairment, use of rescue medication, FeNO, and the occurrence of asthma exacerbations) and asthma-specific QoL.

2. Methods

2.1. Study Design and Patients

Children with persistent asthma aged 6–17 years were included in this one-year longitudinal cohort study (clinicaltrial.gov NCT 01239238) as described previously [14]. Patients were recruited at the outpatient clinics of 2 clinical centers (Sittard and Maastricht) in the Netherlands. All asthmatic children were treated at the outpatient clinic of these 2 specialized pediatric pulmonology centers for at least 6 months and had received inhaled corticosteroids (ICS) in the year preceding the study. All children met the Global Initiative for Asthma (GINA) criteria and the following criteria of the Dutch Society of Pediatrics for an asthma diagnosis: (1) recurrent episodes of wheezing, coughing, breathlessness, or chest tightness [3,5]; (2) reversibility to a bronchodilator defined as an increase in the forced expiratory volume in 1 s (FEV_1) of ≥ 9% of the predicted value [5,15]; and/or (3) bronchial hyperresponsiveness to histamine defined as a 20% drop in the FEV_1 after inhalation of histamine ≤ 8 mg/mL [5]. Patients were excluded in the case of cardiac abnormalities, mental retardation, congenital abnormalities or existence of a syndrome, active smoking, immunotherapy, or no technical satisfactory performance of lung function measurements.

For this study, ethical approval was obtained by the Medical Ethical Committee of the Maastricht University Medical Centre (NL33101.068.10/METC 10-2-064). All parents and children aged twelve years and older signed an informed consent form before the start of the study. All methods and measurement were performed in accordance with the relevant guidelines and regulations.

2.2. Study Parameters

Every 2 months, regular outpatient visits at the hospital took place. During these clinical visits, measurements of asthma control, lung function, FeNO and asthma-specific QoL were taken by a trained research nurse or a medical doctor.

2.3. Questionnaires on Asthma Control, Asthma-Specific QoL, and the International Study of Asthma and Allergies in Childhood (ISAAC)

Asthma control was assessed using 2 methods: (1) an Asthma Control Questionnaire (ACQ) and (2) the GINA criteria [16,17]. The following cut-off points for the level of control were used: ACQ≤0.75 controlled asthma, 0.75< ACQ ≤1.5 partly controlled, and ACQ >1.5 uncontrolled asthma. In addition, the asthma control level during the previous 2 weeks was assessed by scoring symptoms in combination with a FEV_1 assessment, as recommended in the GINA—Asthma Management and Prevention-guidelines [3].

To assess the asthma-specific QoL, children completed the Pediatric Asthma Quality of Life Questionnaire (PAQLQ) [8,11,18]. The standardized version of the PAQLQ contains 23 questions in 3 domains, i.e., activity limitations, symptoms, and emotional function. The range in scores is from 1–7, which represents poor to good asthma-specific QoL [8]. All children completed the ACQ and PAQLQ by themselves, so interference of parents was avoided as much as possible.

2.4. FeNO

Children performed a FeNO online measurement using a NIOX analyzer (NIOX MINO®, Aerocrine, Solna, Sweden) according to American Thoracic Society (ATS) and European Respiratory Society (ERS) standards [19].

2.5. Dynamic Spirometry and Reversibility

Patients were instructed to stop short-acting bronchodilators at least 8 h, and long-acting bronchodilators at least 48 h, before measurement. First, dynamic spirometry was performed by means of the ZAN 100® spirometer, according to ATS/ERS standards (nSpire Health GmbH, Oberthulba, Germany) [20]. The highest value of 3 correctly performed maximal expiratory flow-volume (MEFV) curves was used for analysis. The recorded parameters included the FEV_1, forced vital capacity (FVC), and maximum expiratory flow at 50% of FVC (MEF_{50}), all expressed as a percentage of the predicted value. Second, the patient inhaled 400 µg of salbutamol, and after 15 m lung function measurements were repeated in order to test for reversibility to a bronchodilator.

2.6. Bronchial Hyperresponsiveness

Bronchial hyperresponsiveness at baseline was evaluated by the histamine challenge test [21]. At first, an aerosol of buffered saline was inhaled, followed by aerosols of histamine solutions with a doubling of the concentration from 0.03 to 16 mg/mL at intervals of 5 m. The FEV_1 was measured at 30, 90, and 120 s after completed inhalation. The percentage decline in the FEV_1 was calculated and the test was stopped when a drop of 20% in the FEV_1 occurred (PC_{20}), or the highest concentration of 16 mg/mL was administered. The PC_{20} threshold was calculated from a log concentration versus dose response curve. After reaching the threshold, children inhaled 800 µg of salbutamol, and then 3 MEFV curves were performed.

2.7. Atopy

Sensitization to allergens was objectified by the Phadiatop® (Phadia, Uppsala, Sweden), RAST® (Pharmacia, Uppsala, Sweden) or allergen skin test. These tests were performed preceding the study or at baseline.

2.8. Medication Titration

Patients were treated according to the GINA guidelines [3]. Medication titration was performed on the basis of asthma control levels based on the GINA criteria (Table 1).

Table 1. Criteria for medication titration (step up, no change, or step down).

Step up
Uncontrolled asthma in 1 visit, or partly controlled asthma during 2 consecutive visits.
No change in treatment
One visit with controlled asthma, or one visit with partly controlled asthma.
Step down
Two consecutive visits with controlled asthma.

2.9. Definition of Exacerbation

The definition of an asthma exacerbation was based on the latest ATS/ERS guidelines [22].

2.10. ISAAC Questionnaire and Chronic Rhinitis

At baseline, parents completed electronically the ISAAC (International Study of Asthma and Allergies in Childhood) questionnaire [23]. The items focusing on asthma symptoms were used for statistical analysis. The ISAAC questionnaire was completed by 94% of all parents. A child was considered to have chronic rhinitis in the case of a positive response to 2 ISAAC questions ('chronic rhinitis without a cold' and 'chronic rhinitis in the past 12 months').

2.11. Exposure to Second-Hand Smoke

Parental smoking was assessed using an electronic questionnaire, which was completed by 94% of all parents. Passive smoking or exposure to second-hand smoke was defined as smoking of one or both parents in the presence of the child.

2.12. Data Collection

The collected data were checked and cleaned by an independent monitoring board (Clinical Trial Centre Maastricht). All recorded data during visits were stored in a secured database. In addition, all electronic questionnaires were completed at home.

2.13. Data Analysis

The description of baseline characteristics occurred as follows: numerical variables were expressed as the mean and standard deviation (SD) or as the median and interquartile ranges (IQR, i.e., 25th–75th percentile) and categorical variables were expressed as numbers and percentages. The variation of baseline PAQLQ scores for different asthma control levels was described as the mean and standard deviation. In addition, at baseline the coefficient of variation was calculated for each asthma control level (CV = mean/standard deviation).

To control for interdependency between repeated measurements in the same participant, linear mixed models were used [24]. All participants were included in the analysis, including children who dropped out during the study. In the mixed models, the PAQLQ total scores and, thereafter, the domains were included as the dependent variable. First, the course of the PAQLQ scores during the study was tested for significance in a simple model without the correction of any clinical variable. Second, in order to analyze the association between asthma control and the PAQLQ scores, the ACQ and GINA asthma control levels were included as an independent variable separately. Third, the clinical characteristics, FEV_1 percentage of the predicted value, and β_2-agonist use were included in a new model, while asthma control was excluded. Asthma symptoms represent 1 domain of the PAQLQ; therefore, symptoms were not included as a separate independent variable in any model. Besides, in all models the age, sex, trial site, season, bronchial hyperresponsiveness, atopy, exposure to second-hand smoke, FeNO, and the inhaled daily dose of corticosteroids were included as independent variables. The p-values < 0.05 were considered significant. Data were analyzed using SPSS 20 (SPSS Inc., Chicago, IL, USA).

3. Results

3.1. Patient Characteristics

A total number of 331 children with doctor-diagnosed asthma were asked to participate in the study, of which 96 children actually participated [14]. The majority of subjects were atopic and had severe bronchial hyperresponsiveness despite the use of a moderate daily dose of inhaled corticosteroids. Active parental smoking was reported in the cases of 26% of the children, whereas exposure to second-hand smoke was reported in the cases of 8% of the children (Table 2). There were no clinical important differences in the baseline characteristics between the two centers.

Table 2. Characteristics of the total population at baseline (n = 96).

Parameter	Value
Mean age [range], in years	10 [6–17]
Sex male/female, n	50/46
ACQ score, median [IQR]	0.6 [0.3–1]
PAQLQ total score, median [IQR]	6.4 [5.9–6.7]
Symptoms domain, median [IQR]	6.4 [5.5–6.7]
Activity limitations domain, median [IQR]	6.2 [5.3–6.6]
Emotional functioning domain, median [IQR]	6.9 [6.5–7.0]
FeNO, ppb: median [IQR]	12.5 [8.0–31.0]
FEV_1 % predicted, mean ± SD	96.8 ± 14.2
Reversibility, increase in FEV_1 % predicted: mean ± SD	6.6 ± 8.5
ICS dose of inhaled fluticasone or equivalent, mean ± SD *	269 ± 175
PC_{20}, mg/mL: median [IQR] †	1.2 [0.3–2.9]
Atopic, n % ‡	76
Chronic rhinitis, %	70
Wheezing episodes past year, %	58
Parental smoking, %	26
Exposure to second-hand smoke, %	8

ACQ = Asthma Control Questionnaire, IQR = interquartile range, PAQLQ = Pediatric Asthma Control Quality of Life Questionnaire, FeNO = fractional exhaled nitric oxide, FEV_1: forced expiratory volume in 1 second, SD = standard deviation, ICS = inhaled corticosteroids. * At baseline 94% of the children used ICS. † PC_{20}: concentration of histamine inducing a 20% drop in FEV_1. ‡ Atopy is defined as a positive Phadiatop (Phadia, Uppsala, Sweden), or a positive allergen skin test.

3.2. Influence of Chronic Rhinitis on QoL at Baseline

In comparison with children without chronic rhinitis (n = 27), children with rhinitis (n = 62) had a lower PAQLQ symptoms domain score (mean score (SD) of 5.8 (1.1) versus a score of 6.3 (0.6), p = 0.016), a comparable PAQLQ activity limitation score (mean (SD) of 5.9 (1.0) versus 6.1 (0.7), p = 0.352) or a PAQLQ emotional domain (mean (SD) of 6.5 (1.0) versus 6.6 (0.6), p = 0.516), and a tendency towards a lower PAQLQ total score (mean (SD) of 6.1 (1.0) versus 6.4 (0.5), p = 0.076). A lower PAQLQ score indicates a worse quality of life.

3.3. Course and Variability of Asthma-Specific QoL during the Study

Overall asthma-specific QoL and asthma control improved during the year (p-value < 0.01) (Figure 1). The mean level of the symptoms and activity limitations domain was lower than the level of the emotional functioning domain (Figure 1). In 46% of the children, this emotional functioning domain at baseline showed a maximum score of seven. The variability of the PAQLQ total scores at baseline was larger in the partly or uncontrolled children (coefficient of variation, CV = 19%), than in the controlled children (CV = 6%). This variability is shown in Figure 2, where all the measurements of all the children are included.

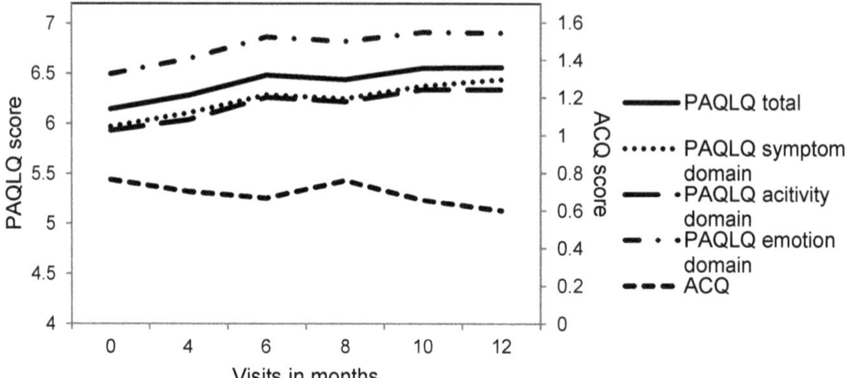

Figure 1. Overview of the course of the PAQLQ and ACQ scores during 12 months. On the right-hand side, the scale and numbers of the ACQ score are given, on the left-hand side, the scale and numbers of the PAQLQ score.

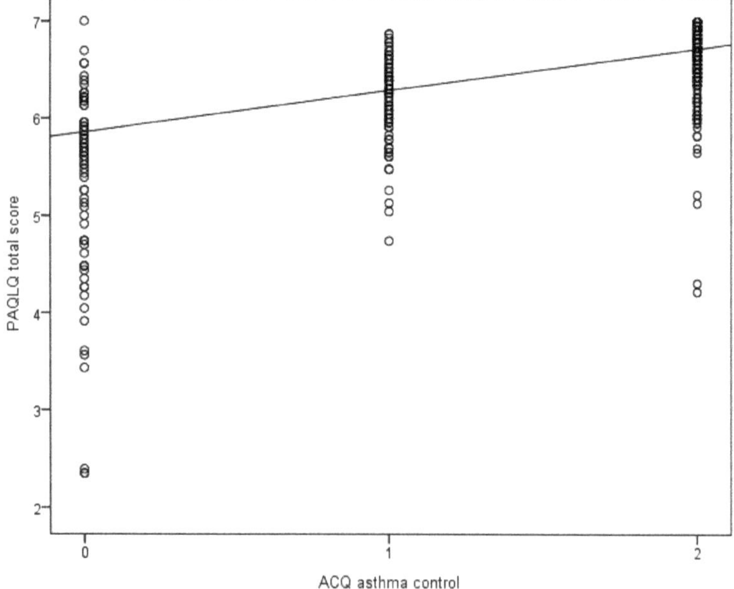

Figure 2. Associations between ACQ asthma control and PAQLQ total scores in a linear mixed model—all measurements taken during one year were included. The regression line is based on a model in which the ACQ level of asthma control is included; the estimates of this model are given in Table 3. For factors in the equation other than ACQ asthma control, mean values were used. ACQ asthma control: 0 = uncontrolled, 1 = partly controlled, and 2 = controlled.

Table 3. Results of the multivariate models with the PAQLQ score as the dependent variable and independent predictors of asthma control (assessed by the ACQ) and other (clinical) parameters (dose of fluticasone or equivalent, age, sex, trial site, season, chronic rhinitis, wheezing episodes in the preceding year, PC_{20} histamine test, atopy, FeNO, exacerbations in the previous 2 months, and exposure to second-hand smoke). Only significant results are shown.

	PAQLQ total score			PAQLQ symptoms domain			PAQLQ activity limitations domain		
	β	CI	P_{value}	β	CI	P_{value}	β	CI	P_{value}
ACQ asthma level of control *	0.43	0.37, 0.50	<0.01	0.63	0.54, 0.71	<0.01	0.60	0.50, 0.69	<0.01
Fluticasone daily dosage or equivalent per 100 μg †	−0.04	−0.07, −0.008	0.01	−0.06	−0.10, −0.02	<0.01	−0.04	−0.08, −0.0004	0.05
Season ‡	‡	‡	0.01			0.01	-	-	-
Sex §	-	-	-	-	-	-	−0.19	−0.36, −0.02	0.03

ACQ = Asthma Control Questionnaire, ICS = inhaled corticosteroids, PAQLQ = Pediatric Asthma Control Quality of Life Questionnaire, β = estimate of corresponding factor in the model, CI = 95% confidence interval of the estimate. The presented data are adjusted for trial site, age, chronic rhinitis, occurrence of wheezing episodes in the preceding year, PC_{20} histamine test, atopy, FeNO, exacerbation in the previous 2 months, and exposure to second-hand smoke. * Increase in the PAQLQ score for an improvement of ACQ asthma control from uncontrolled to partly controlled and partly controlled to controlled. † Decrease in the PAQLQ score per increase of 100 μg fluticasone daily dosage or equivalent. ‡ Decrease in the PAQLQ score for summer versus winter ((estimate) (95% CI) (−0.16) (−0.28, −0.04)) or summer versus spring ((estimate) (95% CI) (−0.17) (−0.28, −0.07)). § Decrease in the PAQLQ score for female versus male. Model with the PAQLQ emotional functioning domain as the dependent variable: of all factors, only the ACQ asthma level of control had a significant association (see text).

3.4. Association between Asthma Control and PAQLQ Scores during a One Year Follow-up

Asthma control based on the ACQ had the strongest longitudinal association with the PAQLQ total scores compared to the occurrence of wheezing episodes in the preceding year and the occurrence of an exacerbation in the previous 2 months (*p*-value (estimate); <0.01 (0.43)) (Table 3). The estimate of 0.43 means that an improvement of asthma control from uncontrolled to partly controlled, or from partly controlled to controlled disease, resulted in an increase of the PAQLQ total score of 0.43. Therefore, deterioration of asthma control from controlled to uncontrolled was associated with a clinically relevant decrease in the PAQLQ total score of 0.86. Additionally, with the PAQLQ subdomains, asthma control had the strongest association of all the clinical characteristics. The estimates for the subdomains were highest for the symptoms and activity limitation and small but significant for the emotional functioning domain (*p*-value (estimate) (95% CI); <0.01 (0.05) (0.03, 0.08)).

We also performed an analysis with asthma control according to the GINA criteria. Similarly to asthma control based on the ACQ, a strong longitudinal association with the PAQLQ total score and a comparable pattern for the PAQLQ domains was found (Table 4). Additionally, the occurrence of wheezing episodes in the preceding year was associated with the PAQLQ total score. Of all the PAQLQ domains, the emotional functioning domain had the smallest association with asthma control based on the GINA criteria (*p*-value (estimate) (95% CI); <0.01 (0.09) (0.05, 0.13). All models were adjusted for clinical characteristics, as described in the method section.

3.5. Factors Independently Related to PAQLQ Scores during One Year Follow-up

Finally, a model consisting of all predefined clinical characteristics (except the ACQ or GINA asthma control) showed that three factors were independently associated with a decrease in the PAQLQ total scores: (1) an increased use of β_2-agonists (Table 5 and Figure 3), (2) the occurrence of wheezing episodes in the year preceding the study, and (3) the occurrence of an asthma exacerbation in the 2 months preceding the PAQLQ assessments (Table 5). Although the FEV_1 percentage of the predicted value was also significantly associated with the PAQLQ total score, the estimates were small (*p*-value (estimate); <0.01 (0.05)) (Table 5, Figure 4). The daily dose of inhaled corticosteroids and FeNO levels showed no longitudinal association with the PAQLQ scores (Table 5). In contrast to the model in which the asthma control was included, no factor in this model was associated with the PAQLQ emotional functioning domain. The presence of chronic rhinitis was not associated with changes in the PAQLQ total score or subdomain scores.

Table 4. Results of the multivariate models with the PAQLQ score as the dependent variable and independent predictors (asthma control according to GINA, dose of fluticasone or equivalent, age, sex, trial site, season, wheezing episodes in the preceding year, PC_{20} histamine test, atopy, FeNO, exacerbations in the previous 2 months, and exposure to second-hand smoke). Only significant results are shown.

	PAQLQ total score			PAQLQ symptoms domain			PAQLQ activity limitations domain		
	β	CI	P_{value}	β	CI	P_{value}	β	CI	P_{value}
GINA asthma level of control*	0.38	0.30, 0.46	<0.01	0.57	0.47, 0.66	<0.01	0.56	0.44, 0.67	<0.01
Wheezing episodes preceding year no/yes†	−0.29	−0.10, −0.49	<0.01	−0.42	−0.16, −0.69	<0.01	−0.36	−0.05, −0.66	0.02
Age in years‡	-	-	-	−0.04	−0.08, <0.01	0.03	−0.05	−0.1, −0.01	0.02
Exacerbation in previous 2 months no/yes§	-	-	-	−0.19	−0.35, −0.02	0.03	-	-	-

GINA = Global Initiative for Asthma, PAQLQ = Pediatric Asthma Control Quality of Life Questionnaire, β = estimate of corresponding factor in the model, CI = 95% confidence interval of the estimate. Adjusted for trial site, sex, season, PC_{20} histamine test, atopy, FeNO, use of fluticasone or equivalent, and exposure to second-hand smoke. * Increase in the PAQLQ score for an increase of the level of control from uncontrolled to partly controlled to controlled based on the GINA criteria. † Decrease in the PAQLQ score in the case of wheezing episodes having occurred in the preceding year. ‡ Decrease in the PAQLQ score when age increase. § Decrease in the PAQLQ score in the case of the occurrence of exacerbations in the preceding 2 months. Model with the PAQLQ emotional functioning domain as the dependent variable: of all factors, only the GINA asthma level of control had a significant association (see text).

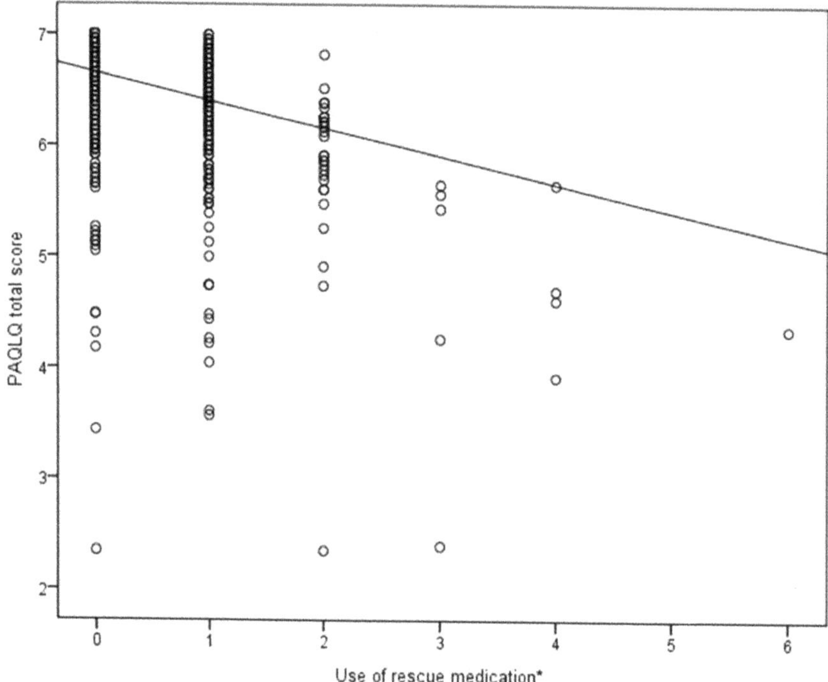

Figure 3. Associations between β_2-agonist use and the PAQLQ total score in a linear mixed model—all measurements taken during one year are included†. * Use of rescue medication during the week preceding the clinical visit: 0 = 0 puffs most days, 1 = 1–2 puffs most days, 2 = 3–4 puffs most days, 3 = 5–8 puffs most days, 4 = 9–12 puffs most days, 5 = 13–16 puffs most days, and 6=more than 16 puffs most days. The regression line is based on the model in which the asthma control levels were excluded, the estimates of this model are given in Table 4. For factors in the equation other than the use of rescue medication, mean values were used.

24. Fitzmaurice, G.M.L.N.; Ware, J.H. *Applied longitudinal analysis*; John Wiley & Sons, Inc.: Hoboken, NJ, USA, 2004.
25. Carranza Rosenzweig, J.R.; Edwards, L.; Lincourt, W.; Dorinsky, P.; ZuWallack, R.L. The relationship between health-related quality of life, lung function and daily symptoms in patients with persistent asthma. *Respir. Med.* **2004**, *98*, 1157–1165. [CrossRef]
26. De Jongste, J.C.; Carraro, S.; Hop, W.C.; Baraldi, E.; CHARISM Study Group. Daily telemonitoring of exhaled nitric oxide and symptoms in the treatment of childhood asthma. *Am. J. Respir. Crit. Care Med.* **2009**, *179*, 93–97. [CrossRef]
27. Luskin, A.T.; Chipps, B.E.; Rasouliyan, L.; Miller, D.P.; Haselkorn, T.; Dorenbaum, A. Impact of asthma exacerbations and asthma triggers on asthma-related quality of life in patients with severe or difficult-to-treat asthma. *J. Allergy Clin. Immunol. Pract.* **2014**, *2*, 544–552.e2. [CrossRef]
28. Petsios, K.T.; Priftis, K.N.; Hatziagorou, E.; Tsanakas, J.N.; Antonogeorgos, G.; Matziou, V.N. Determinants of quality of life in children with asthma. *Pediatric Pulmonol.* **2013**, *48*, 1171–1180. [CrossRef]
29. Mancuso, C.A.; Peterson, M.G. Different methods to assess quality of life from multiple follow-ups in a longitudinal asthma study. *J. Clin. Epidemiol.* **2004**, *57*, 45–54. [CrossRef]
30. Annett, R.D.; Bender, B.G.; DuHamel, T.R.; Lapidus, J. Factors influencing parent reports on quality of life for children with asthma. *J. Asthma* **2003**, *40*, 577–587. [CrossRef]
31. Eiser, C.; Morse, R. Can parents rate their child's health-related quality of life? Results of a systematic review. *Qual. Life Res.* **2001**, *10*, 347–357. [CrossRef]
32. Montalbano, L.; Cilluffo, G.; Gentile, M.; Ferrante, G.; Malizia, V.; Cibella, F.; Viegi, G.; Passalacqua, G.; La Grutta, S. Development of a nomogram to estimate the quality of life in asthmatic children using the Childhood Asthma Control Test. *Pediatric Allergy Immunol.* **2016**, *27*, 514–520. [CrossRef]

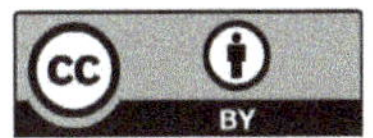

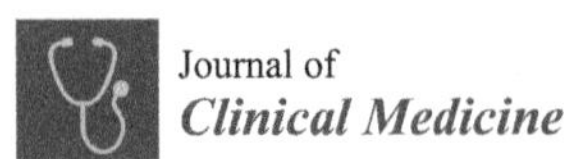
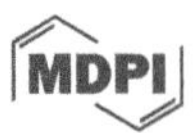

Article

Mitochondrial Function in Peripheral Blood Mononuclear Cells (PBMC) Is Enhanced, Together with Increased Reactive Oxygen Species, in Severe Asthmatic Patients in Exacerbation

Carole Ederlé [1,2], Anne-Laure Charles [2], Naji Khayath [1,2], Anh Poirot [1], Alain Meyer [2,3], Raphaël Clere-Jehl [2], Emmanuel Andres [4], Frédéric De Blay [1,2] and Bernard Geny [2,3,*]

1 Pôle de Pathologie Thoracique, Service de Pneumologie, Nouvel Hôpital Civil, 1, Place de l'Hôpital, FHU OMICARE Université de Strasbourg, 67000 Strasbourg, France; carole.ederle01@gmail.com (C.E.); naji.khayath@gmail.com (N.K.); anh.poirot@chru-strasbourg.fr (A.P.); Frederic.debaly@chru-strasbourg.fr (F.d.B.)

2 Fédération de Médecine Translationnelle de Strasbourg (FMTS), Faculté de Médecine, Equipe d'Accueil 3072, «Mitochondrie, Stress Oxydant, et Protection Musculaire», 11 Rue Humann, Université de Strasbourg, 67000 Strasbourg, France; anne.laure.charles@unistra.fr (A.-L.C.); alain.meyer1@chru-strasbourg.fr (A.M.); Raphael.clere-jehl@chru-strasbourg.fr (R.C.-J.)

3 Service de Physiologie et d'Explorations Fonctionnelles, Hôpitaux Universitaires de Strasbourg, Nouvel Hôpital Civil, 1 Place de l'Hôpital, 67091 Strasbourg CEDEX, France

4 Service de Médecine Interne, Diabète et Maladies Métaboliques, Pôle M.I.R.N.E.D., Hôpitaux Universitaires, 67000 CHRU Strasbourg CEDEX, France; Emmanuel.andres@chru-strasbourg.fr

* Correspondence: bernard.geny@chru-strasbourg.fr

Received: 30 August 2019; Accepted: 27 September 2019; Published: 3 October 2019

Abstract: Asthma is a chronic inflammatory lung syndrome with an increasing prevalence and a rare but significant risk of death. Its pathophysiology is complex, and therefore we investigated at the systemic level a potential implication of oxidative stress and of peripheral blood mononuclear cells' (PBMC) mitochondrial function. Twenty severe asthmatic patients with severe exacerbation (GINA 4–5) and 20 healthy volunteers participated at the study. Mitochondrial respiratory chain complexes activities using different substrates and reactive oxygen species (ROS) production were determined in both groups by high-resolution respirometry and electronic paramagnetic resonance, respectively. Healthy PBMC were also incubated with a pool of plasma of severe asthmatics or healthy controls. Mitochondrial respiratory chain complexes activity (+52.45%, $p = 0.015$ for V_{ADP}) and ROS production (+34.3%, $p = 0.02$) were increased in asthmatic patients. Increased ROS did not originate mainly from mitochondria. Plasma of severe asthmatics significantly increased healthy PBMC mitochondrial dioxygen consumption (+56.8%, $p = 0.031$). In conclusion, such asthma endotype, characterized by increased PMBCs mitochondrial oxidative capacity and ROS production likely related to a plasma constituent, may reflect activation of the immune system. Further studies are needed to determine whether increased PBMC mitochondrial respiration might have protective effects, opening thus new therapeutic approaches.

Keywords: asthma; exacerbation; reactive oxygen species; PBMC; mitochondrial function

---

1. Introduction

Asthma is a common disease that affects 300 million people worldwide (1 in 10 children and 1 in 12 adults) resulting in a substantial morbidity and an important annual healthcare expenditure. The disease is characterized by chronic inflammation of the conducting airway resulting in bronchial obstruction, mucus overproduction, airway remodeling and bronchial hyper-responsiveness [1,2].

Different mechanistic pathways are involved in such complex pathology. Locally, generation of oxidative stress with increased reactive oxygen species (ROS) production and mitochondrial dysfunction have been observed (bronchus, airway epithelium) in murine models of ovalbumin-induced asthma and in bronchial epithelial cell cultures [3–8]. Increased ROS production results in oxidative lipid peroxidation, protein and DNA damages (single-stranded and double-stranded breaks) [9], thought to aggravate the airway inflammation and to play a role in bronchial smooth muscle impairment and mucus secretion. Damaged antioxidant defense mechanisms, altered homeostasis of the airway surface liquid and acute or chronic bacterial airway infections also seem to aggravate oxidative stress in asthma [10]. Several studies highlighted an imbalance between oxidative species and antioxidant mechanisms in asthma. A decrease of superoxide dismutase, gluthation peroxidase or catalase activity was correlated with an aggravation of bronchial obstruction and asthma severity [11–15]. A self-entertaining phenomenon of inflammation and oxidative stress production occurs and damage-associated molecular patterns (so called alarmins), activate immune cells and their specific tissue [16].

In turn, immune cells of asthmatic patients exposed to an allergen, generate ROS, such as hydroxyl radicals, superoxide, peroxydes, peroxynitrite and nitric oxide [9]. This ROS generation was observed in sputum, exhaled breath condensates and bronchoalveolar lavages (BAL) of asthmatic patients, especially in severe asthma [11–14].

Besides this local characterization of the asthma mechanism, there are relatively few data focused on a potential involvement of mitochondrial function of inflammatory circulatory cells. However, dysfunction of the mitochondrial respiratory chain is likely to play a role in the initiation and progression of other inflammatory pathology such as cardiovascular diseases and anaphylactic choc [17–20]. Furthermore, impairments in mitochondrial function and/or elevation of ROS production have been found in allergic diseases such as atopy, atopic dermatitis and allergic rhinitis [3,4,21,22]. Recently, studying systemic involvement in local allergic rhinitis, we observed an impaired mitochondrial function in peripheral blood mononuclear cells (PBMC) 6 hours after an allergen challenge in patients with allergic rhinitis [23].

In the present study, therefore, we tested the hypothesis that peripheral blood mononuclear cell might demonstrate impaired mitochondrial function together with increased ROS production in severe asthmatic patients with severe exacerbation, as compared to healthy subjects.

2. Population and Methods

2.1. Patients and Study Design

Twenty healthy volunteers and 20 severe asthmatic patients experiencing severe exacerbation were enrolled in a prospective and controlled study. Severe asthma was defined as a stage 4 or 5 of GINA classification and severe exacerbation as a need for hospitalization or for systemic steroids (or its increase) for more than 3 days [2]. Exclusion criteria were active smoking, smoking cessation <1 year; ancient smoking >10 packs a year, current depression, cardiovascular insufficiency or severe sepsis.

The study design included the clinical characterization of patients and, peripheral blood mononuclear cells mitochondrial respiratory chain complexes' activities and ROS production in both control subjects and asthmatic patients. Further, after determining an eventual contribution of mitochondria to ROS production, we analyzed the effects of plasma on healthy PBMC. Thus, PBMC from healthy volunteers were placed in contact with heterologous platelet poor plasma of healthy volunteers or severe asthmatics experiencing severe exacerbation.

The study was approved by the ethics committee of the Strasbourg University Hospital (number 2016-69) and informed consent was obtained from each patient.

2.2. Peripheral Blood Mononuclear Cells (PBMC) Isolation

Thirty mL of venous blood was sampled in Sodium Heparinate tubes for each patient. 1mL was kept (on ice) for the study of ROS production. The remaining part of the sample was used to separate peripheral blood mononuclear cells (PBMC) and plasma. Briefly, blood was placed on a ficoll density gradient (Eurobio, Lymphocytes separation medium, Courtabeauf France, France) and centrifuged (2100 rpm, 25 min, 18 °C, without brakes). PBMC (lymphocytes and monocytes) were sampled, washed in a DPBS solution (Dulbecco's Phosphate Buffer Saline 0067M, Hyclone, South Logan, UT, USA) and centrifuged (1600 rpm, 10 min, 18 °C, without brakes). Finally, PBMC were counted by flow cytometry (Muse Cell Analyser, Merck Millipore, Darmstadt, Germany).

2.3. Mitochondrial Respiration

The study of the mitochondrial respiratory chain was performed with a high resolution oxygraph (Oxygraph-2k; Oroboros Instruments, Innsbruck, Austria) at 37 °C. 2.5×10^6 PBMC /mL were introduced in the Oxygraph-2k's chamber with continuous stirring. The dioxygen consumption was analyzed using the DatLab software 4.3 (Oxygraph-2k; Oroboros Instruments, Innsbruck, Austria). At the beginning, cell membranes were permeabilized with saponine (125 µg/mL), and complex I was activated with glutamate (5 mM), and malate (2 mM), this step is the basal dioxygen consumption.

After reaching a steady state for V0, different substrates and inhibitors were introduced in the oxygraph's chamber. ADP (2 mM) induced the activation of ATP synthase (mitochondrial Complex V) and allowed the study of mitochondrial complexes I, III, IV, V. Then, succinate (25 mM) was introduced, an activator of the mitochondrial Complex II, for the study of mitochondrial Complexes I, II, III, IV, V. The addition of rotenone (0.5 µM) allowed analysis of mitochondrial Complexes II, III, IV, V by inhibiting the Complex I. TMPD/ascorbate (0.5 mM/0.5 mM) was then added to give electrons to the Complex IV, so allowed preferentially the complex IV. The result was expressed in pmol/s/10^6cell.

2.4. Reactive Oxygen Species (ROS) Production

2.4.1. Measurement of Superoxide Anions in Blood

ROS production in venous blood was assessed by exploring the superoxide anions production, using electron paramagnetic resonance (EPR), (E-scan, Bruker-Biospin, Rheinstetten, Germany) at 37 °C, as previously described [24]. Briefly, 1 mL venous blood was kept on ice in order to perform the analysis 1 hour after sampling; 25 µL of blood were mixed with spin probe CMH (1-hydroxy-3-methoxycarbonyl-2,2,5,5-tetramethylpyrrolidine HCl, 200 µM). Then, the mixture was introduced in a glass EPR capillary tube (Noxygen Science Transfer & Diagnostics, Elzach, Germany), and then placed inside the cavity of the e-scan spectrometer (Bruker, Rheinstetten, Germany) for data acquisition. Detection of ROS production was conducted using BenchTop EPR spectrometer E-SCAN under the following EPR settings: center field g = 3477,452; sweep width 60 G; microwave power 21.85 mW; modulation amplitude 2.4 G; time constant 40.96 ms; conversion time 10.24 ms; number of lag curve points 6. The EPR signal is proportional to the unpaired electron numbers. The result was expressed in µmol/min.

2.4.2. Mitochondrial ROS Measurement

We determined mitochondrial PBMC ROS production using a fluorescent probe MitoSOX, a red mitochondrial superoxide indicator for live cell imaging (Molecular Probes; Life technologies) [25]. MitoSOX (Invitrogen, Eugene, Oregon, USA) (5 µM) was incubated with 2.5×10^6 PBMC diluted in DPBS, for 10 min at 37 °C. Then, cells were washed and centrifuged (1600 rpm, 10 min). Excitation was set at 510 nm and emission at 580 nm A positive control group of mitochondrial ROS production was elaborated with Antimycin. All the experiments were achieved in a light-protected environment. The result was expressed in AU of fluorescence.

2.5. Mitochondrial Dioxygen Consumption of Healthy PBMC in Contact with Heterologous Plasma

PBMC from 7 healthy volunteers were extracted following the same technique as presented above. Then 2×10^6 cells/mL were placed into each oxygraph's chamber with a pooled heterologous platelet poor plasma. In one chamber, plasma came from a pool of 6 healthy volunteers, and in the other one, plasma came from a pool of 6 severe asthmatics experiencing severe exacerbation.

Before introducing the PBMC, the basal respiration of both pooled plasmas was recorded in the oxygraph's chambers (Oxygraph-2k; Oroboros Instruments, Innsbruck, Austria) at 37 °C.

After 6 h exposure to heterologous plasma, PBMC basal consumption of dioxygen (V0) was measured and different substrates and inhibitors were added in order to study the mitochondrial respiratory chain complexes' activities. Using plasma as the respiratory solution, the uncoupling protocol was more adapted than the classic one. Therefore, an ATP-synthase inhibitor (oligomycine 1.25 μmol/L) was added, to induce a dioxygen consumption mainly due to the leakage of protons through the inner mitochondrial membrane [26]. Then, the uncoupler carbonyl cyanide 4-(trifluoro-methoxy)phenylhydrazone (FCCP 40 μM) was added in order to measure maximal oxygen flux. Rotenone (2 μM) was added to inhibit the complex I. Finally, Complex III was inhibited by antimycine (1.85 μM). Dioxygen consumption was calculated by subtracting the basal plasma respiration as previously described [20,26,27]. The result was expressed in pmol/s/10^6cell.

Simultaneously, ROS production was measured by the evolution of using fluorescent probe Amplex Red (20 μM) and Horseradish peroxidase (HRP, 1 U/mL). We also calculated the free radical leak (FRL) corresponding to the fraction of electrons which reduces O_2 to ROS in the mitochondrial respiratory chain (percentage of free radical leak) instead of reaching cytochrome oxidase to reduce O_2 to water [28]. Because two electrons are needed to reduce one mole of O_2 to H_2O_2, whereas four electrons are transferred in the reduction of one mole of O_2 to water, the FRL (percent) was calculated as the rate of H_2O_2 production divided by twice the rate of O_2 consumption, and the result was multiplied by 100 [29].

2.6. Statistical Analysis

All values are presented as mean ± standard error of the mean (SEM). Qualitative variables were described as numbers and percentages. When values followed the normality curve, Student's test was used. But, if values did not follow the normality curve, a non-parametric Mann–Whitney test was used to compare the control and the asthmatics groups. Concerning data obtained with PBMC exposed to pooled heterogenous control plasma or pooled heterogenous asthmatic plasma, a non-parametric paired test was realized (Wilcoxon test). All analysis were performed with GraphPad Prism 5 (Graph Pad Software, Inc., San Diego, CA, USA). Statistical significance was determined as $p < 0.05$.

3. Results

3.1. Clinical Characteristics of the Subjects

Twenty patients (mean age 50.95 ± 4.06 years, 5 men and 15 women) were admitted for exacerbation of severe asthma at the Strasbourg University Hospital with a need for hospitalization or systemic steroids for more than 3 days. The control group included 20 healthy volunteers (mean age 50.10 ± 3.77 years, 6 men and 14 women) with no medical history of pulmonary or atopic diseases.

Subjects' characteristics are summarized in Table 1. There was no difference in age, sex and smoking between severe asthmatic patients and the control group. Asthmatic patients had a body mass index (BMI) of 28.01 ± 1.47 kg/m^2 versus 23.0 ± 0.72 kg/m^2 in the control group ($p = 0.0040$). Severe asthmatic patients had mainly an uncontrolled allergic asthma. Fourteen patients presented with atopic and eosinophilic asthma whereas 2 patients had a non-atopic and eosinophilic asthma and 4 patients had non-Th_2 mediated asthma. 14 patients had an associated allergic rhinitis, 8 had a basal FEV1 < 80% of the maximal theoretical value. The main cause of exacerbation was bronchial and pulmonary infection and 9 patients were treated by steroids for more than 24 h at the time of inclusion and blood sampling.

Table 1. Demographic, clinical, and biological characteristics of the patients.

	Control Group (n = 20)	Severe Asthmatic Patients (n = 20)
Mean age (years)	50.10 ± 3.77	50.95 ± 4.06
Women	14	15
Male	6	5
Mean body mass index (BMI) (kg/m^2)	23.0 ± 0.72	28.01 ± 1.47
Mean smoking habits (PA)	1.70 ± 0.80	1.90 ± 0.69
Atopy	0	16
Medical history:		
Diabetes	1	4
Arterial hypertension	3	8
Venous thrombosis/pulmonary embolism	0	1
Other lung diseases	0	2
Neoplasia	0	1
Acute coronary syndrom with preserved LVEF	2	1
Blood eosinophil (Normal values: <600/mm^3)		
<300/mm^3		9
300–500/mm^3		2
500–1000/mm^3		9
Blood neutrophils (Normal values: 1500–7500/mm$^{3)}$		
<7500/mm^3		16
>7500/mm^3		4

BMI: Body mass index, PA: packs a year, LVEF: left ventricular ejection fraction.

3.2. *Mitochondrial Respiratory Chain Complexes' Activities Are Enhanced in Asthmatic Patients*

The maximal mitochondrial respiratory chain activity was significantly increased in patients with severe asthma experiencing severe exacerbation in comparison with the control group (Figure 1). Data using specific substrates are presented below.

3.2.1. Basal Consumption of Dioxygen (V_0)

V0 was increased in severe asthmatic patients in comparison with the control group (3.51 ± 0.43 and 2.10 ± 0.22 pmol/s/10^{6}cell respectively, +67.1%, p = 0.005).

3.2.2. Mitochondrial Complexes I + III + IV + Vactivities

V_{ADP} was significantly increased in the severe asthma group compared to the control group (8.78 ± 1.11 vs. 5.76 ± 0.48 pmol/s/10^{6}cell respectively in asthmatic patients and in control subjects, +52.4%, p = 0.015).

3.2.3. Mitochondrial Complexes I + II + III + IV + Vactivities

Vsucc was also significantly increased in the severe asthma group compared to the control group (15.64 ± 2.06 and 9.48 ± 0.91 pmol/s/10^{6}cell, +64.97%, p = 0.007).

3.2.4. Inhibition of the Mitochondrial Complex I by Rotenone

Rotenone injection showed no significant difference between both groups but the combined activity of the Complexes II + III + IV + V tended to be increase in the severe asthmatic patients (10.89 ± 1.70 and 7.22 ± 0.67 pmol/s/10^6cell respectively in asthmatic patients and in control subjects, +50.83%).

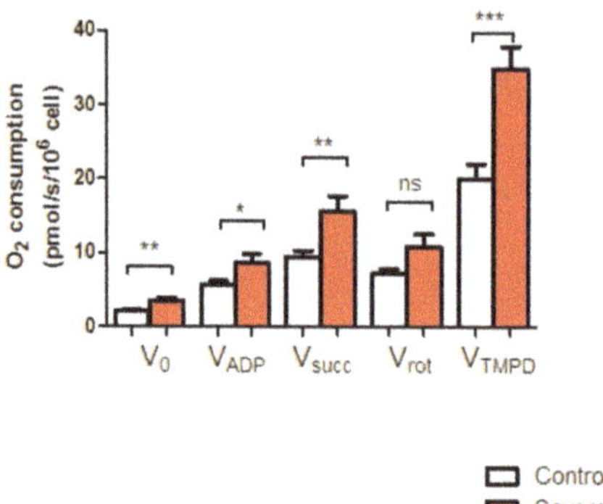

Figure 1. Peripheral blood mononuclear cells (PBMC) mitochondrial respiration in control and severe asthmatic patients. * $p < 0.05$, ** $p > 0.01$, *** $p < 0.001$. ns: non significant.

3.2.5. Complex IV Activity

$V_{TMPD/ascorbate}$ showed an increase of cytochrome C oxidase's activity in asthmatic patients (34.87 ± 2.99 and 20.03 ± 2.02 pmol/s/10^6cell, +74.09%, $p = 0.0003$).

V_0 corresponds to the basal O_2 consumption, with glutamate, and malate as substrates. V_{ADP} corresponds to the ADP-stimulated respiration, with glutamate and malate as substrates. V_{succ} represents the activation of all complexes (I, II, III, IV, V). V_{ROT} represents the complexes II, III, IV, V activities. V_{TMPD} corresponds to the complex IV contribution. Results are expressed as means ± SEM. $n = 20$ per group.

To further investigate a possible effect of corticosteroid or obesity, we analyzed PBMC mitochondrial respiration in asthmatic patients with and without corticosteroid (Figure 2) and with and without a BMI ≥ 30 kg/m^2 (Figure 3).

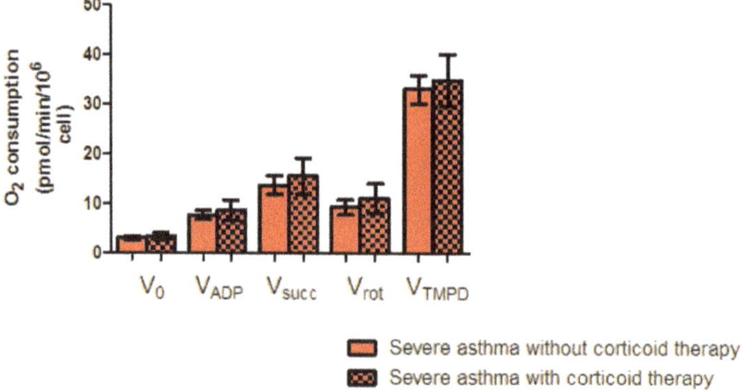

Figure 2. PBMC mitochondrial respiration in severe asthmatic patients treated or not with corticoids.

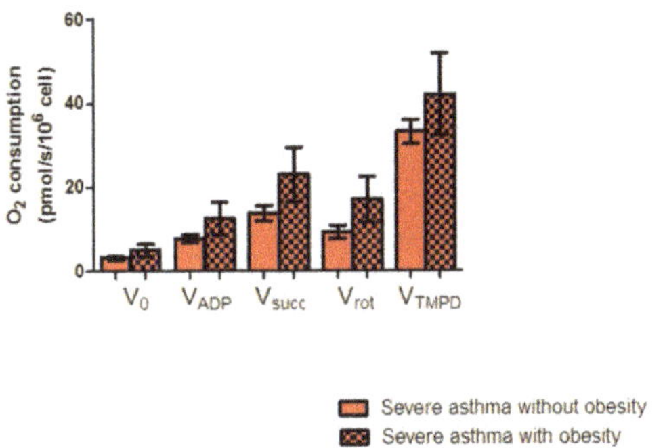

Figure 3. PBMC mitochondrial respiration in severe asthmatic patients, without or with a BMI ≥ 30 kg/m^2.

Concerning the corticosteroids, no significant difference was observed whatever the mitochondrial respiratory chain complex studied between patients treated or not with systemic steroids for more than 24 h.

V_0 corresponds to the basal O_2 consumption, with glutamate, and malate as substrates. V_{ADP} corresponds to the ADP-stimulated respiration, with glutamate and malate as substrates. V_{succ} represents the activation of all complexes (I, II, III, IV, V). V_{ROT} represents the complexes II, III, IV, V activities. V_{TMPD} corresponds to the complex IV contribution. Results are expressed as means ± SEM. $n = 11$ without and 9 with corticoid, respectively.

Moreover, although mitochondrial respiration tended to increase in severe asthmatics patients with a BMI ≥ 30 kg/m^2 as compared to patients with a BMI < 30 kg/m^2, this increase failed to reach statistical significance (23.01 ± 6.43 vs. 13.80 ± 1.88 pmol/s/10^{6}cell, $p = 0.09$ respectively for V_{succ}, and 17.07 ± 5.43 vs. 9.35 ± 1.51 pmol/s/10^{6}cell, $p = 0.08$, for V_{rot}).

V_0 corresponds to the basal O_2 consumption, with glutamate, and malate as substrates. V_{ADP} corresponds to the ADP-stimulated respiration, with glutamate and malate as substrates. V_{succ} represents the activation of all complexes (I, II, III, IV, V). V_{ROT} represents the complexes II, III, IV, V activities. V_{TMPD} corresponds to the complex IV contribution. Results are expressed as means ± SEM. $n = 16$ without and 4 with obesity, respectively.

3.3. Reactive Oxygen Species Are Increased in the Blood of Asthmatic Patients

ROS were significantly increased in the venous blood of severe asthmatic patients in comparison with the control group (0.94 ± 0.08 vs. 0.70 ± 0.07 µmol/min respectively +34.3%, $p = 0.02$, $n = 16$ per group, Figure 4A). To investigate the origin of such ROS, we determined the mitochondrial ROS production.

Mitochondrial ROS production tended to be increased in severe asthmatic patients experiencing severe exacerbation and the control group (2983.0 ± 135.8 and 2571.0 ± 252.2 UA respectively, $p = 0.07$, $n = 8$ per group, Figure 4B).

Systemic steroid treatment > 24 h and obesity did not influence the ROS production.

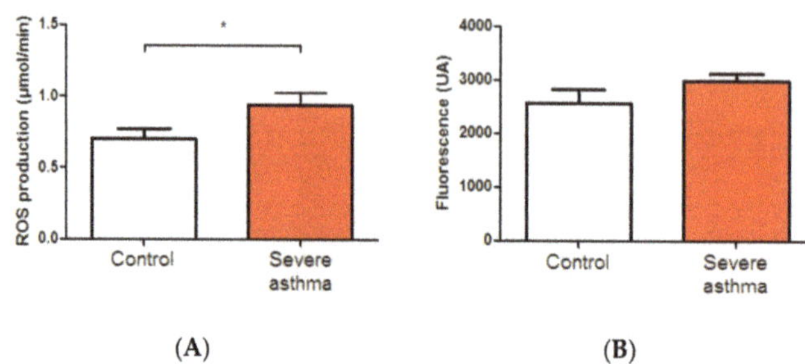

Figure 4. Reactive oxygen species (ROS) in control and severe asthmatic patients experiencing severe exacerbation. (**A**): total ROS level on whole blood was obtained using electron paramagnetic resonance. $n = 16$ per group. (**B**): ROS level on PBMC was detected by MitoSOX-based spectrofluorimetry detection. Results are expressed as means ± standard error of the mean (SEM). $n = 8$ per group. * $p < 0.05$.

3.4. *Effect of Heterologous Plasma of Healthy or Asthmatic Subjects on Mitochondrial Dioxygen Consumption and of Healthy PBMC*

Investigating whether plasma of asthmatic patients *per se* might modulate PBMC mitochondrial function, we observed using different substrates, an enhanced mitochondrial respiration of PBMC in presence of asthmatic plasma as compared to normal plasma ($n = 7$ per group, Figure 5A).

Thus, basal dioxygen consumption Vo was significantly increased in severe asthmatic plasma (1.55 ± 0.29 and 0.64 ± 0.28 pmol/s/10^6 cell, +142.2%, $p = 0.016$).

After ATP synthase inhibition mitochondrial respiration was activated by an uncoupler (FCCP). The Maximal mitochondrial respiratory chain activity was significantly increased in healthy PBMC in contact with pooled plasma from severe asthmatic patients in comparison with healthy PBMC in contact with pooled control plasma (2.87 ± 0.44 and 1.83 ± 0.28 pmol/s/10^6cell, +56.8%, $p = 0.031$).

Similarly, when the complex I was inhibited by rotenone injection mitochondrial activity was significantly increased in healthy PBMC in contact with pooled plasma from severe asthmatic patients in comparison with healthy PBMC (1.82 ± 0.45 and 0.84 ± 0.26 pmol/s/10^6cell, +116.7%, $p = 0.016$).

Finally, when the complex IV was inhibited by antimycin injection, mitochondrial activity tended to increase in healthy PBMC in contact with pooled plasma from severe asthmatic patients as compared to the control group (1.34 ± 0.45 and 0.80 ± 0.26 pmol/s/10^6cell, $p = 0.297$, +67.5%)

The free radical leak was not statistically increased in healthy PBMC in contact with pooled plasma from severe asthmatic patients, in comparison with the control one. These results are presented in Figure 5B.

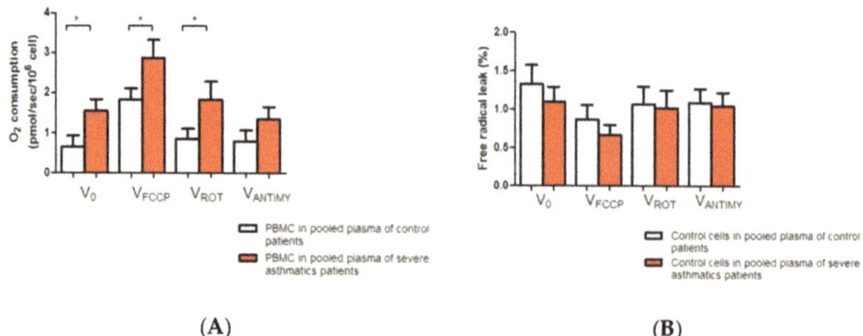

Figure 5. Effect of healthy and asthmatic plasma on PBMC mitochondrial respiration and free radical leak. (**A**) Mitochondrial respiration after different substrates injected. (B) Free radical leak. PBMC: peripheral blood mononuclear cell. FCCP: carbonyl cyanide 4-(trifluoro-methoxy)phenylhydrazone, ROT: rotenone, ANTIMY: antimycin. Results are expressed as means ± SEM. $n = 7$ per group. * $p < 0.05$.

4. Discussion

The main result of this study is to demonstrate that mitochondrial respiratory chain complexes' activities of PBMC are stimulated in severe asthmatic patients with severe exacerbation, and that such enhancement is associated with increased reactive oxygen species. Furthermore, the plasma of asthmatic patients—but not of healthy subjects—appears responsible for PBMC mitochondrial oxidative capacity enhancement.

Asthma is a frequent and severe disease affecting a large proportion of the human population, including children and young people and implying a tremendous socioeconomic burden. The pathophysiology of asthma and the balance between oxidant/antioxidant is the subject of intense ongoing research and some studies have explored the local role of mitochondria in atopic diseases [1–9,16,29]. However, still little is known on the connection between mitochondria and the immune response in asthma, especially in peripheral blood.

Interestingly, our study shows that severe asthmatic patients with severe exacerbation had a significant increase in their PBMC mitochondrial respiratory chain activity, in comparison with the control group. These data contrast with a previous report showing that acute nasal allergen challenge induces mitochondrial dysfunction of peripheral blood mononuclear cells in allergic rhinitis [23] and with the fact that PBMC mitochondrial respiration is generally impaired in cardiovascular diseases [18,19]. Thus, the increase observed in asthmatic patients is particularly interesting. In fact, peripheral blood immune cells like T and B lymphocytes or monocytes (PBMC) were activated in severe asthmatic patients with severe exacerbation [1]. At the mitochondrial level, this activation was expressed by an increased maximal function of the mitochondrial respiratory chain. Interestingly, this is consistent with data obtained on PBMC mitochondrial function in septic shock, often showing an increased mitochondrial respiration after an early impairment [20,30]. Such a response was thought to compensate for the initial mitochondrial dysfunction [30].

The underlying mechanisms still deserve further study but oxidative stress might play a key role. In our study, severe asthmatic patients with severe exacerbation had a significant elevation of ROS in their blood. These ROS did not seem to be mainly produced by mitochondria since the Mitosox analysis was similar in both groups and since the FRL showed no statistically significant difference in the number of O_2 molecules used for the production of ROS in the mitochondria between the two groups. Thus, as previously reported in asthma, reactive oxygen species could have been produced by NADPH-oxidase and/or by xanthine oxidase rather than by the mitochondrion [31,32].

Obesity might also have played a role since there is a link between mitochondrial dysfunction, obesity and asthma or metabolic syndrome [33,34]. Accordingly, PBMC mitochondrial respiration tended to be increased in asthmatic patients presenting with a BMI $\geq$ 30kg/m^2. Although not statistically significant and focused only on several respiratory chain complexes, this result supports further studies on a potential relationship between obesity *per se* and the mitochondrial respiration of circulating cells.

Similarly, corticosteroids might modulate PBMC mitochondrial respiration. Indeed, steroids mediated apoptotic signals in human eosinophils through a mitochondrial pathway [35]. However, in our study, no significant change was observed when comparing asthmatic patients with and without the corticoid therapy.

Finally, we tested whether patients with eosinophilia and hyper-eosinophilia, defined by a blood count of $\geq$300 and $\geq$500/mm^3 respectively, presented with exacerbated PBMC mitochondrial respiration as compared to asthmatic patients without eosinophilia. No difference was observed between both groups, suggesting the eosinophilia might not be a key factor associated with an enhanced PBMC mitochondrial respiration.

The clinical significance of such enhanced mitochondrial respiratory chain complexes' activities in severe asthmatic patients in exacerbation remains to be further investigated. However, recent studies suggest that during the activation of the adaptive immune response, the shift of dendritic cell's mitochondrial respiration toward either a glycolytic or an oxidative metabolism might be related to a pro-inflammatory or to an anti-inflammatory differentiation of T cells, respectively. Thus, a reduced mitochondrial respiration seemed to be associated with pro-inflammatory effects whereas an increased dendritic cell's mitochondrial respiration might antagonize TLR effects [36–38]. Therefore, one might hypothesize that the enhanced mitochondrial respiration we observed could reflect a trend toward a potentially beneficial anti-inflammatory effect.

Accordingly, besides their well-known deleterious effects corresponding to oxidative stress, ROS signaling might also allow protective effects through mitochondrial biogenesis and anti-oxidant system enhancements [39]. In asthma, ROS could have a different role depending on their producing cells. In epithelial and in bronchial smooth muscle cells, ROS likely induce local tissue damages and aggravate inflammation [9,10]. In peripheral blood, the increased ROS was observed without concomitant mitochondrial dysfunction, and could participate in the activation of circulating T lymphocytes, potentially playing a role in the "homing" of immune cells to the inflammatory upper airways [16].

Interestingly, recent data support a link between antigen-specific IgE receptor expression on PBMC and atopic asthma within school-aged children [40]. Furthermore, basophil counts in PBMC populations during childhood acute wheeze/asthma were associated with future exacerbations [41]. Whether the mitochondrial function of PBMC could be used in the future as a biomarker in severe asthma or for a targeted therapy cannot be inferred from our results. But, these data emphasize the potential interest of analyzing PBMC metabolic characteristics, in conjunction with the search of other potential biomarkers in severe asthma [42–44].

Limitations of the Study

Although 20 subjects in each group allowed us to discover interesting characteristics of asthmatic patients, studies with a greater number of subjects will be useful to further investigate the underlying mechanisms. In this context, a study specifically directed toward obese patients and a longer follow-up in order to characterize the patients after the exacerbation will be very interesting for better defining the clinical significance of these data.

5. Conclusions

This study further supports the concept of crosstalk between the mitochondrion and the immune system in asthma. The enhanced mitochondrial respiration observed in the PBMC of patients with severe asthma in exacerbation, likely related to a plasmatic factor potentially including ROS, might participate in the patient's defense mechanisms. However, this issue still has to be investigated and further studies are needed to determine whether circulating cells' mitochondrial function might be used as a biomarker in asthma and whether maintaining healthy mitochondria in asthmatic patients' PBMC might be an interesting therapeutic avenue, as proposed in lung injury [16,45]. Thus, further longitudinal studies exploring the systemic aspects of mitochondrial function and the ROS production in asthma appear warranted.

Author Contributions: Conceptualization: C.E., A.-L.C., N.K., A.M., A.P., F.d.B., B.G.; Methodology: C.E., A.-L.C., N.K., A.P., R.C.-J., F.d.B., B.G.; Validation: all authors; Formal Analysis: C.E., A.-L.C., N.K., F.d.B., B.G.; Writing—Original Draft Preparation: C.E., A.-L.C., B.G.; Writing—Review & Editing: C.E., A.-L.C., N.K., A.M., E.A., F.d.B., B.G.; Supervision: F.d.B., B.G.

Funding: This research received no external funding.

Acknowledgments: We are grateful to AM Kasprowicz for expert secretarial assistance and to L Essari, E Virio, H Yucel and L Kassegne for help in performing the clinical study. We deeply thanks the ARAIRLOR (Association régionale d'aide aux insuffisants respiratoires de Lorraine), and also the ADIRAL (Association D'aide aux Insuffisants Respiratoire d'Alsace Lorraine, France) and the OCOVAS (Association des Opérés du Cœur et des Vaisseaux à Strasbourg, France), for their respective participation in Oroboros and EPR Equipment acquisition.

Conflicts of Interest: The authors declare no conflict of interest.

Abbreviations

ADP	adenosine Di-phosphate
ATP	adenosine Tri-phosphate
AU	Arbitrary unit
FEV1	Forced Expiratory Volume
GINA	global initiative for asthma
NADPH	Nicotinamide adénine dinucléotide phosphate
TMPD	'N, N, N'N'-tétraméthyl-1,4-phénylènediamine

References

1. Lambrecht, B.N.; Hammad, H. The immunology of asthma. *Nat. Immunol.* **2015**, *16*, 45–56. [CrossRef] [PubMed]
2. GINA 2019. Available online: www.ginasthma.org (accessed on 17 June 2019).
3. Reddy, P.H. Mitochondrial Dysfunction and Oxidative Stress in Asthma: Implications for Mitochondria-Targeted Antioxidant Therapeutics. *Pharmaceuticals* **2011**, *4*, 429–456. [CrossRef] [PubMed]
4. Aguilera-Aguirre, L.; Bacsi, A.; Saavedra-Molina, A.; Kurosky, A.; Sur, S.; Boldogh, I. Mitochondrial dysfunction increases allergic airways inflammation. *J. Immunol.* **2009**, *183*, 5379–5387. [CrossRef] [PubMed]
5. Mabalirajan, U.; Dinda, A.K.; Kumar, S.; Roshan, R.; Gupta, P.; Sharma, S.K.; Ghosh, B. Mitochondrial structural changes and dysfunction are associated with experimental allergic asthma. *J. Immunol.* **2008**, *181*, 3540–3548. [CrossRef]
6. Boldogh, I.; Bacsi, A.; Choudhury, B.K.; Dharajiya, N.; Alam, R.; Hazra, T.K.; Mitra, S.; Goldblum, R.M.; Sur, S. ROS generated by pollen NADPH oxidase provide a signal that augments antigen-induced allergic airway inflammation. *J. Clin. Investig.* **2005**, *115*, 2169–2179. [CrossRef]
7. Dharajiya, N.; Choudhury, B.K.; Bacsi, A.; Boldogh, I.; Alam, R.; Sur, S. Inhibiting pollen reduced nicotinamide adenine dinucleotide phosphate oxidase-induced signal by intrapulmonary administration of antioxidants blocks allergic airway inflammation. *J. Allergy Clin. Immunol.* **2007**, *119*, 646–653. [CrossRef]
8. Bacsi, A.; Choudhury, B.K.; Dharajiya, N.; Sur, S.; Boldogh, I. Subpollen particles-carriers of allergenic proteins and oxidases. *J. Allergy Clin. Immunol.* **2006**, *118*, 844–850. [CrossRef]
9. Chan, T.K.; Loh, X.Y.; Peh, H.Y.; Tan, W.N.F.; Tan, W.S.D.; Li, N.; Tay, I.J.J.; Wong, W.S.F.; Engelward, B.P. House dust mite-induced asthma causes oxidative damage and DNA double-strand breaks in the lungs. *J. Allergy Clin. Immunol.* **2016**, *138*, 84–96. [CrossRef]
10. Antus, B. Oxidative Stress Markers in Sputum. *Oxid. Med. Cell Longev.* **2016**. [CrossRef]
11. Sahiner, U.M.; Birben, E.; Erzurum, S.; Sackesen, C.; Kalayci, O. Oxidative stress in asthma. *World Allergy Organ. J.* **2011**, *4*, 151–158. [CrossRef]
12. Aldakheel, F.M.; Thomas, P.S.; Bourke, J.E.; Matheson, M.C.; Dharmage, S.C.; Lowe, A.J. Relationships between adult asthma and oxidative stress markers and pH in exhaled breath condensate: A systematic review. *Allergy* **2016**, *71*, 741–757. [CrossRef]
13. Louhelainen, N.; Myllärniemi, M.; Rahman, I.; Kinnula, V.L. Airway biomarkers of the oxidant burden in asthma and chronic obstructive pulmonary disease- current and future perspectives. *Int. J. Chron. Obstruct. Pulmon. Dis.* **2008**, *3*, 585–603.
14. Comhair, S.A.; Ricci, K.S.; Arroliga, M.; Lara, A.R.; Dweik, R.A.; Song, W.; Hazen, S.L.; Bleecker, E.R.; Busse, W.W.; Chung, K.F.; et al. Correlation of systemic superoxide dismutase deficiency to airflow obstruction in asthma. *Am. J. Respir. Crit. Care Med.* **2005**, *172*, 306–313. [CrossRef]
15. Comhair, S.A.; Erzurum, S.C. Antioxidant responses to oxidant mediated lung diseases. *Am. J. Physiol. Lung Cell Mol. Physiol.* **2002**, *283*, L246–L255. [CrossRef]
16. Iyer, D.; Mishra, N.; Agrawal, A. Mitochondrial Function in Allergic Disease. *Curr. Allergy Asthma Rep.* **2017**, *17*, 29. [CrossRef]
17. Ijsselmuiden, A.J.; Musters, R.J.; de Ruiter, G.; van Heerebeek, L.; Alderse-Baas, F.; van Schilfgaarde, M.; Leyte, A.; Tangelder, G.J.; Laarman, G.J.; Paulus, W.J. Circulating white blood cells and platelets amplify oxidative stress in heart failure. *Nat. Clin. Pract. Cardiovasc. Med.* **2008**, *5*, 811–820. [CrossRef]

18. Li, P.; Wang, B.; Sun, F.; Li, Y.; Li, Q.; Lang, H.; Zhao, Z.; Gao, P.; Zhao, Y.; Shang, Q.; et al. Mitochondrial respiratory dysfunctions of blood mononuclear cells link with cardiac disturbance in patients with early-stage heart failure. *Sci. Rep.* **2015**. [CrossRef]
19. Coluccia, R.; Raffa, S.; Ranieri, D.; Micaloni, A.; Valente, S.; Salerno, G.; Scrofani, C.; Testa, M.; Gallo, G.; Pagannone, E.; et al. Chronic heart failure is characterized by altered mitochondrial function and structure in circulating leucocytes. *Oncotarget* **2018**, *9*, 35028–35040. [CrossRef]
20. Clere-Jehl, R.; Helms, J.; Kassem, M.; Le Borgne, P.; Delabranche, X.; Charles, A.L.; Geny, B.; Meziani, F.; Bilbault, P. Septic Shock Alters Mitochondrial Respiration of Lymphoid Cell-Lines and Human Peripheral Blood Mononuclear Cells: The Role of Plasma. *Shock* **2019**, *51*, 97–104. [CrossRef]
21. Kaminski, M.M.; Sauer, S.W.; Klemke, C.D.; Suss, D.; Okun, J.G.; Krammer, P.H.; Gulow, K. Mitochondrial reactive oxygen species control T cell activation by regulating IL-2 and IL-4 expression: Mechanism of ciprofloxacin-mediated immunosuppression. *J. Immunol.* **2010**, *184*, 4827–4841. [CrossRef]
22. Pattnaik, B.; Bodas, M.; Bhatraju, N.K.; Ahmad, T.; Pant, R.; Guleria, R.; Ghosh, B.; Agrawal, A. IL-4 promotes asymmetric dimethylarginine accumulation, oxo-nitrative stress, and hypoxic response-induced mitochondrial loss in airway epithelial cells. *J. Allergy. Clin. Immunol.* **2016**, *138*, 130–141. [CrossRef] [PubMed]
23. Qi, S.; Barnig, C.; Charles, A.L.; Poirot, A.; Meyer, A.; Clere-Jehl, R.; de Blay, F.; Geny, B. Effect of nasal allergen challenge in allergic rhinitis on mitochondrial function of peripheral blood mononuclear cells. *Ann. Allergy Asthma. Immunol.* **2017**, *118*, 367–369. [CrossRef] [PubMed]
24. Marchandot, B.; Kibler, M.; Charles, A.L.; Trinh, A.; Petit Eisenmann, H.; Zeyons, F.; Von Hunolstein, J.J.; Reyde, A.; Matsushita, K.; Kindo, M.; et al. Does Transcatheter Aortic Valve Replacement Modulate the Kinetic of Superoxide Anion Generation? *Antioxid. Redox. Signal* **2019**, *31*, 420–426. [CrossRef] [PubMed]
25. Mukhopadhyay, P.; Rajesh, M.; Yoshihiro, K.; Haskó, G.; Pacher, P. Simple quantitative detection of mitochondrial superoxide production in live cells. *Biochem. Biophys. Res. Commun.* **2007**, *358*, 203–208. [CrossRef] [PubMed]
26. Anderson, E.J.; Neufer, P.D. Type II skeletal myofibers possess unique properties that potentiate mitochondrial H(2)O(2) generation. *Am. J. Physiol. Cell Physiol.* **2006**, *290*, C844–C851. [CrossRef] [PubMed]
27. Wolff, V.; Schlagowski, A.I.; Rouyer, O.; Charles, A.L.; Singh, F.; Auger, C.; Schini-Kerth, V.; Marescaux, C.; Raul, J.S.; Zoll, J.; et al. Tetrahydrocannabinol induces brain mitochondrial respiratory chain dysfunction and increases oxidative stress: A potential mechanism involved in cannabis-related stroke. *Biomed. Res. Int.* **2015**. [CrossRef]
28. Sumbalova, Z.; Droescher, S.; Hiller, E.; Chang, S.C.; Garcia-Souza, L.F.; Calabria, E.; Volani, C.; Krumschnabel, G.; Gnaiger, E. O2k-Protocols: Isolation of peripheral blood mononuclear cells and platelets from human blood for HRR. *Mitochondr. Physiol. Network.* **2018**, *21*, 1–16.
29. Bonato, M.; Tiné, M.; Bazzan, E.; Biondini, D.; Saetta, M.; Baraldo, S. Early Airway Pathological Changes in Children: New Insights into the Natural History of Wheezing. *J. Clin. Med.* **2019**, *8*, 1180. [CrossRef]
30. Maestraggi, Q.; Lebas, B.; Clere-Jehl, R.; Ludes, P.O.; Chamaraux-Tran, T.N.; Schneider, F.; Diemunsch, P.; Geny, B.; Pottecher, J. Skeletal Muscle and Lymphocyte Mitochondrial Dysfunctions in Septic Shock Trigger ICU-Acquired Weakness and Sepsis-Induced Immunoparalysis. *Biomed. Res. Int.* **2017**. [CrossRef]
31. Rahman, I.; MacNee, W. Oxidative stress and regulation of glutathione in lung inflammation. *Eur. Respir. J.* **2000**, *16*, 534–554. [CrossRef]
32. Dikalov, S. Cross talk between mitochondria and NAPH oxidases. *Free Radic. Biol. Med.* **2011**, *51*, 1289–1301. [CrossRef] [PubMed]
33. Bhatraju, N.K.; Agrawal, A. Mitochondrial Dysfunction Linking Obesity and Asthma. *Ann. Am. Thorac. Soc.* **2017**, *14*, S368–S373. [CrossRef] [PubMed]
34. Létuvé, S.; Druilhe, A.; Grandsaigne, M.; Aubier, M.; Pretolani, M. Critical role of mitochondria, but not caspases, during glucocorticosteroid-induced human eosinophil apoptosis. *Am. J. Respir. Cell Mol. Biol.* **2002**, *5*, 565–571. [CrossRef] [PubMed]
35. Agrawal, A.; Mabalirajan, U.; Ahmad, T.; Ghosh, B. Emerging interface between metabolic syndrome and asthma. *Am. J. Respir. Cell Mol. Biol.* **2011**, *44*, 270–275. [CrossRef] [PubMed]
36. Meyer, A.; Laverny, G.; Bernardi, L.; Charles, A.L.; Alsaleh, G.; Pottecher, J.; Sibilia, J.; Geny, B. Mitochondria: An Organelle of Bacterial Origin Controlling Inflammation. *Front. Immunol.* **2018**, *9*, 536. [CrossRef] [PubMed]

37. Mildner, A.; Jung, S. Development and function of dendritic cell subsets. *Immunity* **2014**, *40*, 642–656. [CrossRef]
38. Krawczyk, C.M.; Holowka, T.; Sun, J.; Blagih, J.; Amiel, E.; DeBerardinis, R.J.; Cross, J.R.; Jung, E.; Thompson, C.B.; Jones, R.G.; et al. Toll-like receptor-induced changes in glycolytic metabolism regulate dendritic cell activation. *Blood* **2010**, *115*, 4742–4749. [CrossRef]
39. Lejay, A.; Meyer, A.; Schlagowski, A.I.; Charles, A.L.; Singh, F.; Bouitbir, J.; Pottecher, J.; Chakfé, N.; Zoll, J.; Geny, B. Mitochondria: Mitochondrial participation in ischemia-reperfusion injury in skeletal muscle. *Int. J. Biochem. Cell Biol.* **2014**, *50*, 101–105. [CrossRef]
40. Leffler, J.; Read, J.F.; Jones, A.C.; Mok, D.; Hollams, E.M.; Laing, I.A.; Le Souef, P.N.; Sly, P.D.; Kusel, M.M.H.; de Klerk, N.H.; et al. Progressive increase of FcεRI expression across several PBMC subsets is associated with atopy and atopic asthma within school-aged children. *Pediatr. Allergy Immunol.* **2019**, *30*, 646–653. [CrossRef]
41. Leffler, J.; Jones, A.C.; Hollams, E.M.; Prastanti, F.; Le Souëf, P.N.; Holt, P.G.; Bosco, A.; Laing, I.A.; Strickland, D.H. Basophil counts in PBMC populations during childhood acute wheeze/asthma are associated with future exacerbations. *J. Allergy Clin. Immunol.* **2018**, *142*, 1639–1641. [CrossRef]
42. Price, D.B.; Rigazio, A.; Campbell, J.D.; Bleecker, E.R.; Corrigan, C.J.; Thomas, M.; Wenzel, S.E.; Wilson, A.M.; Small, M.B.; Gopalan, G.; et al. Blood eosinophil count and prospective annual asthma disease burden: A UK cohort study. *Lancet Respir. Med.* **2015**, *3*, 849–858. [CrossRef]
43. Sidhu, S.S.; Yuan, S.; Innes, A.L.; Kerr, S.; Woodruff, P.G.; Hou, L.; Muller, S.J.; Fahy, J.V. Roles of epithelial cell-derived periostin in TGF-beta activation, collagen production, and collagen gel elasticity in asthma. *Proc. Natl. Acad. Sci. USA* **2010**, *107*, 14170–14175. [CrossRef] [PubMed]
44. Takayama, G.; Arima, K.; Kanaji, T.; Toda, S.; Tanaka, H.; Shoji, S.; McKenzie, A.N.J.; Nagai, H.; Hotokebuchi, T.; Izuhara, K. Periostin: A novel component of subepithelial fibrosis of bronchial asthma downstream of IL-4 and IL-13 signals. *J. Allergy Clin. Immunol.* **2006**, *118*, 98–104. [CrossRef] [PubMed]
45. Islam, M.N.; Das, S.R.; Emin, M.T.; Wei, M.; Sun, L.; Westphalen, K.; Rowlands, D.J.; Quadri, S.K.; Bhattacharya, S.; Bhattacharya, J. Mitochondrial transfer from bone-marrow-derived stromal cells to pulmonary alveoli protects against acute lung injury. *Nat. Med.* **2012**, *18*, 759–765. [CrossRef] [PubMed]

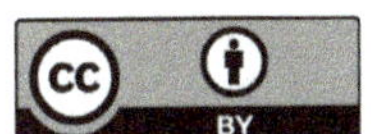

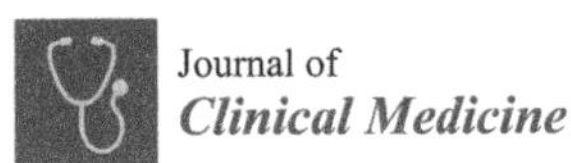
Journal of
Clinical Medicine

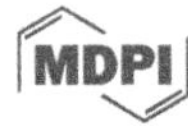

Review

Acid-Base Disturbances in Patients with Asthma: A Literature Review and Comments on Their Pathophysiology

Ioannis Vasileiadis [1,*], Emmanouil Alevrakis [2], Sevasti Ampelioti [3], Dimitrios Vagionas [1], Nikoletta Rovina [1] and Antonia Koutsoukou [1]

1 Intensive Care Unit, 1st Department of Respiratory Medicine, National and Kapodistrian University of Athens, Sotiria Hospital, 115 27 Athens, Greece; vagionasdimitrios@gmail.com (D.V.); nikrovina@med.uoa.gr (N.R.); koutsoukou@yahoo.gr (A.K.)
2 4th Department of Respiratory Medicine, Sotiria Hospital, 115 27 Athens, Greece; m.alevrakis@gmail.com
3 5th Department of Respiratory Medicine, Sotiria Hospital, 115 27 Athens, Greece; sevi.ampelioti@gmail.com
* Correspondence: ioannisvmed@yahoo.gr or ivasileiadis@med.uoa.gr; Tel: +30-697-764-4866 or +30-210-7763725 ; Fax: +30-210-778-1250

Received: 27 March 2019; Accepted: 23 April 2019; Published: 25 April 2019

Abstract: Asthma is a common illness throughout the world that affects the respiratory system function, i.e., a system whose operational adequacy determines the respiratory gases exchange. It is therefore expected that acute severe asthma will be associated with respiratory acid-base disorders. In addition, the resulting hypoxemia along with the circulatory compromise due to heart–lung interactions can reduce tissue oxygenation, with a particular impact on respiratory muscles that have increased energy needs due to the increased workload. Thus, anaerobic metabolism may ensue, leading to lactic acidosis. Additionally, chronic hypocapnia in asthma can cause a compensatory drop in plasma bicarbonate concentration, resulting in non-anion gap acidosis. Indeed, studies have shown that in acute severe asthma, metabolic acid-base disorders may occur, i.e., high anion gap or non-anion gap metabolic acidosis. This review briefly presents studies that have investigated acid-base disorders in asthma, with comments on their underlying pathophysiology.

Keywords: asthma; lactic acidosis; hyperchloremic acidosis; hypocapnia; hypercapnia

1. Introduction

Asthma is a common yet complex airway disease, characterized mainly by chronic airway inflammation and temporal variability in symptoms and expiratory airflow limitation. A complete analysis of the pathophysiology of the disease is beyond the scope of this paper, but a brief review of the main mechanisms involved in disease exacerbations is necessary to better grasp the acid-base derangements often encountered in these patients. Although asthma is increasingly being recognized as a heterogeneous disease with many different phenotypes, the mechanics of disease exacerbation seem to be common amongst patients. In acute asthma exacerbations, exposure to a precipitating factor leads to an exaggerated inflammatory response in the airways owing to an innate airway hyperresponsiveness in these patients. The immediate result of this inflammatory response is contraction of bronchial smooth muscles, bronchial edema, and mucus hypersecretion leading to mucus plugging. The consequent narrowing of airway diameter leads to increases in airway resistance and limitation of expiratory flow, and hence to air trapping and dynamic hyperinflation. As tidal breathing then starts taking place within the flat portion of the pressure-volume curve, the elastic work of breathing is dramatically increased. Hyperinflation essentially leads to the generation of an inspiratory threshold, which is reflected by the presence of positive end-expiratory pressure (auto-PEEP). This inspiratory threshold must be overcome by the inspiratory muscles during each breath in order for inspiratory flow to begin. Another deleterious factor is the disadvantageous positioning of respiratory muscle length-tension curves in these large lung volumes, necessitating the recruitment of accessory inspiratory and expiratory muscles, further contributing to respiratory muscle fatigue [1].

The aforementioned pathophysiological mechanisms eventually lead the deteriorating patient towards ventilatory failure. Nonetheless, acute respiratory failure is a far more common event in acute asthma. Indeed, hypoxemia is widely prevalent, with PaO_2 levels of less than 60 mmHg even in non-severe asthma [2] having being reported in several studies [3]. Even though this effect was attributed to ventilation/perfusion (V_A/Q) inequalities owing to regional differences in airflow, it was not until the advent of the multiple inert gas elimination technique that this phenomenon was adequately demonstrated [4].

The pathophysiological disorders in asthma result in various acid-base disturbances; these are summarized in Figure 1 and are briefly discussed below.

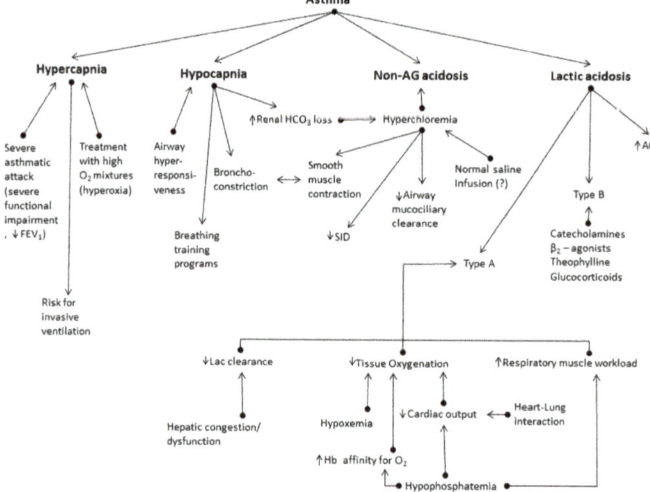

Figure 1. Acid-base disorders in asthma. FEV_1 = forced expiratory volume in 1 s. AG = anion-gap.

2. Respiratory Alkalosis

Acute asthmatic crisis is usually accompanied by hyperventilation and hypocapnia with respiratory alkalosis [3,5]. However, it seems that mild, asymptomatic asthma is also associated with hypocapnia. Studies that have demonstrated hypocapnia in asymptomatic asthmatics, as well as during asthmatic attacks, are presented in Table 1.

Table 1. Respiratory alkalosis.

Study	Study Design	Study Population	Methods	Significant Findings
Osborne C.A. et al., 2000 [6]	Case-Control Study	23 asymptomatic asthmatics, 17 healthy subjects	Measured various stable state parameters	$PaCO_2$ and $P_{ET}CO_2$ lower in asymptomatic asthmatics
Van den Elshout et al., 1991 [7]	Case- Control Study	30 asthmatics, 17 healthy subjects	Induction of hypercapnia and hypocapnia	Hypocapnia induced increases in airway resistance in asthmatic patients
Raimondi et al., 2013 [8]	Case series	314 patients admitted for ASA	ABGs, electrolytes and spirometry results documented	Hypocapnia was prominent in less severe asthma exacerbations

Abbreviations used: ASA = acute severe asthma, ABGs = arterial blood gases, $PETCO_2$ = end-tidal carbon dioxide.

In a study, asymptomatic patients with asthma had significantly lower partial pressure of carbon dioxide (PCO_2) in arterial blood and end-tidal PCO_2 ($P_{ET}CO_2$) values compared to normal subjects, with no difference in the ventilatory pattern [6]. To note, there was no statistically significant difference in the other acid-base variables between asthma patients and healthy controls, i.e., the pH values were similar in both groups. Hypocapnia was attributed to airway hyperresponsiveness. In another study, similar results were found; normal subjects had higher $P_{ET}CO_2$ at rest compared to asthmatic patients. This study evaluated the effect of hypocapnia and hypercapnia in patients with asthma and in healthy subjects. It was found that while the fall of PCO_2 increased airway resistance in asthmatic patients, it did not significantly change the respiratory resistance in normal individuals [7]. It was suggested that hypocapnia is probably associated with the airway obstruction observed in asthmatics, thus having an important role in the pathophysiology of asthma. Low PCO_2 has been demonstrated to increase airway smooth muscle tension in animal models, as well; the proposed mechanism by which hypocapnia affects smooth muscle contraction is the alteration of calcium uptake due to an increase in intracellular pH [9,10]. Corroborating the above findings, it has further been shown that high PCO_2 values cause bronchodilation and reduce airway resistance in both asthma patients and normal subjects [7,11]. As hypocapnia has been implicated in the pathophysiology of asthma, training techniques have been proposed to improve patients' respiratory pattern, reduce hyperventilation, and increase PCO_2, in an attempt to reverse the bronchoconstrictive effect of hypocapnia. Breathing retraining has been used in the management of asthma. The Buteyko breathing technique, an innovative treatment approach for asthma, named after Professor Konstantin Buteyko, has been widely applied [12]. In a recent trial, breathing training programs improved disease-related quality of life in adult asthmatic patients [13].

3. Respiratory Acidosis

Respiratory acidosis is a very common acid base disturbance in acute severe asthma and is widely considered to be an ominous finding. Its early recognition and treatment is important and decisive for the final outcome, as it can lead to respiratory failure and arrest if prolonged. Studies relating hypercapnia during asthmatic attacks are presented in Table 2.

Table 2. Respiratory acidosis.

Study	Study Design	Study Population	Methods	Significant Findings
Mountain et al., 1988 [14]	Retrospective	61 patients with hypercapnic ASA, 168 with nonhypercapnic ASA	Various outcomes documented	Hypercapnic patients had more severe airway obstruction, symptoms
Lee K.H. et al., 1997 [15]	Retrospective	48 patients with 49 admissions to the ICU due to ASA	Various outcomes documented	Respiratory acidosis linked to higher mortality
Raimondi et al., 2013 [8]	Case series	314 patients admitted for ASA	ABGs, electrolytes and spirometry results documented	Inverse correlation between FEV_1 and respiratory acidosis. Inability to perform spirometry linked to high pCO_2
Cham et al., 2002 [16]	Prospective observational	127 patients with severe exacerbation of asthma and COPD in the ED	Acute respiratory acidosis documented and linked to clinical presentation	Drowsiness linked to sevenfold likelihood of respiratory acidosis. Flushing and intercostal retractions good predictors of respiratory acidosis

Abbreviations used: ICU = intensive care unit, COPD = chronic obstructive pulmonary disease, pCO_2 = partial carbon dioxide pressure, ED = emergency department.

In asthmatic patients, hypercapnia and respiratory acidosis occur in clinical exacerbations characterized by severe airway obstruction [14]. Simpson et al., in one of the earliest published studies, noted that hypoxemia and respiratory acidosis are common in children with acute severe asthma, as in 10 out of the 24 acute attacks that were studied CO_2 retention was observed, while three patients developed carbon dioxide narcosis [17]. On the other hand, Weng et al. found that the degree of hypoxemia correlated with the degree of airway obstruction, but neither $PaCO_2$ nor pH did. This study reported 177 events in 139 asthmatic children, both symptomatic and asymptomatic. Respiratory acidosis or mixed acidosis was present in severely dyspneic patients [18]. Lee et al. noted that $PaCO_2$ was significantly higher and the arterial blood pH lower in asthmatics who died, and delays in providing mechanical ventilation led to worse outcomes [15]. Several studies have attempted to find clinical signs that could be correlated to the presence of respiratory acidosis. Cham et al. tried to find clinical predictors for acute respiratory acidosis in 141 episodes in patients with either asthma or chronic obstructive pulmonary disease (COPD). A total of 41 patients had hypercapnia (32.3%), and acidosis was present in 27 (65.9%). The frequency of acute respiratory acidosis was 0.39 in COPD and 0.10 in asthma. Drowsiness, flushing, and intercostal retractions were strong predictors for acute respiratory acidosis [16]. It has also been reported that the absence of pulsus paradoxus makes the presence of hypercapnia unlikely, although it is noted that clinical signs and symptoms during acute severe asthma often are not correlated with the severity of the functional impairment [19]. Raimondi et al. performed a case series study exploring acid-base patterns in patients admitted for acute severe asthma, in correlation with forced expiratory volume in 1 s (FEV_1) values [8]. Airway obstruction severity did not seem to correlate significantly with PaO_2 values, a finding also reported in several other studies in the past [18,20,21] and thought to be due to V_A/Q mismatch not being connected to air flow rates; moreover, treatment with β-agonists may lead to further widening of V_A/Q mismatch. A statistically significant reverse correlation was demonstrated between FEV_1 and $PaCO_2$ levels. Inability to complete spirometry was shown to be accompanied with a significantly higher frequency of respiratory acidosis, with some patients being deemed unable to undergo a spirometry maneuver by the attending physician. Less severe cases of acute asthma presented mostly with respiratory alkalosis.

Hypercapnia in asthma, in addition to the severity of the disease, is also associated with the therapeutic administration of oxygen. Thus, in patients with severe asthma exacerbation, significant increase (≥4 mmHg) in transcutaneous PCO_2 ($PtCO_2$) was observed in a higher proportion in those receiving high oxygen mixtures (>8 L/min), compared to those who received titrated oxygen (to achieve oxygen saturation of 93–95%) [22]. Hypercapnia induced by hyperoxia has been known for quite some time, and has been mainly studied in patients with COPD. For the pathophysiological interpretation of the mechanism involved, the simplistic view of Campbell (1960) had prevailed, who assumed that in chronic COPD patients with hypercapnia, respiratory control is based only on hypoxic drive as their hypercapnic respiratory drive is blunted [23]. Subsequent studies, mainly in patients with COPD, did not confirm this hypothesis. It was found that oxygen-induced hypercapnia does not indicate a deficiency/impairment of the respiratory control system for CO_2 homeostasis and is not correlated with changes in ventilation. Instead, the reduction of V_A/Q matching was proposed as the cause, due to the release of hypoxic pulmonary arterial vasoconstriction, with a consequent increase in functional dead space ventilation [24–28]. However, in another study in COPD patients, oxygen-induced hypercapnia was characterized by reduction in ventilation; the increased dead-space ventilation in the group of patients where PCO_2 increased more than 3 mmHg (retainers) was attributed to bronchodilation due to the higher CO_2 tension [29]. Another mechanism implicates the Haldane effect, in which oxygen displaces the CO_2 dissociation curve to the right, increasing $PaCO_2$, which cannot be normalized as patients with severe COPD are unable to increase ventilation [25,30].

4. Metabolic acidosis

Non-anion gap (non-AG) metabolic acidosis as well as increased AG acidosis may occur in asthma (Table 3).

Table 3. Metabolic acidosis.

Study	Study Design	Study Population	Methods	Significant Findings
Mountain, R.D. et al., 1990 [31]	Retrospective	229 acute asthma episodes in 170 patients (Hospital Admissions)	Clinical features and arterial blood gases examined	Simple or mixed metabolic acidosis in 28% of the episodes.
Rashid, A.O. et al., 2008 [32]	Retrospective	109 patients hospitalized for asthma exacerbations	Acid-base, electrolyte status and outcomes	10.1% AG acidosis, 29.4% NAG acidosis. NAG acidosis patients had significantly higher intubation rates

Table 3. *Cont.*

Study	Study Design	Study Population	Methods	Significant Findings
Rabbat, A. et al., 1998 [33]	Prospective	29 non-intubated patients admitted to the ICU for ASA	Serial lactate measurements during treatment, correlation with outcomes	Hyperlactatemia a common finding on admission (59%) or during treatment (100%). No prognostic value, no correlation with $PaCO_2$ or PEF
Meert, K.L. et al., 2012 [34]	Prospective observational	105 children with ASA admitted to a PICU	Blood lactate measurements followed by lactate/pyruvate ration measurements	Primarily type B lactic acidosis (associated with normal oxygen delivery). Presumed to be due to β-adrenergic stimulation
Raimondi et al., 2013 [8]	Case Series	314 patients admitted for ASA	ABGs, electrolytes and spirometry results documented	Most cases of metabolic acidosis attributed to chronic hypocapnia. Hyperlactatemia attributed mostly to adrenergic stimulation

Abbreviations used: AG = anion-gap, NAG = non-anion gap, PEF = peak expiratory flow, PICU: pediatric intensive care unit, $PaCO_2$ = partial carbon dioxide tension.

4.1. Non-Anion Gap Metabolic Acidosis

Although metabolic acidosis in asthma is often considered to be secondary to hyperlactatemia, non-anion gap (non-AG) metabolic acidosis has also been reported. The presence (and absence thereof) of non-AG in patients with acute asthma has been a subject of debate in medical literature, with many studies [3,4] reporting no such findings, and others [35,36] documenting simple or mixed metabolic acidosis in as many as 38% of the study population. Mountain et al. noted that metabolic acidosis in acute asthma was more likely to occur in male patients and in patients with greater airflow obstruction and lower FEV_1 [31]. Rashid et al. studied the clinical outcome in 109 adult patients hospitalized for asthma exacerbations. These patients were divided in three groups: group I included those patients who did not present with metabolic acidosis, group II those with AG metabolic acidosis, and group III those with non-AG metabolic acidosis. Out of these, 32 (29.4%) developed non-AG metabolic acidosis, while metabolic acidosis with elevated anion gap occurred in 11 patients (10.1%) [32]. The group of patients with non-AG metabolic acidosis had significantly higher chloride anion (Cl^-) concentrations, with a tendency to hyperchloremia, while sodium (Na^+) and potassium (K^+) concentrations were not different compared to patients without acidosis or with elevated AG acidosis. The patients with non-AG acidosis were also at increased risk of respiratory failure and need for invasive, mechanical ventilation. Another study evaluated the acid-base status in 22 patients with acute severe asthma [36]. Ten patients had metabolic acidosis, defined by a base deficit > 2 mEq/L. None of these patients had an elevated AG. The most likely explanation for the observed metabolic acidosis in these patients, as in the previous study, was the renal loss of bicarbonates (HCO_3^-) due to renal compensation for preexistent, sustained hypocapnia. The HCO_3^- levels were low-normal or decreased in these patients, while the pH values ranged from alkaline to moderately acidotic. It appears that non-AG acidosis is a frequent acid-base disorder in asthmatic exacerbations, due to the excretion of HCO_3^-, in response to chronic, sustained hypocapnia. Hypocapnia immediately shifts the dissociation reaction of H_2CO_3 to the left

$$CO_2 + H_2O \leftrightarrow H_2CO_3 \leftrightarrow H^+ + HCO_3^- \tag{1}$$

reducing H^+ and HCO_3^- concentrations and increasing pH. In the short term, the decrease in $PaCO_2$ alkalinizes the extracellular fluid, to the extent predicted by the Henderson–Hasselbalch equation. Persistent hypocapnia causes a further decrease in HCO_3^- concentration, due to suppression of renal acid secretion/increase of HCO_3^- excretion [37,38]. By definition, the primary metabolic acidosis of this type, i.e., with non-elevated AG, is accompanied by an increase in the concentration of Cl^-, i.e., hyperchloremic acidosis [39]. Hyperchloremic, non-AG acidosis, secondary to chronic hypocapnia, was also noted in the study of Rashid et al. [32], in asthmatic patients. However, in an earlier animal study it was found that, during compensation for hypocapnia, the reduction in renal proton excretion was associated with increased Na^+ excretion and not with Cl^- retention and hyperchloremia [40]. Furthermore, in another study, chronic hypocapnia was found to suppress renal acid secretion while inducing renal K^+ wasting [41]. Interestingly, in a recent study [42], ascent to high altitude elicited a hypoxic ventilatory response in normal adults, resulting in increased ventilation and decreased $PaCO_2$; hypocapnia was accompanied by strong ion difference (SID) reduction, signaling metabolic acidosis according to Stewart's view [43]. Concerning the non-AG metabolic acidosis in patients with asthma, as a compensatory response to chronic hypocapnia, we should comment on the following issues:

1. Insofar as chronic hypocapnia in these patients is accompanied by hyperchloremia, the role of Cl^- channels in vascular and non-vascular smooth muscle contraction, as in the human airways, must be stressed, e.g., an alteration of Cl^- concentration changes the myogenic tone in the blood vessels [44,45]. Additionally, Cl^- channels in epithelial cells may affect mucus hydration on the airway surfaces [46]. Overall, Cl^- may have a critical role in asthma pathophysiology.
2. In conditions like asthma exacerbations, where an acute acid-base disorder complicates a chronic respiratory disorder, such as chronic hypocapnia in asthmatics, the use of base excess (or base deficit) method [47] to assess the severity of metabolic acidosis can lead to 'erroneous assessment' of the patient's acid-base status, lacking any clinical relevance. Thus, in the study of Okrent et al. [36], in patients with acute severe asthma, metabolic acidosis was diagnosed by the increase of base deficit > 2 mEq/L. In this study, authors supported that this indicated a true loss of the body's alkaline reserve. Nevertheless, one of the patients with the more severe metabolic acidosis, diagnosed with the base excess criterion (−4.9 mEq/L), had hypocapnia (PCO_2 = 27 mmHg), pH higher than the mean physiological value (7.43), and HCO_3^- concentration lower than the normal value (19 mEq/L), for which, however, no treatment is indicated, and which actually corresponds to the expected metabolic compensation for a chronic respiratory alkalosis (the expected HCO_3^- concentration reduction ($\Delta(HCO_3^-)$) equals $0.4 \times \Delta PCO_2$, i.e., $(HCO_3^-) = 18.8$ mEq/L) [37]. Thus, the physiologic compensation for an uncomplicated acid-base disturbance has been viewed as a serious metabolic acidosis superimposed on the chronic respiratory disorder. Overall, caution is needed in assessing the metabolic component of these acid-base disorders by utilizing the base excess values; diagnostic errors and therapeutic ill-practices may occur when they are not considered alongside the required clinical information. Criticism on the subject has long been made by Schwartz and Relman [48], which even took the form of a 'transatlantic debate' with arguments from both sides [49].
3. Finally, regarding the increased clinical risk demonstrated in asthmatics with non-AG acidosis (accompanied by hyperchloremia) [32], it should be noted that there are several studies suggesting that hyperchloremia per se is associated with poor outcome in hospitalized and critically ill patients [50–52]. Hyperchloremia induced by intravenous administration of crystalloid solutions with high Cl^- concentration is not to be overlooked [53,54], although there is no study investigating this issue exclusively in patients with acute severe asthma. In addition, hypocapnia, besides the acid-base balance, can have serious effects on the organs and systems in the body, and can adversely affect outcome in the critically ill [55].

4.2. Lactic Acidosis

Hyperlactatemia is a very common finding in patients with acute severe asthma. Lactic acidosis has two types: type A, which is associated with impaired oxygen delivery; and type B, where the oxygen delivery is normal but cellular function is impaired. The exact cause of lactic acidosis in these patients remains elusive, and several possible mechanisms have been proposed over the years. Acute severe asthma is characterized by hypoxemia [3,56] and may be accompanied by functional cardiac disorders (heart-lung interaction); increased right ventricular (RV) afterload during acute severe asthma, with increased impedance to RV ejection, and reduction of left ventricular (LV) preload and LV compliance due to leftward septal shift may reduce cardiac output [57,58]. Thus, lactate increase may result from severe hypoperfusion and decrease in oxygen supply to the tissues. In addition, respiratory muscle fatigue, due to increased respiratory muscle work load, can also increase lactate levels [59,60], especially under hypoxic conditions along with compromised tissue perfusion. In patients with acute severe asthma, a negative correlation between the peak lactate levels and the phosphate levels on admission was found [33]. In this study, hypophosphatemia preceded the increase in lactate levels in most patients. Hypophosphatemia may complicate treatment with bronchodilators in acute severe asthma patients [61]. Low phosphate levels in the blood may lead to reduced ATP synthesis in the muscles, accounting for muscle weakness and respiratory and heart failure [62]. Additionally, hypophosphatemia is known to impair the contractile properties of the diaphragm [63] and increase the hemoglobin affinity for oxygen due to a decrease in 2,3-diphosphoglycerate (2,3-DPG) [64], compromising tissue oxygenation. In a state of low cardiac output, hepatic perfusion decreases; also, the RV function disorder can increase the right heart filling pressures and lead to hepatic congestion [65–67]. Thus, hepatic dysfunction during acute severe asthma may result in impaired lactate clearance and hyperlactatemia [68,69]. An increase in lactate levels can also be observed during clinical improvement after bronchodilator treatment. It has been suggested that reperfusion of the previously ischemic organs, e.g., respiratory muscles, can lead to lactate release [70,71]. That is, the increase in lactate intracellular levels during the period of ischemia and anaerobic respiration may not be reflected in the lactate circulating levels in the serum. Serum lactate concentration can be increased after restoring tissue perfusion. Increased catecholamines in plasma may increase metabolic rate and lactate production without coexisting cell hypoxia. Increased levels of catecholamines in the blood have been found in patients with asthma, especially norepinephrine [72]. Additionally, catecholamines are used therapeutically during acute severe asthma, to promote bronchodilatation [73] and/or hemodynamic support. However, catecholamines have marked metabolic effects and may cause hyperlactatemia [74]. Treatment with bronchodilators has also been implicated in the lactate increase, i.e., the use of β_2-adrenergic agonists, such as salbutamol [75]. In animals, β_2-adrenoreceptor stimulation after salbutamol administration induced a significant increase in plasma lactate concentration; lactate increase was inhibited by clonidine (α_2-adrenoreceptor agonist), a drug with opposite effects on the system of adenylate cyclase [76]. Stimulation of β_2-adrenergic receptors increases glycogenolysis in the liver and muscle as well as lipolysis, through the increase of intracellular cAMP [77]. Free fatty acids liberated during lipolysis inhibit the oxidation of pyruvate by pyruvate dehydrogenase and may further increase lactate production [78]. Finally, theophylline and glucocorticoids may have a role in the increased lactate production during acute severe asthma. Theophylline is a non-selective 5′-phosphodiesterase inhibitor and potentiates the activity of β-adrenergic agents by increasing the intracellular concentration of cAMP [79–81]. Glucocorticoids are also known to increase the β-receptor's sensitivity to β-adrenergic agonists [82]. Thus, when treating severe asthma attack, despite improvement in bronchospasm, a patient may hyperventilate and look more dyspneic; this may be a compensatory mechanism for lactic acidosis induced by therapy, to maintain pH within normal limits, and should not be seen as a worsening of airway obstruction [83]. In order to distinguish the type of lactic acidosis (A and B), the ratio of the concentration of lactate to the concentration of pyruvate in the blood can be used. Under aerobic conditions, this ratio is normally low, whereas under anaerobic conditions, due to the inability of cells to further metabolize pyruvate in mitochondria, this ratio increases to levels > 25:1 [84,85]. Thus, in a study concerning children with asthma, lactic acidosis was found to be predominantly of type B, with normal oxygen supply to the tissues, and was attributed to β-adrenergic stimulation [34].

5. Conclusions

Various acid-base disorders, of complex etiology, have been observed in asthma. Airway hyperresponsiveness leads to hyperventilation and chronic hypocapnia with a consequent increase in renal bicarbonate loss. This results in hyperchloremic acidosis, which becomes more clinically evident-with a clear effect on blood acidity-during severe asthma attacks, in case PCO_2 normalizes or increases. Hypocapnia, and possibly hyperchloremia, may be related to the pathogenicity of the disease. Hypercapnia characterizes severe asthma attacks, with imminent risk for intubation and mechanical ventilation. Hypercapnia has been attributed to both the severity of the functional respiratory disorder and treatment with high oxygen mixtures (hyperoxia induced). Finally, increased AG metabolic acidosis has also been observed in asthma, i.e., lactic acidosis. Its etiology includes: **a.** disturbance of tissue oxygenation, e.g., by cardiac output reduction and hypoxemia or increased oxygen demands of respiratory muscles due to increased workload, **b.** reduced lactate clearance due to liver congestion and dysfunction, and **c.** treatment effect, e.g., β-agonists, on cellular metabolism, resulting in increased lactate production. The thorough and careful evaluation of acid-base disorders in asthma will serve the differential diagnostic approach concerning the underlying pathogenetic disorder and its treatment.

Author Contributions: Conceptualization, I.V.; Investigation, I.V., E.A., and S.A.; Writing-Original Draft Preparation, I.V., E.A., S.A., and N.R.; Review and Editing, D.V., I.V., and A.K.; Supervision, I.V., N.R., and A.K.; Funding Acquisition, N.R.

Acknowledgments: In this section you can acknowledge any support given which is not covered by the author contribution or funding sections. This may include administrative and technical support, or donations in kind (e.g., materials used for experiments).

Conflicts of Interest: The authors declare no conflict of interest.

References

1. McFadden, E. Acute Severe Asthma. *Am. J. Respir. Crit. Care Med.* **2003**, *168*, 740–759. [CrossRef]
2. Tai, E.; Read, J. Blood-gas tensions in bronchial asthma. *Lancet* **1967**, *1*, 644–646. [CrossRef]
3. McFadden, E.R., Jr.; Lyons, H.A. Arterial blood gas tensions in asthma. *N. Eng. J. Med.* **1968**, *278*, 1027–1032. [CrossRef] [PubMed]
4. Rodriguez-Roisin, R.; Roca, J. Contributions of multiple inert gas elimination technique to pulmonary medicine. 3. Bronchial asthma. *Thorax* **1994**, *49*, 1027–1033. [CrossRef]
5. Rodriguez-Roisin, R. Gas exchange abnormalities in asthma. *Lung* **1990**, *168*, 599–605. [CrossRef]
6. Osborne, C.A.; O'Connor, B.J.; Lewis, A.; Kanabar, V.; Gardner, W.N. Hyperventilation and asymptomatic chronic asthma. *Thorax* **2000**, *55*, 1016–1022. [CrossRef]
7. Van den Elshout, F.J.; van Herwaarden, C.L.; Folgering, H.T. Effects of hypercapnia and hypocapnia on respiratory resistance in normal and asthmatic subjects. *Thorax* **1991**, *46*, 28–32. [CrossRef] [PubMed]
8. Raimondi, G.A.; Gonzalez, S.; Zaltsman, J.; Menga, G.; Adrogué, H.J. Acid–base patterns in acute severe asthma. *J. Asthma* **2013**, *50*, 1062–1068. [CrossRef] [PubMed]
9. Twort, C.H.; Cameron, I.R. Effects of PCO_2, pH and extracellular calcium on contraction of airway smooth muscle from rats. *Respir. Physiol.* **1986**, *66*, 259–267. [CrossRef]
10. Lindeman, K.S.; Croxton, T.L.; Lande, B.; Hirshman, C.A. Hypocapnia-induced contraction of porcine airway smooth muscle. *Eur. Respir. J.* **1998**, *12*, 1046–1052. [CrossRef] [PubMed]
11. D'Angelo, E.; Calderini, I.S.; Tavola, M. The effects of CO_2 on respiratory mechanics in anesthetized paralyzed humans. *Anesthesiology* **2001**, *94*, 604–610. [CrossRef] [PubMed]
12. Bruton, A.; Lewith, G.T. The Buteyko breathing technique for asthma: A review. *Complement. Ther. Med.* **2005**, *13*, 41–46. [CrossRef]
13. Bruton, A.; Lee, A.; Yardley, L.; Raftery, J.; Arden-Close, E.; Kirby, S.; Zhu, S.; Thiruvothiyur, M.; Webley, F.; Taylor, L.; et al. Physiotherapy breathing retraining for asthma: A randomised controlled trial. *Lancet Respir. Med.* **2018**, *6*, 19–28. [CrossRef]
14. Mountain, R.D.; Sahn, S.A. Clinical features and outcome in patients with acute asthma presenting with hypercapnia. *Am. Rev. Respir. Dis.* **1988**, *138*, 535–539. [CrossRef] [PubMed]
15. Lee, K.H.; Tan, W.C.; Lim, T.K. Severe asthma. *Singap. Med. J.* **1997**, *38*, 238–240, 243.
16. Cham, G.W.; Tan, W.P.; Earnest, A.; Soh, C.H. Clinical predictors of acute respiratory acidosis during exacerbation of asthma and chronic obstructive pulmonary disease. *Eur. J. Emerg. Med.* **2002**, *9*, 225–232. [CrossRef] [PubMed]
17. Simpson, H.; Forfar, J.O.; Grubb, D.J. Arterial blood gas tensions and ph in acute asthma in childhood. *Br. Med. J.* **1968**, *3*, 460–464. [CrossRef] [PubMed]
18. Weng, T.R.; Langer, H.M.; Featherby, E.A.; Levison, H. Arterial blood gas tensions and acid-base balance in symptomatic and asymptomatic asthma in childhood. *Am. Rev. Respir. Dis.* **1970**, *101*, 274–282.

19. Rosenzweig, J.R.C.; Edwards, L.; Lincourt, W.; Dorinsky, P.; ZuWallack, R.L. The relationship between health-related quality of life, lung function and daily symptoms in patients with persistent asthma. *Respir. Med.* **2004**, *98*, 1157–1165. [CrossRef]
20. Waddell, J.A.; Emerson, P.A.; Gunstone, R.F. Hypoxia in bronchial asthma. *Br. Med. J.* **1967**, *2*, 402–404. [CrossRef]
21. Miyamoto, T.; Mizuno, K.; Furuya, K. Arterial blood gases in bronchial asthma. *J. Allergy* **1970**, *45*, 248–254. [CrossRef]
22. Perrin, K.; Wijesinghe, M.; Healy, B.; Wadsworth, K.; Bowditch, R.; Bibby, S.; Baker, T.; Weatherall, M.; Beasley, R. Randomised controlled trial of high concentration versus titrated oxygen therapy in severe exacerbations of asthma. *Thorax* **2011**, *66*, 937–941. [CrossRef]
23. Tobin, M.J. *Principles and Practice of Mechanical Ventilation*, 3rd ed.; McGraw Hill Professional: New York, NY, USA, 2012; p. 87.
24. Aubier, M.; Murciano, D.; Fournier, M.; Milic-Emili, J.; Pariente, R.; Derenne, J.P. Central respiratory drive in acute respiratory failure of patients with chronic obstructive pulmonary disease. *Am. Rev. Respir. Dis.* **1980**, *122*, 191–199. [CrossRef]
25. Aubier, M.; Murciano, D.; Milic-Emili, J.; Touaty, E.; Daghfous, J.; Pariente, R.; Derenne, J.P. Effects of the administration of O_2 on ventilation and blood gases in patients with chronic obstructive pulmonary disease during acute respiratory failure. *Am. Rev. Respir. Dis.* **1980**, *122*, 747–754. [CrossRef]
26. Sassoon, C.S.; Hassell, K.T.; Mahutte, C.K. Hyperoxic-induced hypercapnia in stable chronic obstructive pulmonary disease. *Am. Rev. Respir. Dis.* **1987**, *135*, 907–911. [CrossRef]
27. Dick, C.R.; Liu, Z.; Sassoon, C.S.; Berry, R.B.; Mahutte, C.K. O_2-induced change in ventilation and ventilatory drive in COPD. *Am. J. Respir. Crit. Care Med.* **1997**, *155*, 609–614. [CrossRef] [PubMed]
28. Abdo, W.F.; Heunks, L.M. Oxygen-induced hypercapnia in COPD: Myths and facts. *Crit. Care* **2012**, *16*, 323. [CrossRef] [PubMed]
29. Robinson, T.D.; Freiberg, D.B.; Regnis, J.A.; Young, I.H. The role of hypoventilation and ventilation-perfusion redistribution in oxygen-induced hypercapnia during acute exacerbations of chronic obstructive pulmonary disease. *Am. J. Respir. Crit. Care Med.* **2000**, *161*, 1524–1529. [CrossRef]
30. Luft, U.C.; Mostyn, E.M.; Loeppky, J.A.; Venters, M.D. Contribution of the Haldane effect to the rise of arterial Pco2 in hypoxic patients breathing oxygen. *Crit. Care Med.* **1981**, *9*, 32–37. [CrossRef]
31. Mountain, R.D.; Heffner, J.E.; Brackett, N.C.; Sahn, S.A. Acid-base disturbances in acute asthma. *Chest* **1990**, *98*, 651–655. [CrossRef] [PubMed]
32. Rashid, A.O.; Azam, H.M.; DeBari, V.A.; Blamoun, A.I.; Moammar, M.Q.; Khan, M.A. Non-anion gap acidosis in asthma: Clinical and laboratory features and outcomes for hospitalized patients. *Ann. Clin. Lab. Sci.* **2008**, *38*, 228–234.
33. Rabbat, A.; Laaban, J.P.; Boussairi, A.; Rochemaure, J. Hyperlactatemia during acute severe asthma. *Intensive Care Med.* **1998**, *24*, 304–312. [CrossRef] [PubMed]
34. Meert, K.L.; McCaulley, L.; Sarnaik, A.P. Mechanism of lactic acidosis in children with acute severe asthma. *Pediatr. Crit. Care Med.* **2012**, *13*, 28–31. [CrossRef] [PubMed]
35. Roncoroni, A.; Adrogué, H.; De Obrutsky, C.W.; Marchisio, M.L.; Herrera, M. Metabolic acidosis in status asthmaticus. *Respiration* **1976**, *33*, 85–94. [CrossRef]
36. Okrent, D.G.; Tessler, S.; Twersky, R.A.; Tashkin, D.P. Metabolic acidosis not due to lactic acidosis in patients with severe acute asthma. *Crit. Care Med.* **1987**, *15*, 1098–1101. [CrossRef]
37. Adrogué, H.J.; Madias, N.E. Secondary responses to altered acid-base status: The rules of engagement. *J. Am. Soc. Nephrol.* **2010**, *21*, 920–923. [CrossRef]
38. Madias, N.E.; Adrogué, H.J. Cross-talk between two organs: How the kidney responds to disruption of acid-base balance by the lung. *Nephron Physiol.* **2003**, *93*, 61–66. [CrossRef]
39. Kraut, J.A.; Madias, N.E. Differential diagnosis of non-gap metabolic acidosis: Value of a systematic approach. *Clin. J. Am. Soc. Nephrol.* **2012**, *7*, 671–679. [CrossRef]
40. Gennari, F.J.; Goldstein, M.B.; Schwartz, W.B. The nature of the renal adaptation to chronic hypocapnia. *J. Clin. Investig.* **1972**, *51*, 1722–1730. [CrossRef]
41. Krapf, R.; Beeler, I.; Hertner, D.; Hulter, H.N. Chronic respiratory alkalosis. The effect of sustained hyperventilation on renal regulation of acid-base equilibrium. *N. Engl. J. Med.* **1991**, *324*, 1394–1401. [CrossRef]

42. Zouboules, S.M.; Lafave, H.C.; O'Halloran, K.D.; Brutsaert, T.D.; Nysten, H.E.; Nysten, C.E.; Steinback, C.D.; Sherpa, M.T.; Day, T.A. Renal reactivity: Acid-base compensation during incremental ascent to high altitude. *J. Physiol.* **2018**, *596*, 6191–6203. [CrossRef] [PubMed]
43. Stewart, P.A. Independent and dependent variables of acid-base control. *Respir. Physiol.* **1978**, *33*, 9–26. [CrossRef]
44. Kitamura, K.; Yamazaki, J. Chloride channels and their functional roles in smooth muscle tone in the vasculature. *Jpn. J. Pharmacol.* **2001**, *85*, 351–357. [CrossRef] [PubMed]
45. Bulley, S.; Jaggar, J.H. Cl^- channels in smooth muscle cells. *Pflugers Arch.* **2014**, *466*, 861–872. [CrossRef] [PubMed]
46. Wang, W.; Ji, H.L. Epithelial sodium and chloride channels and asthma. *Chin. Med. J. (Engl.)* **2015**, *128*, 2242–2249. [CrossRef] [PubMed]
47. Berend, K. Diagnostic use of base excess in acid-base disorders. *N. Engl. J. Med.* **2018**, *378*, 1419–1428. [CrossRef] [PubMed]
48. Schwartz, W.B.; Relman, A.S. A critique of the parameters used in the evaluation of acid-base disorders. "Whole-blood buffer base" and "standard bicarbonate" compared with blood pH and plasma bicarbonate concentration. *N. Engl. J. Med.* **1963**, *268*, 1382–1388. [CrossRef]
49. Severinghaus, J.W. Siggaard-andersen and the "great trans-atlantic acid-base debate". *Scand. J. Clin. Lab. Investig. Suppl.* **1993**, *214*, 99–104.
50. Neyra, J.A.; Canepa-Escaro, F.; Li, X.; Manllo, J.; Adams-Huet, B.; Yee, J.; Yessayan, L.; Acute Kidney Injury in Critical Illness Study Group. Association of hyperchloremia with hospital mortality in critically Ill septic patients. *Crit. Care Med.* **2015**, *43*, 1938–1944. [CrossRef]
51. Thongprayoon, C.; Cheungpasitporn, W.; Cheng, Z.; Qian, Q. Chloride alterations in hospitalized patients: Prevalence and outcome significance. *PLoS ONE* **2017**, *12*, e0174430. [CrossRef]
52. Huang, K.; Hu, Y.; Wu, Y.; Ji, Z.; Wang, S.; Lin, Z.; Pan, S. Hyperchloremia is associated with poorer outcome in critically Ill stroke patients. *Front. Neurol.* **2018**, *9*, 485. [CrossRef]
53. Semler, M.W.; Self, W.H.; Wanderer, J.P.; Ehrenfeld, J.M.; Wang, L.; Byrne, D.W.; Stollings, J.L.; Kumar, A.B.; Hughes, C.G.; Hernandez, A.; et al. Balanced crystalloids versus saline in critically Ill adults. *N. Engl. J. Med.* **2018**, *378*, 829–839. [CrossRef]
54. Krajewski, M.L.; Raghunathan, K.; Paluszkiewicz, S.M.; Schermer, C.R.; Shaw, A.D. Meta-analysis of high-versus low-chloride content in perioperative and critical care fluid resuscitation. *Br. J. Surg.* **2015**, *102*, 24–36. [CrossRef]
55. Laffey, J.G.; Kavanagh, B.P. Hypocapnia. *N. Engl. J. Med.* **2002**, *347*, 43–53. [CrossRef]
56. Rudolf, M.; Riordan, J.F.; Grant, B.J.; Maberly, D.J.; Saunders, K.B. Arterial blood gas tensions in acute severe asthma. *Eur. J. Clin. Investig.* **1980**, *10*, 55–62. [CrossRef]
57. Buda, A.J.; Pinsky, M.R.; Ingels, N.B., Jr.; Daughters, G.T., 2nd; Stinson, E.B.; Alderman, E.L. Effect of intrathoracic pressure on left ventricular performance. *N. Engl. J. Med.* **1979**, *301*, 453–459. [CrossRef]
58. Jardin, F.; Farcot, J.C.; Boisante, L.; Prost, J.F.; Gueret, P.; Bourdarias, J.P. Mechanism of paradoxic pulse in bronchial asthma. *Circulation* **1982**, *66*, 887–894. [CrossRef]
59. Grassino, A.; Macklem, P.T. Respiratory muscle fatigue and ventilatory failure. *Annu. Rev. Med.* **1984**, *35*, 625–647. [CrossRef]
60. Freedman, S.; Cooke, N.T.; Moxham, J. Production of lactic acid by respiratory muscles. *Thorax* **1983**, *38*, 50–54. [CrossRef]
61. Brady, H.R.; Ryan, F.; Cunningham, J.; Tormey, W.; Ryan, M.P.; O'Neill, S. Hypophosphatemia complicating bronchodilator therapy for acute severe asthma. *Arch. Intern. Med.* **1989**, *149*, 2367–2368. [CrossRef]
62. Pesta, D.H.; Tsirigotis, D.N.; Befroy, D.E.; Caballero, D.; Jurczak, M.J.; Rahimi, Y.; Cline, G.W.; Dufour, S.; Birkenfeld, A.L.; Rothman, D.L.; et al. Hypophosphatemia promotes lower rates of muscle ATP synthesis. *FASEB J.* **2016**, *30*, 3378–3387. [CrossRef] [PubMed]
63. Aubier, M.; Murciano, D.; Lecocguic, Y.; Viires, N.; Jacquens, Y.; Squara, P.; Pariente, R. Effect of hypophosphatemia on diaphragmatic contractility in patients with acute respiratory failure. *N. Engl. J. Med.* **1985**, *313*, 420–424. [CrossRef] [PubMed]
64. Sheldon, G.F. Hyperphosphatemia, hypophosphatemia, and the oxy-hemoglobin dissociation curve. *J. Surg. Res.* **1973**, *14*, 367–372. [CrossRef]

65. Henrion, J.; Minette, P.; Colin, L.; Schapira, M.; Delannoy, A.; Heller, F.R. Hypoxic hepatitis caused by acute exacerbation of chronic respiratory failure: A case-controlled, hemodynamic study of 17 consecutive cases. *Hepatology* **1999**, *29*, 427–433. [CrossRef] [PubMed]
66. Ford, R.M.; Book, W.; Spivey, J.R. Liver disease related to the heart. *Transplant. Rev. (Orlando)* **2015**, *29*, 33–37. [CrossRef]
67. Waseem, N.; Chen, P.H. Hypoxic hepatitis: A review and clinical update. *J. Clin. Transl. Hepatol.* **2016**, *4*, 263–268. [PubMed]
68. Sterling, S.A.; Puskarich, M.A.; Jones, A.E. The effect of liver disease on lactate normalization in severe sepsis and septic shock: A cohort study. *Clin. Exp. Emerg. Med.* **2015**, *2*, 197–202. [CrossRef]
69. De Jonghe, B.; Cheval, C.; Misset, B.; Timsit, J.F.; Garrouste, M.; Montuclard, L.; Carlet, J. Relationship between blood lactate and early hepatic dysfunction in acute circulatory failure. *J. Crit. Care* **1999**, *14*, 7–11. [CrossRef]
70. Gillani, S.; Cao, J.; Suzuki, T.; Hak, D.J. The effect of ischemia reperfusion injury on skeletal muscle. *Injury* **2012**, *43*, 670–675. [CrossRef]
71. Kalogeris, T.; Baines, C.P.; Krenz, M.; Korthuis, R.J. Ischemia/Reperfusion. *Compr. Physiol.* **2016**, *7*, 113–170.
72. Ind, P.W.; Causon, R.C.; Brown, M.J.; Barnes, P.J. Circulating catecholamines in acute asthma. *Br. Med. J. (Clin. Res. Ed.)* **1985**, *290*, 267–269. [CrossRef]
73. Papiris, S.A.; Manali, E.D.; Kolilekas, L.; Triantafillidou, C.; Tsangaris, I. Acute severe asthma: New approaches to assessment and treatment. *Drugs* **2009**, *69*, 2363–2391. [CrossRef]
74. Stratakos, G.; Kalomenidis, J.; Routsi, C.; Papiris, S.; Roussos, C. Transient lactic acidosis as a side effect of inhaled salbutamol. *Chest* **2002**, *122*, 385–386. [CrossRef]
75. Barth, E.; Albuszies, G.; Baumgart, K.; Matejovic, M.; Wachter, U.; Vogt, J.; Radermacher, P.; Calzia, E. Glucose metabolism and catecholamines. *Crit. Care Med.* **2007**, *35*, S508–S518. [CrossRef] [PubMed]
76. Reverte, M.; Moratinos, J. Effects of salbutamol and BRL 37344 on diastolic arterial blood pressure, plasma glucose and plasma lactate in rabbits. *Fundam. Clin. Pharmacol.* **1994**, *8*, 417–424. [CrossRef]
77. Haffner, C.A.; Kendall, M.J. Metabolic effects of beta 2-agonists. *J. Clin. Pharm. Ther.* **1992**, *17*, 155–164. [CrossRef]
78. Batenburg, J.J.; Olson, M.S. Regulation of pyruvate dehydrogenase by fatty acid in isolated rat liver mitochondria. *J. Biol. Chem.* **1976**, *251*, 1364–1370. [PubMed]
79. Kovacevic, A.; Schwahn, B.; Schuster, A. Hyperlactic acidosis as metabolic side-effect of albuterol and theophylline in acute severe asthma. *Klin. Padiatr.* **2010**, *222*, 271–272. [CrossRef] [PubMed]
80. Barnes, P.J. Theophylline. *Am. J. Respir. Crit. Care Med.* **2013**, *188*, 901–906. [CrossRef] [PubMed]
81. Sturney, S.; Suntharalingam, J. Treating acute asthma-salbutamol may not always be the right answer. *Clin. Med. (Lond.)* **2012**, *12*, 181–182. [CrossRef]
82. Stiles, G.L.; Caron, M.G.; Lefkowitz, R.J. Beta-adrenergic receptors: Biochemical mechanisms of physiological regulation. *Physiol. Rev.* **1984**, *64*, 661–743. [CrossRef] [PubMed]
83. Dodda, V.R.; Spiro, P. Can albuterol be blamed for lactic acidosis? *Respir. Care* **2012**, *57*, 2115–2118. [CrossRef] [PubMed]
84. Vernon, C.; Letourneau, J.L. Lactic acidosis: Recognition, kinetics, and associated prognosis. *Crit. Care Clin.* **2010**, *26*, 55–83. [CrossRef] [PubMed]
85. Gutierrez, G.; Wulf, M.E. Lactic acidosis in sepsis: A commentary. *Intensive Care Med.* **1996**, *22*, 6–16. [CrossRef] [PubMed]

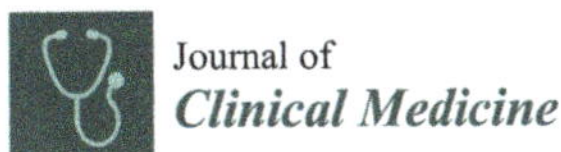
Journal of
Clinical Medicine

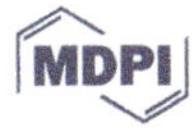

Review

Acute Severe Asthma in Adolescent and Adult Patients: Current Perspectives on Assessment and Management

Eirini Kostakou [1,†], Evangelos Kaniaris [1,†], Effrosyni Filiou [1], Ioannis Vasileiadis [1], Paraskevi Katsaounou [2], Eleni Tzortzaki [3], Nikolaos Koulouris [1], Antonia Koutsoukou [1] and Nikoletta Rovina [1,*]

1. ICU, 1st Department of Pulmonary Medicine, "Sotiria" Hospital, Athens School of Medicine, National and Kapodistrian University of Athens, 11527 Athens, Greece
2. 1st ICU, Evangelismos Hospital, Athens School of Medicine, National and Kapodistrian University of Athens, 11527 Athens, Greece
3. Respiratory Outpatient Clinic, 71305 Heraklion, Greece

* Correspondence: nikrovina@med.uoa.gr
† These authors contributed equally to this work.

Received: 6 July 2019; Accepted: 19 August 2019; Published: 22 August 2019

Abstract: Asthma is a chronic airway inflammatory disease that is associated with variable expiratory flow, variable respiratory symptoms, and exacerbations which sometimes require hospitalization or may be fatal. It is not only patients with severe and poorly controlled asthma that are at risk for an acute severe exacerbation, but this has also been observed in patients with otherwise mild or moderate asthma. This review discusses current aspects on the pathogenesis and pathophysiology of acute severe asthma exacerbations and provides the current perspectives on the management of acute severe asthma attacks in the emergency department and the intensive care unit.

Keywords: acute severe asthma exacerbation; near fatal asthma

---

1. Introduction

Asthma is a chronic inflammatory disorder of the airways, a common and potentially serious chronic disease that is associated with variable expiratory flow, airway wall thickening, respiratory symptoms, and exacerbations (flare-ups), which sometimes require hospitalization and may be fatal [1]. In reference to asthma, an exacerbation is defined as an event characterized by change from the patient's previous status, including a progressive increase in relevant symptoms and a decrease in respiratory function. The latter can be quantified by respiratory function measurements such as peak expiratory flow (PEF), and forced expiratory volume in 1 s (FEV_1), which when compared with the patient's previous or predicted values, reflect the deterioration in expiratory airflow, the prominent pathophysiological effect of an asthma attack.

The most common causes of these exacerbations are exposure to external agents, such as indoor and outdoor allergens [2–4], air pollutants [5], and respiratory tract infections (primarily viral mainly human rhinovirus (HRV) [6,7]. The mechanisms by which these environmental stimuli and viruses initiate asthma or cause worsening of the disease are under research.

Asthma exacerbations may also be triggered by exercise [8], weather changes [9], foods [10,11], additives, drugs [1–14], and extreme emotional expressions [15,16]. The physiological hallmarks of asthma are airway inflammation, airway remodeling and bronchial hyperresponsiveness (BHR) [17]. Exposure to the above-mentioned external stimuli and specifically to inhaled allergens is capable of inducing an inflammatory response in sensitized individuals and as a result to lead to exacerbations [18,19]. A hypothesis explaining this fact is that the inflammatory response resulting from inhaled allergen may drive BHR directly, or induce structural changes in the airway leading to persistent BHR [17,20]. Experimental mouse models of asthma have shown that allergen exposure protocols induce immune-mediated airway inflammation defined by: elevated levels of asthma biomarkers (IgE, the T-helper cell 2 (Th2) cytokines, interleukins (IL)-4, -5 and -13, and eosinophils), induction of airway remodeling (increases in airway smooth muscle, collagen deposition and goblet cell hyperplasia), and BHR that is sustained after the resolution of eosinophilic inflammation [21–23].

Other factors that may cause exacerbations are rhinitis [24] or sinusitis [25], polyposis [26], gastroesophageal reflux [27], menstruation [28,29], or even pregnancy [30,31]. They can happen either to patients with known asthma of any level of severity, or less frequently as a first presentation. Exacerbations vary in severity, as well as in response to therapy. This has led to an effort of categorize the severity of these exacerbations. The most frequently proposed categories include elements of the clinical presentation of the asthma patient, as well as a measurement of their respiratory function at the time of the exacerbation. It is of paramount importance for the clinician to distinguish the severe exacerbations, because these are the ones that correlate with worse consequences.

2. Definition of Acute Severe Asthma

The Global Initiative for Asthma guidelines refers to a severe asthma exacerbation describing a patient who talks in words, leans forward, is agitated, uses accessory respiratory muscles, has a respiratory rate > 30/min, heart rate > 120/min, O_2 saturation on air < 90% and PEF ≤ 50% of their best or predicted value [1]. According to the 2014 British Guidelines for Asthma, acute severe asthma is defined as the asthma exacerbation that presents with any of the following: PEF 33–50% best or predicted, respiratory rate ≥ 25/min, heart rate ≥ 110/min and inability to complete sentences in one breath [32]. The ATS/ERS task force defines a severe asthma exacerbation by the fact that they require urgent action in order to prevent a serious outcome, such as hospitalization or death from asthma [33]. This task force recommends that the definition of a severe asthma exacerbation for clinical trials should include at least one of the following: (a) use of systemic corticosteroids (tablets, suspension, or injection), or an increase from a stable maintenance dose, for at least three days; and (b) a hospitalization or emergency department visit because of asthma, requiring systemic corticosteroids. Although these definitions are not identical, the point remains that identifying this condition is important as it is correlated with worse outcomes and greater risk of needing mechanical ventilation.

There are other entities similar but not identical to that of acute severe asthma that also require precise definitions. Kenyon et al. proposed the term Critical Asthma Syndromes (CAS) to identify any child or adult who is at risk of fatal asthma [34]. This term includes acute severe asthma, refractory asthma, status asthmaticus, and near fatal asthma, all of them conditions that can lead to respiratory exhaustion and arrest. Refractory asthma is, according to a definition set by the Unbiased Biomarkers for the Prediction of Respiratory Disease Outcomes (U-BIOPRED) consortium in 2011, patients with asthma in whom after excluding any alternative diagnoses, after treating comorbidities and removing trigger factors cannot maintain good asthma control, despite high-intensity treatment and confirmed compliance with treatment. These patients have frequent severe exacerbations (≥2 per year), or can only be well when receiving systemic corticosteroids [35]. Near fatal asthma (NFA) is defined as an asthma exacerbation resulting in respiratory arrest requiring mechanical ventilation or a $pCO_2 \geq 45$ mm Hg. Some writers tend to recognize status asthmaticus and acute severe asthma as the same condition and define it mainly by its response to treatment, thus referring to it as an exacerbation that does not respond to repeated courses of β2-agonist therapy [36].

3. Epidemiology

According to the Global Asthma Report, approximately 334 million people in the world suffer from asthma, thus being the most prevalent chronic respiratory disease, with chronic obstructive pulmonary disease (COPD) affecting only half of the aforementioned number of people [37]. However, according to Eurostat [38], in most European countries age standardized asthma admission rates declined from 2001–2005 to 2011–2015, with an over two-fold reduction in some countries. (Figure 1) The latest World Health Organization (WHO) estimates, released in December 2016, present that there were 383,000 deaths due to asthma in 2015. There has been a decrease of almost 26% in the asthma deaths, when comparing 2015 to 1990 [37]. However, international mortality statistics for asthma are limited to those countries reporting detailed causes of death. Figure 2 depicts the age-standardized mortality rates for asthma among countries reporting asthma separately in two recent five-year periods (2001–2005 and 2011–2015) [38].

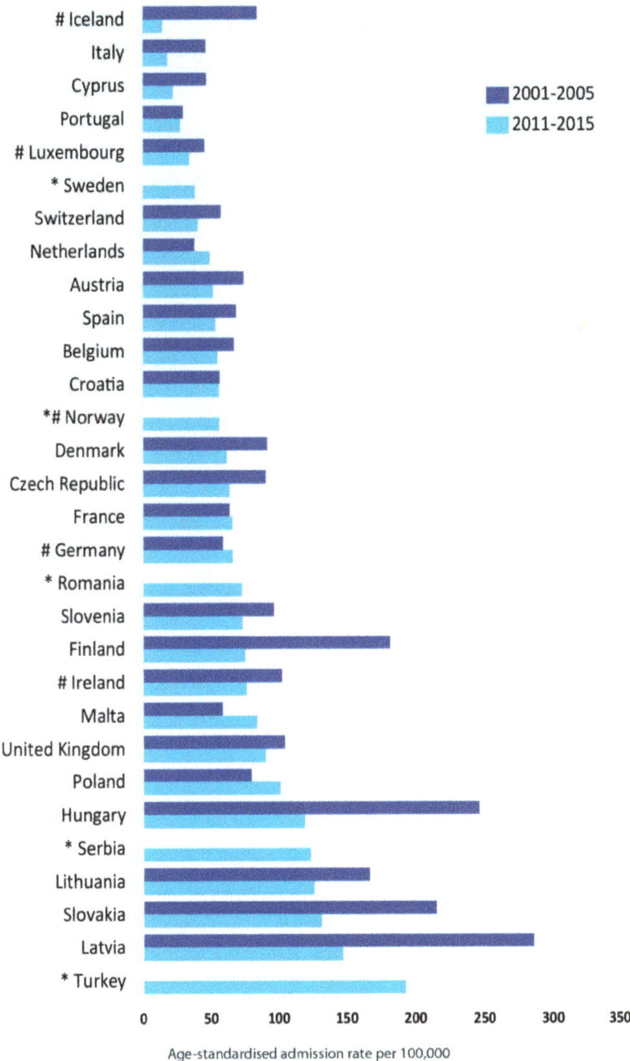

Figure 1. Age-standardized admission rates for asthma (all ages) in 30 European countries in two time periods: 2001–2005 and 2011–2015. Source: Eurostat updated from ec.europa.eu/Eurostat/web/health/health-care/data/database (version dated November 2017).

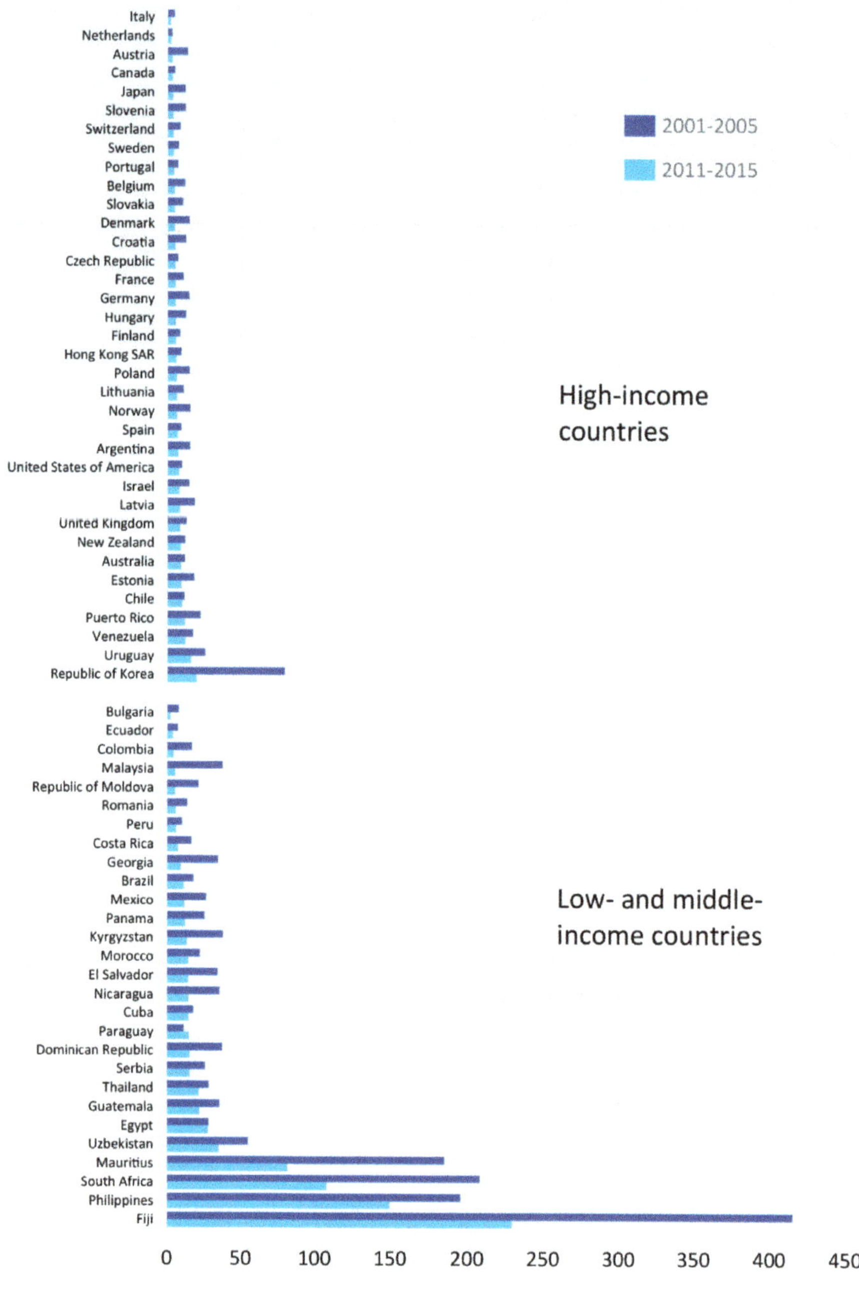

Figure 2. Age-standardized mortality rates for asthma (all ages) by country in two time periods: 2001–2005 and 2011–2015. Source: Eurostat updated from ec.europa.eu/Eurostat/web/health/health-care/data/database (version dated November 2017).

Although asthma is a disease not only of low- and lower-middle-income countries, most asthma-related deaths occur in those areas [38]. There is an established connection between asthma deaths and the Socio-Demographic Index (SDI), but interestingly not with SDI and asthma prevalence. A recent study in Brazil demonstrated that urbanization has affected public health, resulting in higher asthma related morbidity and mortality, despite the fact that the urbanized population now has improved access to the health system [39]. There are no accurate figures describing the rate of acute severe asthma, but there are sufficient data regarding the asthma related hospitalizations and asthma related mortality. Recent studies estimate the risk of death of the patients who are hospitalized as a result of asthma exacerbation as less than 0.5% [40,41]. That risk is greater when the patient requires intubation and mechanical ventilation, which underlines the importance of identifying and promptly treating acute severe asthma. Four percent of asthma related hospitalizations result in mechanical ventilation. There is a substantial economic burden associated with asthma hospitalizations, and it has been demonstrated that in the US in 2012 the overall cost was more than 2 billion dollars, which is a significant percentage (more than 1/3) of the annual asthma related expenditure [41]. Middle aged women are more likely to get hospitalized with asthma related morbidities [41].

With regards to the identified phenotypes of asthma, data from a recent cluster analysis from Japan revealed a wide heterogeneity among asthma patients who presented and were admitted with severe and life-threatening asthma in 17 institutions across the country [42]. Another recent group-based trajectory analysis on patients with problematic and uncontrolled asthma, showed that near fatal events were noted in all groups, but were more frequent in patients with persistent frequent exacerbations [43]. It is not only patients with severe and poorly controlled asthma who are at risk for having an acute severe asthma exacerbation, but this has been observed as well in patients with otherwise mild or moderate asthma. The current literature describes two distinct clinico-pathophysiological entities of acute severe asthma attacks that present at the emergency department: the slow onset, late arrival and the sudden onset fatal asthma. It has been estimated that the majority (80–85%) of asthma-related fatalities belong to the slow onset group. These patients may have symptoms and uncontrolled disease for several days prior to the presentation with acute severe asthma. Sudden onset has been defined as severe airflow obstruction established after 1–3 h of symptom presentation. Barr et al. reported that patients presenting with sudden onset asthma, were more likely to have been exposed to an exacerbation trigger such as a respiratory allergen, exercise and psychosocial stress and less often respiratory infection and had greater improvement when compared with the slow onset cohort [44]. A retrospective cohort study in the United States demonstrated evidence that the sudden-onset patients were older, were more likely to present during the night and early morning hours at the emergency department, more often required intubation and mechanical ventilation, and had higher rate of ICU admission, but, on the other hand, had shorter hospital stay [45]. In this study the sudden onset cohort was only 6% of 1260 patients in 30 hospitals.

4. Risk Factors for Asthma Exacerbations

Many factors have been studied regarding their correlation with acute severe asthma and asthma related death (Table 1). In adults, asthma exacerbations are more often in females [46,47]. This is difficult to be explained since female asthmatics have lower levels of total serum IgE [48] and the incidence of atopy is actually lower in comparison to males [49]. A possible explanation could have to do with the connection between asthma worsening and the menses, which is a recognized contributing factor of asthma worsening [50]. Furthermore, pregnancy in asthmatic women is a condition that requires special considerations, considering the effect of the disease, as well as the medication on the mother and the fetus. Pregnancy is not always correlated with worse asthma control, although there seems to be a correlation between asthma severity and morbidities and exacerbations during pregnancy [51]. There has been reported a cluster of obese females with late-onset corticosteroid asthma with frequent exacerbations although they preserve a relatively good baseline lung function [52].

Table 1. Risk factors for fatal asthma exacerbations.

A History of Near Fatal Asthma Requiring Intubation and Mechanical Ventilation
Hospitalization or emergency care visits for asthma in the past year Currently using or having recently stopped using oral steroids Not currently using inhaled steroids SABA over-use (more than one canister of salbutamol/month (or equivalent)) History of psychiatric disease or psychosocial problems
Female Sex
Age > 40 years
Smoking history
Poor perception of airflow limitation
Hyperinflation in chest radiograph Poor adherence with asthma medications and/or poor adherence
(or lack of) with a written asthma action plan Food allergy

SABA, short acting beta agonist. Adapted from Global Initiative for Asthma (GINA) guidelines 2018 [1].

Obesity per se has also been correlated with worse asthma control, as well as more frequent and severe exacerbations. This correlation is strengthened by the apparent effect of weight loss and bariatric surgery on better control and less exacerbations and hospitalizations [53].

Ethnicity and socioeconomic status [54,55] are robust determinants of asthma exacerbation rates. African Americans have 4.2- and 2.8-fold higher rates of emergency room visits and hospitalizations for asthma exacerbation, respectively, compared to Caucasians, followed by Hispanics [39]. A possible explanation for these differences could be the poorer adherence to treatment [56] and the poorer quality of healthcare in ethnic minorities [57]. A significant genetic component might also contribute, since an increased risk of exacerbations has been documented in males with African ancestry [58].

Severe exacerbations may occur in patients with mild or well controlled asthma [59,60]. However, poor asthma control is an independent risk factor for future acute exacerbations [61–65]. A history of a recent exacerbation is the strongest predictor of future exacerbations in children and adults with asthma [66–69]. A small percentage of asthmatics exhibit severe disease exacerbations, despite the fact that they are already under treatment with high doses of inhaled and/or systemic corticosteroids [70,71]. These patients suffering from severe asthma (SA) that is poorly controlled and in some cases life-threatening [34,35], although comprising a small percentage of the total asthma population (5–10%), they denote 50% of total healthcare costs, rendering SA a substantial health and socio-economic burden [36,37].

Finally, poor perception of airflow limitation may affect patients with a history of near-fatal asthma and appears to be more common in males [72,73]. On the other hand, regular or overuse of short acting beta agonists (SABA) causes down regulation of beta receptors and leads to lack of response, leading in turn to overuse [74]. Overuse may also be habitual. Dispensing ≥3 SABA canisters/year (average 1.5 puffs/day or more) is associated with increased risk of emergency department visits or hospitalizations no matter what the severity of asthma is [75], while dispensing ≥12 canisters/year (1/month) increases the risk of death [76]. Incorrect inhaler technique (seen in up to 80% of asthma patients) [77], as well as suboptimal adherence to treatment (seen in up to 75% of patients) are important modifiable factors contributing to symptoms and exacerbations [77].

There has been a lot of interest regarding the effect of psychological factors on the risk for fatal or near fatal asthma, this however has not been established, as shown in a 2007 systematic review by Alvarez et al. [78]. Anxiety, depression and socio-economic problems are very common in patients with difficult to treat asthma and contribute to poor symptom control, poor adherence to treatment and impaired quality of life [79].

Obesity and other comorbidities other than the psychiatric conditions already mentioned that contribute to persistent symptoms, exacerbations and poor quality of life include chronic rhinosinusistis [80], inducible laryngeal obstruction (often referred as vocal cord dysfunction, VCD), gastroesophageal regurgitation disorder (GERD), chronic obstructive pulmonary disease (COPD), obstructive sleep apnea, bronchiectasis, cardiac disease, and kyphosis due to osteoporosis (followed by corticosteroid overuse) [80].

5. Factors that Trigger Asthma Exacerbations

Severe exacerbations usually occur in response to a variety of external agents (e.g., respiratory pathogens, allergens, air pollutants, smoke, and cold or dry air).

5.1. Respiratory Pathogens

Viral respiratory infections are the most common triggers for a severe asthma exacerbation, comprising up to 76–80% of the causes of an acute asthma exacerbation in adults [81]. Human rhinovirus (RV) (types A and C), influenza virus (types A and B), para-influenza virus, and respiratory syncytial virus (RSV) are frequent causes of an acute exacerbation and hospitalization [56,82]. Coronaviruses, meta-pneumoviruses, bocaviruses, and adenoviruses may also trigger a severe acute exacerbation, however to a lesser extent [57]. During the 2009 H1N1 influenza A pandemic, mortality and admissions to the ICU with H1N1 infections were frequently associated with asthma [82,83]. In contrast to other respiratory viruses (i.e., RSV and Influenza Virus), RV does not exert a definite cytopathic effect [84]; instead, it compromises the function of the epithelial barrier through the release of reactive oxygen species during viral replication [85]. During this process, the induction of immune and adaptive immune response activates the synthesis and early secretion of IFNs and other pro-inflammatory cytokines (i.e., IL-10, IL-6, IL-8, RANTES, and ENA-78) [86], which play a significant role in the protective mechanisms against viral infection [87,88]. There is evidence that in asthmatic patients there is dysregulated immune response against RV [89]. Several studies have demonstrated the implication of interferons in the susceptibility to asthma exacerbations in children and adults in the context of a viral respiratory infection. Miller et al. [90] showed that RV was related to asthma exacerbation with the implication of IFN III. Similarly, Jones et al. [91] documented an increased susceptibility to severe respiratory viral infections during the first years of life through dysregulated type III IFN responses, while recent studies [92,93] document a varying susceptibility to asthma exacerbations depending on the type and level of expression of cytokines and IFNs upon viral infection. Finally, Fedele et al. [94] documented that RV infection more frequently induces a Th2-mediated immune response than RSV infection, justifying the higher incidence of asthma prevalence after RV infections.

Bacterial infections may also trigger acute exacerbations, usually on the basis of impaired anti-bacterial defense after a viral respiratory infection [95]. There are bidirectional interactions between viruses and bacteria that seem to have an impact on the severity of asthma as well as the likelihood of an acute exacerbation. Viral infections facilitate the disruption of airway epithelial layers and the expression of airway receptors that bacteria use in order to invade [96]. Furthermore, in the presence of co-infection, an increased release of inflammatory cytokines and mediators is induced, heightening the burden of inflammation and predisposing to a higher risk of exacerbations [97]. Specifically, co-infections of respiratory viruses and *Moraxella catarrhalis*, *Hemophilus influenza*, and/or *Streptococcus pneumonia* have a greater impact on the risk for more severe acute asthma exacerbations [97]. The clarification of the mechanisms implicate the case of co-infections on inter-relationship for providing evidence for potential novel therapeutic targets that may prevent acute asthma exacerbations.

5.2. Allergen Sensitization and Viral Infections

Evidence support the theory that allergic sensitization increases the susceptibility for viral infections and probably their ability to provoke further inflammation [98].

For example, it has been shown that the combination of RV infection and direct exposure to allergens cause epithelial cell production of IL-25 and IL-33 in the airways, mediators involved in Th2 type inflammation and remodeling [99,100]. Moreover, in a murine model of asthma RV infection acquired in early life stages in mice induced an IL-13- and IL-25-mediated Th2 immune response with parallel suppression of IFN-γ, IL-12, and TNF-α [101], with detrimental changes in airway homeostasis, consisting of innate lymphoid cell expansion, mucous hypersecretion, and airway responsiveness. Furthermore, recurrent RV infections stimulate airway remodeling by upregulating molecules such as VEGF and TGF-β, as well as chemoattractants for airway smooth muscles (i.e., CCL5, CXCL8, and CXCL10) [102,103].

Other data show that the occupancy of the IgE membrane receptors inhibits antiviral induction of interferon-a from plasmacytoid dendritic cells leading to subsequent increased susceptibility to viral infections and asthma exacerbations. It is noteworthy that an inverse correlation between interferon levels and airway eosinophilia, IL-4 levels, and total serum IgE was observed [104].

5.3. Allergen Exposure, Tobacco Smoke, and Environmental Pollutants

Indoor or outdoor exposure to allergens may lead to poor asthma control and severe asthma exacerbations in sensitized patients [105–109]. Allergens activate mast cells to release histamine, prostaglandin D2, and cysteinyl leukotrienes. These induce inflammatory responses, airway smooth muscle constriction, increased microvascular permeability, and mucus secretion, diminishing at the same time the innate immune responses and subsequently increasing the susceptibility to viral infections [106,107]. Of great importance is the mold sensitization, which has been associated with the phenotype of severe asthma and with severe asthma attacks. High airborne concentrations of mold have been associated with increased emergency visits for asthma exacerbations [108]. Specifically, Alternaria is associated with highly increased risk (almost 200-fold) of severe exacerbations and need for ICU admittance in both children and adults [109]. Furthermore, cockroach and mouse antigens are associated with early wheeze and atopy in an inner-city birth cohort [110].

Exposure to multiple allergens has been documented as being a common feature in several studies of indoor exposure [111,112]. Salo et al. [112] showed that more than 50% of subjects were sensitized at least to six detectable allergens, while 45% were sensitized at least to three allergens. In a study from China, Kim et al. [111] showed sensitization to one or more allergens in almost 50% of the subjects with most common sensitizers being shellfish, dust mites, and cockroaches. However, less than 1% of these subjects had clinically important food allergy or asthma.

Indoor exposure to endotoxin and pollutants (such as particulate matter and nitrogen dioxide) has also been found to increase the risk of severe exacerbations in children with asthma and the use of particulate filters seem effective in reducing exposure levels and therefore, asthma control [113,114]. Differences in allergic sensitizations by race and genetic ancestry have also been documented [115], and along with the location of residence seem to be more important predictors of allergic sensitization than genetic ancestry. This fact points out the hypothesis that disparities in allergic sensitization by race may be observed as an effect of environmental rather than genetic factors.

Tobacco smoke remains one of the most significant triggers of disease, despite increased public awareness of the detrimental effects of smoking. Asthma patients who smoke have more frequent emergency department visits and hospitalizations for an exacerbation than asthma patients who do not smoke [116]. Several studies of patients with allergic rhinitis have shown the significant effect of smoking on the development of asthma. Polosa et al. [117] showed that in a 10-year period smoking had a dose-related effect on the development of asthma in allergic rhinitic patients resulting in an odds ratio of 2.05 for incident asthma for smoking 10 pack-years, and 3.7 and 5.05 for 11–20 and >20 pack-years, respectively.

Second-hand smoke is also associated with deteriorated lung function, poor treatment response, and frequent emergency department visits for asthma [118–120]. The measurement and monitoring of cotinine levels in serum, urine, and saliva have become a useful tool in determining passive smoke exposure as well as in evaluating uncontrolled asthma. Hassanzad et al. demonstrated that higher cotinine levels were associated with a higher risk for severe asthma. [121]. Increasing interest has also raised on the potential hazards of third-hand smoke (THS) in children. THS is residual nicotine and other chemical pollutants remaining in the indoor environment and on household surfaces for weeks to months after active tobacco smoking has stopped. It seems that young children may be more susceptible to the adverse effects of THS exposure since they crawl and tend to ingest several items from the surrounding [122]. However, more research is needed to assess the real extent of the hazards arising from THS.

Environmental pollutants, such as particulate matter, ozone, sulfur dioxide, nitrogen dioxide, and diesel exhaust, may act synergistically with viral infections to cause asthma exacerbations [123] The effects of air pollution on severe asthma exacerbations may be affected by other exposures, such as stress, vitamin D insufficiency, and seasonality [4,5]. This was demonstrated in a study of children aged 0–18 years in California, where particulate matter (size, 2.5 mm; $PM_{2.5}$) and ozone were associated with severe asthma exacerbations in the warm season, while in the cool season exacerbations were associated with articulate matter of $PM_{2.5}$, carbon monoxide, and NOx (NO_1NO_2) [124,125].

6. Genetic Associations with Asthma Exacerbations

Genome-wide association studies of asthma in children and adults have identified polymorphisms for IL33, IL1RL1/IL18R1, HLA-DQ, SMAD3, and IL2RB9 and the locus on chromosome 17q21 including the genes ZPBP2, GSDMB, and ORMDL3 that are implicated in epithelial barrier function and innate and adaptive immune responses in asthma [126,127]. Genetic variants in the class I major histocompatibility complex-restricted T cell-associated molecule gene (CRTAM) was associated with an increased rate of asthma exacerbations in children with low circulating vitamin D levels [128]. One of the most well replicated genetic regions affecting asthma risk is the 17q12–21 locus, which includes ORMDL3 and GSDMB. The TT allele at rs7216389 is associated with an odds ratio of 1.6 of having an asthma exacerbation when compared with the CC allele [129].

Furthermore, polymorphisms for FCER2 have been associated with decreased FCER2 gene expression, increased serum IgE levels and risk of severe exacerbations [130]. Association was also found between variants in chitinase 3-like 1 (CHI3L1; YKL-40) and asthma exacerbations and hospitalizations [131,132]. Specifically, studies in murine models of asthma implicate YKL-40 in IgE induction, antigen sensitization, dendritic cell accumulation and activation, and alternative macrophage activation [133], while purified YKL-40 induces interleukin-8 secretion in bronchial epithelial cells [134].

7. Pathogenesis-Immunobiology

Asthma is a heterogeneous condition with complex observable characteristics (phenotype) and their underlying mechanisms (endotype), resulting from complex host–environment interactions (Figure 3). Usually, inflammatory cells are present and activated in the airways of severe asthmatics and persist despite treatment, but their relevance to lack of control and disease severity is largely unknown. These cells include not only eosinophils and neutrophils, but also T-lymphocytes, mast cells, macrophages and airway structural cells which are also crucially involved in the inflammatory reaction and remodeling in asthma. Although it is well accepted that asthma is characterized by eosinophilic infiltration, inflammatory phenotypes of severe asthma can be characterized by persistence of eosinophilic or neutrophilic infiltration, as well as by absence of inflammatory infiltration (paucigranulocytic) [135,136]. Depending on the type of immune cell responses implicated in disease pathogenesis, asthma endotypes are categorized as type 2 asthma, characterized predominantly by T helper type 2 (Th2) cell-mediated inflammation and non-type 2 asthma, associated with Th1 and/or Th17 cell inflammation [137,138]. Eosinophilic, Th2 airway inflammation is present in around 50% of adults with asthma, and is estimated to be higher in the absence of corticosteroids [139].

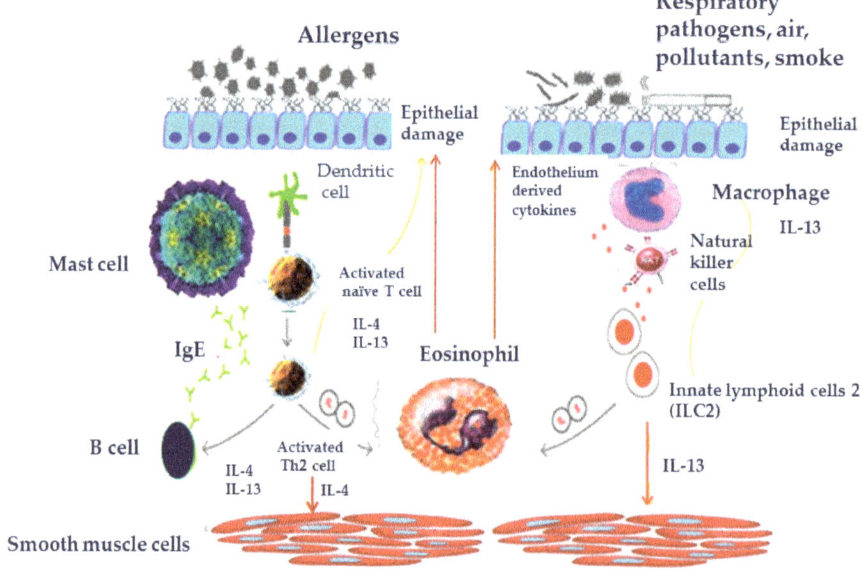

Figure 3. Pathogenesis of acute exacerbations in asthma.

Th2 mediated airway inflammation plays a central role in the pathophysiology of allergic eosinophilic asthma. The allergic sensitization of dendritic cells (DCs) in the presence of thymic stromal lymphopoietin (TSLP), induces Th2 lymphocytes to produce cytokines such as interleukins IL-4, IL-5, and IL-13 [140]. Chemokines such as eotaxin 1, 2, 3 (CCL11, CCL24 and CCL26, respectively) induce through their receptors (chemokine receptor 3, CCR3) [141] and other chemoattractant agents, such as mast cell derived prostaglandin D2 (PGD2) eosinophil recruitment in the mucosa. Furthermore, IL-4 and IL-13 activate B lymphocytes to produce allergen specific IgE, which binds to the high affinity mast cell receptors, leading to their activation [140].

In non-allergic eosinophilic asthma, airway epithelial damage caused by pollution and pathogens leads to IL-5 and IL-13 production by innate lymphoid cells (ILC2s), in response to PGD2, TSLP, IL-25 and IL-33 [142]. ILC2s and Th2 cells are a significant source of type 2 cytokines and play a role in eosinophilic inflammatory response, allergy and remodeling in asthma [143,144]. Increased circulating and sputum IL-5 and IL-13-producing ILC2s were detected in severe asthma compared to mild asthma patients [145]. Furthermore, increased numbers of IL-5$^+$ and IL-13$^+$ ILC2s were found in sputum after allergen challenge in asthma patients [146]. IL-13-expressing ILC2 and Th2 cells are also responsible for bronchial epithelial tight junction barrier leakiness in asthma patients [147,148].

Chronic inflammation that characterizes severe asthma leads to tissue remodeling, fixed airway obstruction, and no response to bronchodilatory treatment [149]. It seems that chronic persistent inflammation and the release of a plethora of cytokines (IL-5, IL-9, IL-13, osteopontin, and activin-A9), chemokines (CCR3 dependent) and growth factors (TGF-β1 and VEGF) from inflammatory and epithelial cells play a central role in the establishment of airway remodeling [150].

Physiologically, airway inflammation is counteracted by inhibitory molecules and suppressor cells including CD4$^+$ regulatory T cells (Tregs) [151,152] which becomes visible upon Treg depletion which causes spontaneous asthma-like airway pathology [153]. Patients suffering from allergic asthma have reduced numbers of Tregs that furthermore show impaired suppressive capacity [154–157]. Some currently applied therapies aim at enhancing Treg cell number and function [154,158], whereas adoptive transfer of Tregs can suppress both the priming and the effector phase of allergic airway inflammation in experimental models of murine asthma [159–161].

Mixed eosinophilic and neutrophilic inflammation of the airways are commonly found in severe asthma [162] and this mixed inflammatory pattern can be a biomarker of the most severe types of the disease [163]. Elevated sputum neutrophil counts were found to be associated with more severe asthma phenotypes and with poor response to treatment with steroids in a cluster analysis from the Severe Asthma Research Program (SARP) [164]. Airway neutrophilia has been associated with persistent airflow obstruction in patients with refractory asthma and a progressive loss of lung function [165] Furthermore, it is associated with higher bronchial hyperresponsiveness independent of eosinophilia [166].

It is suggested that increased neutrophil counts in peripheral blood and sputum could be secondary to the treatment with corticosteroids, since the anti-apoptotic effect of corticosteroids on neutrophils is well established [167]. However, neutrophilic inflammation may be observed regardless of corticosteroid treatment in patients with refractory asthma or in patients experiencing acute severe exacerbations [168–170].

Neutrophil recruitment and activation into the airways have been associated with stimulation of toll-like receptors (TLR) signaling and activation of innate immunity, causing a shift toward Th1 and Th17 responses. This process leads to increased production of interleukin (IL)-8, IL-17A, neutrophil elastase, and matrix metalloproteinase 9 [171]. Neutrophils are triggered by IL-8 to produce enzymes and other factors that contribute to eosinophil activity [171]. Evidence suggests that neutrophil subsets may mediate differential effects on immune surveillance and microbial killing. A variety of epithelial insults (ozone, bacteria, and viruses) induce secretion of chemokines and cytokines that promote neutrophil trafficking. Neutrophils primarily traffic to inflamed sites and then secrete granular enzymes, reactive oxygen species, and proteins to eliminate invading bacteria, fungal elements, and viruses. Undoubtedly, neutrophils play pivotal roles in innate immunity [172]. During asthma exacerbations, the presence of chemokines and cytokines (IL-8 and IL-17A) prolongs neutrophils' lifespan thus enabling them to migrate from tissue to the systemic circulation or to lymph nodes to modulate adaptive immune responses, Figure 4. The combined functions of these cytokines and activated enzymes promote airway structures to contribute to the lower FEV_1, remodeling and fixed airway obstruction seen in adult patients with severe neutrophilic asthma [173].

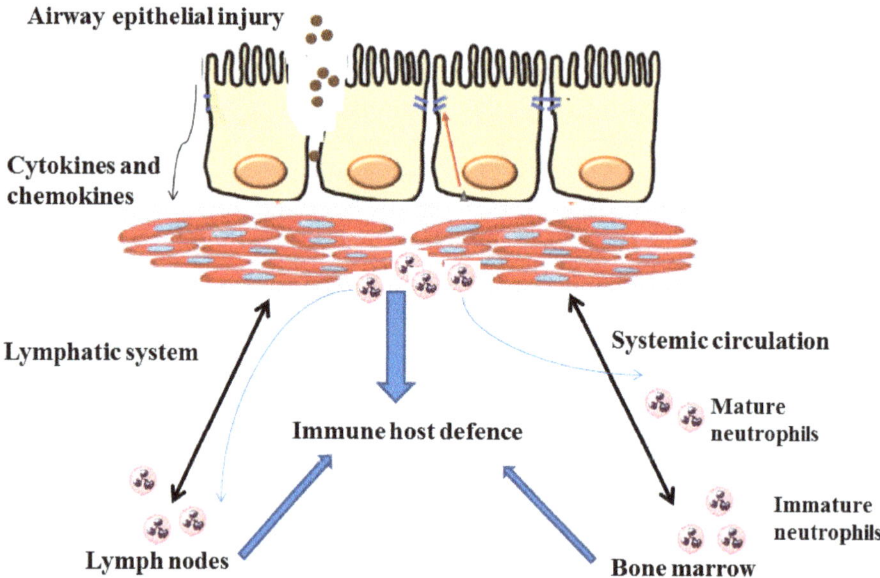

Figure 4. The role of the neutrophil in modulating local inflammatory responses.

8. Biomarkers Correlating with Risk of Asthma Exacerbations

The better understanding of the pathophysiology of asthma has led to the recognition of biomarkers with a potential to predict severe exacerbations. Among T2-high asthma biomarkers sputum and blood eosinophil count, serum IgE, serum periostin levels, and levels of nitric oxide in exhaled breath (FeNO) seem to associate with the severity of asthma and the rate and severity of exacerbations.

Sputum eosinophils have been correlated with increased asthma severity and airway responsiveness. Increased sputum eosinophil counts have been used as a measure of better response to corticosteroid treatment, in terms of reducing exacerbations. In the systematic review by Petsky et al. [174] it was demonstrated that asthma treatment guided by sputum eosinophil counts led to a significant reduction in the exacerbation rate. In children, elevated blood eosinophil count is associated with persistent asthma symptoms, and responsiveness to treatment can be predicted by the number of eosinophils without having set though a validated cut-off point [175]

Baseline blood eosinophil count is being used as a biomarker that predicts the clinical efficacy of anti-IL5 therapy in patients with severe eosinophilic asthma with a history of exacerbations [176–178], with eosinophil cut-offs set to ≥150 to ≥300 cells/μL [179] in mepolizumab trials. It has been demonstrated, however, that higher eosinophil counts than these cut-offs are associated with poor asthma control and more severe exacerbations [180]. In the study of Zieger et al. [181], a blood eosinophil count > 400 cells/μL was found to be an independent risk factor for exacerbations, emergency department visits or hospitalizations for asthma. Although blood eosinophil count levels predict the rate of exacerbations, this is not the case with sputum eosinophil count [179,182].

Total serum IgE level is a biomarker used in severe allergic asthma for the treatment with anti-IgE antibody (omalizumab). In association with elevated levels of fractional exhaled nitric oxide (FENO) (>19.5 parts per billion) and blood eosinophil count (>260/μL), it significantly predicts which patients with severe allergic asthma will respond to omalizumab, reducing the exacerbation rate [183].

The production of nitric oxide in the airways indicates Th2 type inflammation [184,185] and FeNO is a noninvasive biomarker of eosinophilic airway inflammation. There are contradictory data on whether FeNO has the ability to classify asthma severity [186–188]. Studies have shown that FeNO can predict accelerated decline of lung function [189], asthma relapse after corticosteroid treatment discontinuation [184], and degree of airway inflammation [190]. However, its ability to be used as a biomarker to predict exacerbations seems to be limited, even when combined with clinical features [191]. In the study by van der Valk et al. [192], repeated measurements of FENO predicted moderate asthma exacerbations (not requiring systemic corticosteroids or hospitalizations) but not severe asthma exacerbations.

Exhaled breath condensate (EBC) has been used in assessing exacerbations. Low EBC pH, various cytokines, chemokines, NO-related products, leukotrienes, and volatile organic compounds, better in combination, have been used as biomarkers associated with clinical characteristics and exacerbations [193].

Serum periostin is a biomarker of allergic eosinophilic asthma and has been used in the identification of patients who will respond to Th2-directed therapies [194]. However, limited data suggest that the serum periostin level predicts asthma exacerbations [195]. Sputum periostin, on the other hand, is associated with persistent airflow limitation, eosinophilic asthma refractory to ICS [196], while it is a potential marker for airway remodeling, as well [197,198].

There is an increasing need for developing biomarkers that will guide clinicians in the management of asthma, in terms of better and easier phenotyping asthma, predicting exacerbations, and treatment response.

9. Pathophysiology

Acute severe asthma commonly presents with abnormal arterial gas exchange. Arterial hypoxemia is largely attributed to ventilation/perfusion mismatch (V/Q mismatch). Hypercapnia, on the other hand, is not only present due to V/Q mismatch, but also due to respiratory muscle fatigue leading to alveolar hypoventilation. Trying to assess the exact profile of the V/Q mismatch that characterizes acute severe asthma, studies have demonstrated that although in asthma patients there is a wide spectrum of V/Q abnormalities, the most common in acute severe asthma (ASA) patients is having increased blood flow, in the context of high cardiac output, distributed in alveolar spaces with low ventilation and remarkably low V/Q ratios [199]. The pattern of ventilation-perfusion is bimodal in acute severe asthma, ranging from normally perfused areas to areas of hypoxic pulmonary vasoconstriction.

With regards to the mechanics of the respiratory system, acute asthma exacerbation is characterized by reversible bronchoconstriction and increased airway resistance, followed by low flow rates, premature small airway closure, decreased elastic recoil, pulmonary hyperinflation and increased work of breathing. There is a substantial decrease in the FEV_1 and the PEF of the patients, whereas the residual volume may increase as much as 400% of the normal and the functional residual capacity may even reach double the normal values [199]. In severe asthma exacerbations, total lung capacity (TLC) is also increasing. These changes in lung volumes help constricted airways remain open. During passive expiration of the lungs, the driving forces of the respiratory system are the elastic forces. The lower the elastic forces are, or the higher the resistive forces, the longer will the time needed to full expiration of the inspired tidal volume be, characteristic that may be quantified by a long expiratory time constant of the respiratory system. Incomplete exhalation of delivered tidal volume makes inspiration begin at a volume at which respiratory system exhibits a positive recoil pressure. The presence of flow at the end of the expiration is due to the presence of positive alveolar pressure at the end of expiration. This process is called dynamic hyperinflation and the positive end-expiratory alveolus pressure associated with higher relaxation volume is called intrinsic (auto) Positive End Expiratory Pressure (PEEP) [200] (Figure 5). Dynamic hyperinflation depends on the expiratory time constant, expiratory flow limitation, expiratory time, inspiratory muscle activity during exhalation, tidal volume, and external flow resistance [201]. Although this initially may act in favor of the patient, by reducing the resistive work of breathing, the thorax and lungs increase in volume, length–tension relationships of the respiratory muscles shorten and the strength of contraction eventually diminishes. As the severe exacerbation remains unresponsive, expiratory and accessory muscles become active, the work of breathing increases and fatigue is a serious and potentially fatal possibility, as it further compromises respiratory function and deteriorates respiratory failure. Bronchospasm and increased resistance, mucous and compression of the peripheral airways from auto-PEEP, lead to significant heterogeneity of the lung. Normal lung units coexist with pathological lung units creating a variety of many different time constants across the lung.

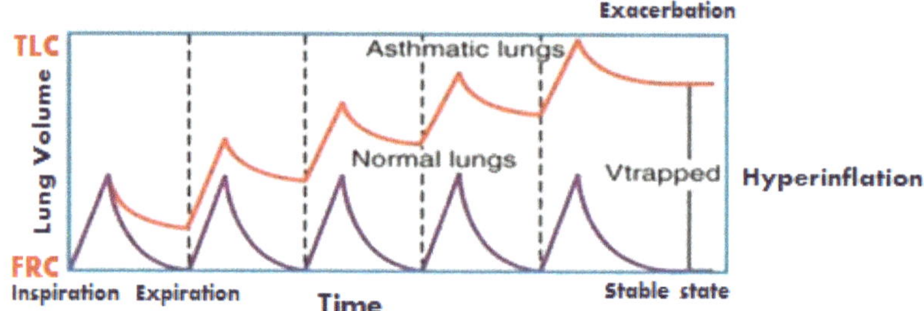

Figure 5. Dynamic hyperinflation during exacerbation.

Hemodynamic compromise is another important feature of a severe asthma attack that leads to significant dynamic hyperinflation. The development of positive intrathoracic pressures lead to decrease of the right heart output by decreasing right heart preload (venous return and end–diastolic volume of the right heart) and increasing right heart afterload (vascular pulmonary resistance). The decreased right heart output in parallel with the diastolic dysfunction of the left heart (caused by shifting the intraventricular septum towards the left ventricle) and its incomplete filling, lead to a significant reduction of the arterial systolic pressure in inspiration and the presence of pulsus paradoxus sign [202] (Figure 6).

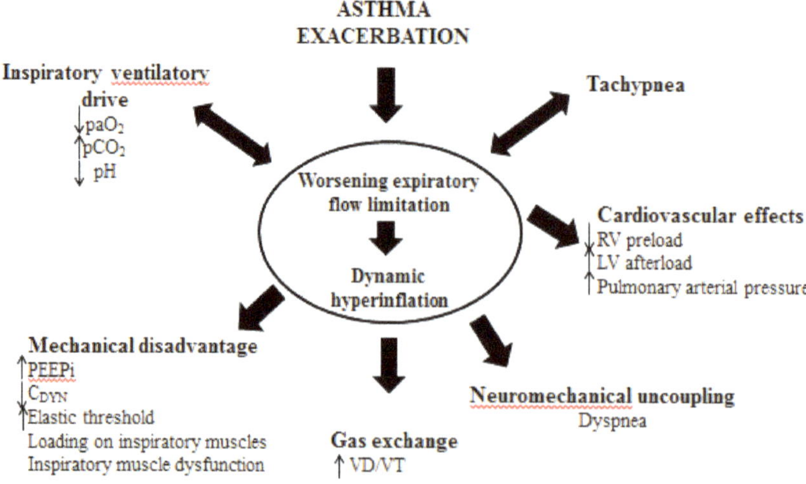

Figure 6. Pathophysiological changes due to dynamic hyperinflation.

Thus, due to uncontrolled or difficult to treat dynamic hyperinflation, a patient with asthma can be drowsy, confused or agitated, or may present with paradoxical thoracic-abdominal movement, with absent of wheeze in lung auscultation, bradycardia or with pulsus paradoxus. This patient is near respiratory arrest status and endotracheal intubation. Mechanical ventilation and admission to an ICU may be imminent [203].

10. Clinical Assessment

Identification of severe asthma exacerbations is of outmost importance, as they are related with worse outcomes and require close observation and aggressive management. A brief interview with the patient is necessary to determine certain features in the patient's history that need to be looked into closely, because current literature identifies them as factors that increase asthma-related death. Hospital and Intensive Care Unit (ICU) admission, as well as mechanical ventilation due to an asthma exacerbation has been shown to significantly increase the risk for a new episode of near fatal and fatal asthma [204]. It is also very important to obtain a detailed description of the patient's medication history. Medications that play a significant role in the prediction of asthma related morbidities and death are inhaled and systematic corticosteroids, as well as the use of beta agonists. In this context, not currently using inhaled corticosteroids (ICS), currently using or having recently discontinued treatment with oral corticosteroids (OCS), as well as documented overuse of short acting β agonists (SABAs) are all factors related with an increased risk for asthma associated morbidity and mortality [205,206]. Elements from the medication history may also conceal clues that may suggest inadequate treatment, or even poor adherence to a prescribed treatment plan. The lack of a written asthma plan and socioeconomic factors are also associated with a greater risk for a severe exacerbation [207].

Patients suffering from an asthma exacerbation may present with a variety of signs and symptoms [208] (Figure 7). Dyspnea, chest tightness, cough and wheezing are few of those, but there is wide heterogeneity in the asthmatic patient presentation. Features that characterize acute severe asthma are agitation, drowsiness or signs of confusion, significant breathlessness at rest, with the patient talking in words, tachypnea of more than 30 breaths per minute, use of accessory respiratory muscles, tachycardia of >120 beats per minute and pulsus paradoxus. Moreover, it is crucial to identify signs that indicate an imminent respiratory arrest, such as paradoxical thoraco-abdominal movement, silent chest with absence of wheeze, bradycardia, while the absence of pulsus paradoxus might imply muscle fatigue [208]. Upon examining the patient with acute severe asthma, apart from recognizing the signs that indicate severity, it is imperative to diagnose any pathology that might attenuate the exacerbation and requires specific treatment. Such entities are pneumothorax and pneumo-mediastinum, and pneumonia. At the same time, the clinician needs to exclude conditions that may mimic the symptoms of an asthma attack, such as cardiogenic pulmonary edema, exacerbation of chronic obstructive disease, airway obstruction caused by a foreign body or an intraluminal mass, pulmonary embolism, hyperventilation syndrome and vocal cord dysfunction [209–211].

Although lung function measurements are less sensitive than the history of symptoms, during an asthma exacerbation, serial PEF and FEV_1 measurements are more objective and reliable indicators of severity and should remain part of the initial assessment of an asthma patient presenting to the emergency department according to current guidelines [1,2]. Regarding PEF, the cut-off value of 50% of the patient's best or predicted value is within the definition of an acute severe asthma episode, and requires greater attention and action. Moreover, a value of less than 33% of their best or predicted value is an indicator of life-threatening asthma. Serial monitoring of PEF may also assist the decision of either discharging the patient, should this be accompanied with a clinical improvement, or for ICU referral if the values are continuously deteriorating despite initial appropriate treatment. There is certainly a concern regarding the safety of this test in the setting of an acute exacerbation in the emergency department, and it should be performed with caution and continuous observation of the patient.

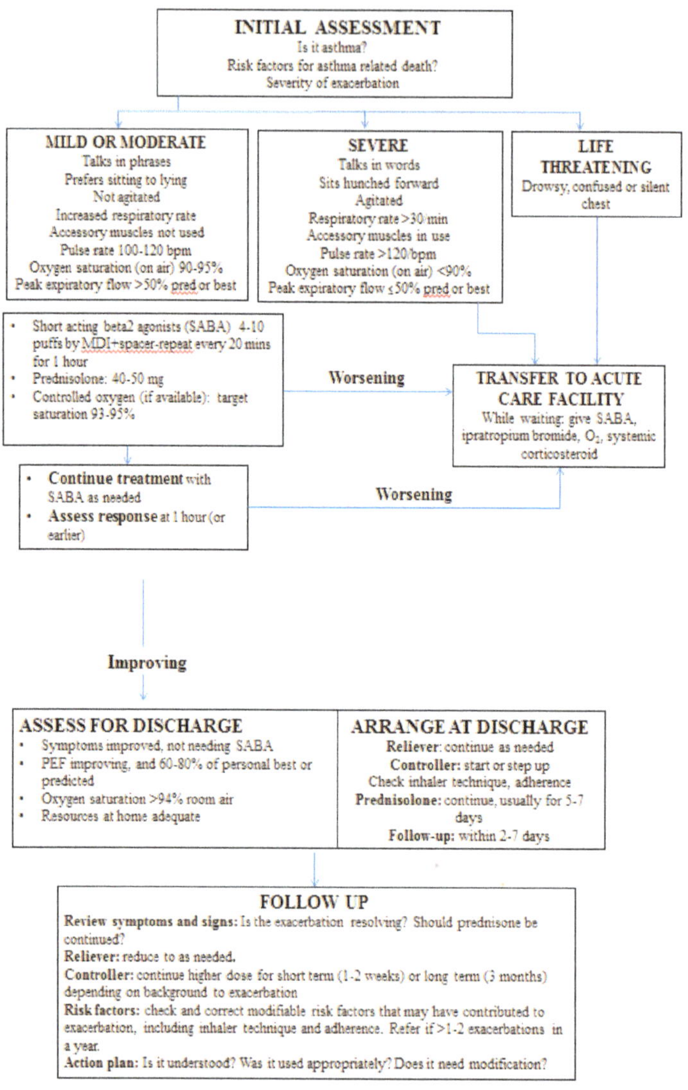

Figure 7. Global Initiative for Asthma (GINA) recommendations for the management of asthma exacerbations in acute care facility. PEF: Peak expiratory flow; FEV_1: Forced expiratory volume in one second; SABA, short acting beta 2 agonists; ICU, Intensive Care Unit.

Further laboratory testing is not necessary for every patient that presents to the emergency department with an exacerbation. Chest radiographs are advised when the clinician needs to exclude conditions such as pneumonia, pneumothorax or atelectasis, but not for all patients. Arterial blood gas analysis should be performed on all patients that are critically ill, and/or are desaturating less than 92% despite treatment [212]. By performing arterial blood gas analysis, the clinician will be able to assess not only hypoxemia and the trend of $PaCO_2$, but also acid base disturbances, such as respiratory acidosis and lactic acidosis which are common on acute severe asthma [213]. Further investigations may include total white blood cell count, to evaluate the potential of infection, levels of brain natriuretic peptide to exclude the presence of congestive heart failure and electrolyte level measurement.

11. Pharmacological and Non-Pharmacological Management

Most current guidelines regarding asthma exacerbations highlight the necessity of supplying the asthma patient with a written plan of action appropriate for their level of control, which will lead to early recognition and management of their exacerbations [1,2]. It is of outmost importance that the patients become educated on when to seek help, during the event of an acute exacerbation. In primary care and further in the emergency department or the hospital ward, a severe asthma attack needs to be identified within a short time period in order for the correct action to be taken. A severe exacerbation of asthma is a life-threatening medical emergency, thus being crucial to transfer the patient to an acute care facility, once such a condition is identified, ensuring the patient's safety. During the transfer, it is required to provide controlled oxygen therapy, inhaled SABA, ipratropium bromide, and systemic corticosteroids. In the emergency department the pharmacological therapy of acute severe asthma should consist of SABA, ipratropium bromide, systemic corticosteroids (oral or iv), controlled oxygen therapy, and the clinician should consider the use of iv magnesium sulfate and high dose ICS [1]. (Figure 7, Table 2)

11.1. *β2-Adrenergic Receptor Agonists*

The cornerstones of acute asthma medication are bronchodilators and especially short acting beta agonists (SABA). It is recommended that in acute severe asthma SABAs are administered repetitively or continuously. These substances activate the β2 adrenoreceptors (β2ARs), which are located mainly on the smooth airway muscle cells, but are also found on other airway cells even on the inflammatory cells. Their very important characteristic is that they have a rapid onset of action, while at the same time being well tolerated, despite high doses. Although the β2 AR agonists are substances known for centuries, the great challenge remains improving their selectivity, in order to benefit from their desired effect, while at the same time reducing their adverse effects. All current asthma guidelines introduce short acting β2 agonists (SABAs), as the first line treatment for acute severe asthma. In the first steps of escalating therapy during an exacerbation, the patient is advised to increase their use "as needed". That is also the recommendation for the primary care setting, as well as for the emergency department, where repeated inhaled administration of SABA is advised. Studies on the efficacy of nebulizers vs. metered dose inhalers (MDIs) have not proven superiority of nebulized administration. In a recent review, nebulized delivery did not improve hospital admission, length of stay in the emergency department or pulmonary function [214]. According to GINA 2018, the preferred method of administration is with strong evidence (Evidence A) pMDI with a spacer [1]. This evidence becomes less strong when referring to severe and near fatal asthma. Although continuous nebulization of SABAs was initially a very promising perspective, several studies and meta-analyses have failed to clearly demonstrate strong evidence on favor of continuous nebulized SABAs for acute asthma. Rodrigo et al. in 2002 performed a systematic review and meta-analysis that showed no difference in respiratory function measured in the first hours of administration or on the rate of hospital admissions [215]. A Cochrane systematic review on the subject, including few more studies, showed significant difference on both respiratory function and hospital admissions, in favor of the continuous use of SABA, while at the same time demonstrating a good tolerance from the patients who did not present more adverse effects with this method of administration [216]. The most commonly used SABA is salbutamol or albuterol as named in the United States, which has an onset of action of less than 10 min and duration of approximately 6 h. Lebalbuterol is a recent addition to the choices of SABAs, with its benefit of a lower than salbutamol dose that provides similar effect. There is currently evidence about its efficacy in acute severe asthma as an intermittent regimen, but not as a continuous nebulization strategy [217,218]. Continuous intravenous infusion of β2 agonists has also been proposed as a therapy, especially in patients who did not respond to intensive bronchodilation. There is no evidence to support the use of intravenous β2 agonists [219,220] or the method of continuous, subcutaneous infusions of terbutaline [221]. Epinephrine has been studied, as a nebulized, subcutaneous, intramuscular and intravenous administration, but, in current guidelines, its use is restricted for acute asthma related with anaphylaxis and angioedema [1,222,223].

11.2. Anticholinergics

Anticholinergic agents act as inhibitors of acetylcholine at the muscarinic cholinergic receptor. Therefore, they inhibit parasympathetic nerve impulses and they produce a beneficial effect in acute asthma, by causing airway smooth muscle relaxation. Furthermore, they enhance β2-agonist-induced bronchodilation via intracellular processes and they prolong their bronchodilator effect [61,224]. The anticholinergic agent used primarily is ipratropium bromide due to its selectivity for airway smooth muscle receptors, which reduces the systemic adverse effects. Their use is included in current guidelines for moderate to severe acute and life-threatening asthma, as well as for patients who show poor response to initial SABA therapy [1,2]. It is not recommended to use anticholinergics as a single therapy for acute asthma. It has been demonstrated that the addition of inhaled ipratropium bromide to therapy with SABAs improve hospitalization rates, relapse rates and are associated with lung function improvement [62–64]. This combination therapy benefit is greater for the patients who present with acute severe asthma and are at a higher risk of hospitalization. There is an increased rate of adverse effects, which are of mild nature, such as mouth dryness and tremor.

11.3. Corticosteroids

Within the asthma setting, it has been well established that inhaled corticosteroids reduce the rates of hospitalization and mortality for patients with asthma [65,225]. In the event of acute exacerbation, there is a different approach of their use. Current recommendations suggest that high dose ICS given within the first hour of the patient's presentation in the emergency department, reduce the rate of hospital admissions, for patients who are not on systemic corticosteroid therapy [1]. Recent evidence however seems to be conflicting regarding their performance without the use of systemic corticosteroids, when rate of hospital admissions or changes in lung function has been studied [226,227].

Systemic corticosteroids, due to their significant anti-inflammatory properties, have a fundamental role in the management of acute asthma, and particularly for patients who present with exacerbation while receiving oral corticosteroids (OCS), or have previous history of exacerbation that required use of OCS. They are also recommended for patients who did not respond to initial SABA therapy with a prolonged effect. Apart from their role against asthma associated inflammation, they seem to increase the number and sensitivity of β-adrenergic receptors, and also restrain the migration and function of eosinophils and other inflammatory cells. On the other hand, their lack of bronchodilatory effects prohibits their use for acute asthma as a monotherapy [74]. A recent multi-center study showed that there is a significant percentage of patients who get admitted to hospital with acute asthma and do not receive systemic corticosteroids, despite the clear suggestion of current guidelines [228]. With regards to the root of administration, intravenous administration seems to not provide additional efficacy to the use of oral therapy [229,230]. Intramuscular regimens seem to be as effective as oral in reducing the risk for relapse [231]. The oral route is better tolerated and preferred, because it is quicker and less expensive. Identifying groups of patients where intravenous administration could be more beneficial is a recent field of study, and guidelines support that they should be considered for patients who may be unable to swallow due to breathlessness, or may not absorb efficiently the medication due to gastro-enteral disturbances, such as vomiting [1]. There is a lack of robust evidence to clarify the superiority of longer or higher dose OCS, thus the literature suggests a 5–7-day regimen of 50 mg prednisolone as a single dose, or 200 mg hydrocortisone in divided doses [1,2,232].

11.4. Magnesium Sulfate

Magnesium has been proven to be an important co-factor in enzymatic reactions and changes of its concentrations may result in different response from the smooth muscles. Hypomagnesemia may cause contraction, whereas hypermagnesemia causes relaxation of the smooth muscles and bronchodilation, possibly through inhibition of calcium influx into the muscles.

Recent recommendations include magnesium sulfate, at dose of 2 g infused over 20 min, as a second line intervention for acute severe asthma exacerbation [1,233]. It has been shown to reduce the rate of hospitalization in adults with FEV_1 of 25–30% at presentation and those who are unresponsive to initial treatment, and have persistent hypoxemia, and correlates with improvement in lung function [234,235]. Its infusion has not been correlated with severe adverse events; it is however contra-indicated for patients with renal insufficiency, hypermagnesemia and myasthenia Gravis. Magnesium has also been tried in its nebulized form for asthma exacerbation, with very few data to support it. A recent systematic review, which examined the efficacy and safety of inhaled administration of magnesium, concluded that, although safe, it has not shown significant benefits when compared with the first line inhaled agents, thus it is not routinely recommended [236]. The current literature is reluctant to fully support the use of magnesium, mainly because of the heterogeneity of the severity of asthma attacks it has been used on in trials, especially in the context of optimized first line treatment with β2-agonists and corticosteroids [237]. A 2014 randomized controlled trial failed to show any evidence of clear benefit in the use of either intravenous or inhaled magnesium [238]. Further prospective trials are necessary to provide accurate evidence on this treatment option.

11.5. Methylxanthines

On the ground of their anti-inflammatory properties, methylxanthines (aminophylline and theophylline) used to be included in the primary treatment for acute asthma. Their poor safety profile, which includes significant side effects, in combination with the inability to provide evidence of improved outcomes, such as improved pulmonary function or rate of hospitalization when given for severe acute asthma, has excluded them from current guidelines [1,239]. A more recent review and meta-analysis, however, has supplied some evidence of aminophylline's efficacy, when combined with other bronchodilators, but more data are needed on this direction [240].

11.6. Leukotriene Modulators

Although leukotriene receptor antagonists (LTRAs) are included as a controller agent in the asthma management, there are limited data on the efficacy of intravenous or oral antileukotriene drugs in acute asthma. Montelukast and zafirlukast were studied on patients with acute asthma and demonstrated some evidence of lung function improvement [241,242]. A review of the literature, however failed to provide robust evidence of the effectiveness of this medication category on lung function or on the outcomes of the patients [243].

11.7. Oxygen Supply

Although asthma exacerbations are not usually accompanied with severe hypoxemia, acute severe asthma often presents with arterial PO_2 derangements, due to extensive V/Q mismatch as explained above. Oxygen should be administered via nasal cannula or mask, with a target of arterial oxygen saturation of 93–95%, or to those patients where saturation monitoring is not available [1]. Although not all guidelines agree on the level of the desirable target saturation, studies have shown that, in severe acute asthma, oxygen therapy with controlled low flow administration, with a target SpO_2, is correlated with better outcomes than the use of per se high flow 100% oxygen delivery, as it has been shown to correlate with increases in $PaCO_2$, as well as with decreased values of PEF [244,245]. There is also some evidence about the use of oxygen driven nebulization with SABAs, because of the pulmonary vasodilation caused by the β2-agonist, which results in increasing perfusion of poorly ventilated areas, thus resulting in deterioration of the V/Q abnormalities [246].

Table 2. Pharmacological management of patients with acute severe exacerbation in the emergency department.

Medication	Dosing	References
Salbutamol (albuterol) solution for nebulization: single dose 2.5 mg/2.5 mL	Continuous nebulization for an hour and re-assess clinical response	[214–221,223]
Ipratropium bromide	Nebulization of 0.5 mg/2.5 mL/4–6 h in combination with salbutamol (same nebulizer)	[61–63,224]
Corticosteroids	Methylprednisolone iv infusion of 40 mg or hydrocortisone iv, 200 mg or oral prednisone 40 mg	[65,225–232]
Magnesium sulfate	Single iv infusion of 2 gr/20 min	[233–238]
Methylxanthines	Not recommended as first line; poor response and potential serious adverse events	[239,240]
Leukotriene receptor antagonists	Single iv infusion of 7–14 mg over 5 min	[241–243]
Epinephrine (adrenaline)	0.3–0.4 mL sc of a 1:1000 (1 mg/mL) solution/20 min for 3 doses in case of no response	[222]
Terbutaline (1 mg/mL)	0.25 mg sc/20 min for 3 doses in case of no response (preferred in pregnancy)	[221,223]
Heliox	Helium/oxygen mixture in a 80:20 or 70:30 ratio	[247–249]

iv, intravenous; sc, subcutaneous.

11.8. Heliox

Heliox is a mixture of helium (70–80%) with oxygen (20–30%). Heliox can be used for severe asthma exacerbations that are unresponsive to standard therapy or in patients having an upper airway obstruction component. Heliox, with density less than air, leads to lower Reynolds number, thus decreasing resistance to airflow under conditions of turbulent flow, as are prominent in the central airways and at the branch points. This effect can potentially decrease the work of breathing and improve ventilation. On the contrary, airflow in smaller airways, which are mainly affected during an asthma exacerbation, will not improve with heliox, as it is typically laminar, depending on gas viscosity rather than density.

Despite the theoretical benefits of heliox, and while a few case series have suggested a beneficial effect in acute asthma, no studies in adults have demonstrated an advantage of heliox above and beyond standard oxygen therapy. In asthma exacerbation either without or with intubation, heliox has not demonstrated consistent benefit [247,248].

Heliox has demonstrated greatest benefit for improving symptoms when used as a nebulizing gas for a beta-2 agonist medication. Benefit is generally seen within minutes after the initiation of therapy [247]. Another study has shown that using heliox as a carrier gas increase gas delivery up to 50% in a mechanical model for both MDIs and nebulizers [249]. Given that its effect is based on the percentage of helium, it should not be administrated to patients requiring $FiO_2 > 40\%$.

11.9. Ketamine

Ketamine is well known drug that has been in use since circa 1960. It is a dissociative anesthetic drug that has the potential to have different actions, depending on the dose used. It may work as a potent analgesic and as an anesthetic agent, but may also have secondary effects as a bronchodilator, while at the same time preserving airway reflexes and sympathetic nervous system tone, with no effects on the cardiovascular system. A dose of 1–2 mg/kg dose has been described as an inductive agent in rapid sequence intubation (RSI) of asthma patients [250]. In doses lower than this it does not have sedative effects, whereas in higher doses it can cause laryngospasm and apnea. Its psychoactive effects make it even less popular for use. In the context of asthma, there are no large randomized trials to examine its effect. There is some evidence of its bronchodilatory effect, especially in mild and moderate asthma exacerbations, and in doses lower than 1 mg/kg, but larger trials would be necessary to establish its role for asthma [251,252].

11.10. Antibiotics

There is no evidence supporting the use of antibiotics per se for severe acute asthma, unless the patient's history and clinical assessment indicate the presence of infection. In a recent retrospective cohort study, it has been demonstrated that, in patients hospitalized with acute asthma and receiving OCS, antibiotic use was associated with longer hospital length of stay and hospital cost, whereas it held similar risk of treatment failure [253]. In a previous study in the US, 60% of the patients who were admitted to hospital with asthma exacerbation, received antibiotics, with no clear indication accompanying this decision [254]. Current guidelines suggest against their use and that they should be considered after optimizing other treatment options and when there is clear evidence of infection [1].

11.11. Non-Invasive Mechanical Ventilation

Although the benefits of non-invasive mechanical ventilation (NIMV) are well recognized in the acute exacerbation of chronic obstructive pulmonary disease and pulmonary edema, its usage for asthma exacerbation remains controversial. Despite the lack of supporting evidence, NIMV is commonly used in patients with severe asthma exacerbation as a mean to obviate the need for intubation and mechanical ventilation and its detrimental effects.

In the absence of clinical guidelines that recommend the use of NIMV for the management of acute asthma, evidence suggests that a trial of NIMV (for one or two hours) may be beneficial for a low risk group of patients [255], particularly those unresponsive to medical therapy. Prolonged trials of NIMV are not recommended. Suggested criteria for an NIMV trial include RR > 25 breaths per minute, heart rate > 110 beats per minute, hypoxemia with PaO_2/FiO_2 ratio greater than 200, hypercapnia with $PaCO_2 < 60$ mmHg, $FEV_1 < 50\%$ less than predicted and use of accessory respiratory muscles. A trial of NIMV should not be undertaken if there is any absolute criterion for endotracheal intubation (respiratory arrest, hemodynamic instability or shock, GSC < 8), excessive respiratory secretions and risk of aspiration, severe agitation and poor patient collaboration and any cause that precludes the right mask fitting (facial surgery) [256].

In a trial of 30 patients who presented to the emergency department with a severe asthma exacerbation that was not responding to inhaled bronchodilator therapy, NIMV was associated with reduction in the rate of hospitalization and increased lung function. Improvements in respiratory rate and dyspnea appear to be influenced by the amount of pressure support above expiratory positive airway pressure (EPAP) provided. The use of NIMV has been associated with reduction in endotracheal intubation, improvement in oxygenation, decrease in carbon dioxide retention, and improvement in airflow obstruction. Studies are controversial regarding the mortality and ICU length stay [86]. NIMV can also be used in the asthmatic patients who are at risk for intubation, following extubation [257].

11.12. Invasive Mechanical Ventilation

The decision to intubate and mechanically ventilate a near-fatal asthma patient is considered a challenging task and should be based primary on a series of clinical evaluations. Major indications for initiation of invasive mechanical ventilation (IMV) are: (1) cardiac arrest; (2) respiratory arrest or bradypnea; (3) respiratory insufficiency with $PaO_2 < 60$ mmHg on 100% FiO_2 and $PaCO_2 > 50$ mmHg; (4) physical exhaustion; and (5) compromised level of consciousness. Relative indications for IMV are: (1) hypercapnia $PaCO_2 > 50$ mmHg or $PaCO_2$ increased by 5 mmHg per hour; (2) worsening respiratory acidosis;, (3) inability to treat patient appropriately; (4) failure to improve with proper therapy; and (5) clinical signs of deterioration and respiratory fatigue such as tachypnoea of >40 breaths per minute, severe hypoxemic respiratory insufficiency, hemodynamic instability, paradoxical thoracic movement, and silent chest [258].

The decision to intubate and mechanically ventilate a patient with acute asthma exacerbation is a clinical one and may be made urgently. When the clinician decides that respiratory failure is progressing, and is unlikely to be reversed by further pharmacologic therapy, intubation should be performed as quickly as possible by a skilled intensivist or anesthesiologist, who has extensive experience in intubation and airway management, using rapid sequence intubation (RSI) protocol suitable for asthmatic patients (good preparation, sufficient pre-oxygenation, suitable induction to anesthesia agents suitable for asthma, and placement of the endotracheal tube) [259]. Regarding the preferred method of intubation, oral endotracheal intubation is preferred, although the literature also includes awake nasotracheal intubation, which may be complicated by the fact that many asthmatic patients also have nasal polyps [203]. Additionally, oral intubation allows the use of an endotracheal tube of a larger diameter, facilitating secretion removal and bronchoscopy, if needed, while at the same time decreasing inspiratory airway resistance. It should be noted that unlike other conditions in which intubation and mechanical ventilation can solve problems, the dynamic hyperinflation that mechanical ventilation can create or even exacerbate can have devastating consequences for a severe asthmatic patient, such as cardiovascular collapse and/or barotrauma and ventilator induced lung injury. Therefore, there are certain considerations to be made before and during RSI. During RSI in such patients one should anticipate rapid oxygen desaturation despite maximal effort at pre-oxygenation especially in those patients who do not achieve a SpO_2 above 93%, so adequate pre-oxygenation is advised. Bag mask ventilation should be done using small tidal volume and high inspiratory flow rate with a prolonged expiratory phase, attempting with this way to mimic the approach used during mechanical ventilation. Excessive mag mask ventilation should be avoided because of the risk of pneumothorax [260,261]. Manipulation of the airway can cause laryngospasm and worsening of bronchoconstriction, so one could consider the use of atropine to attenuate vagal reflexes [203]. The literature suggests the bolus use of intravenous ketamine for RSI taking advantage of its bronchodilatory effect, while propofol is also considered a safe approach. Opiates and barbiturates should be avoided due to the risk of histamine release that can exacerbate bronchoconstriction [262]. If muscle relaxants are needed, non-depolarizing muscle relaxants (except maybe atracurium and mivacurium) and succinylcholine are suitable in asthmatic patients [263].

11.13. Goals of Mechanical Ventilation

Near fatal asthma is characterized by severe dynamic hyperinflation of the lung with severe respiratory and circulatory consequences. The aim of mechanical ventilation is to maintain adequate oxygenation, to reduce the work of breathing and to prevent and confront further hyperinflation without any circulatory compromise or ventilator induced lung injury [264]. The intubation and post-intubation period is often complicated with severe cardio-respiratory derangement. Hypotension, the most common post-intubation complication, may be caused due to dynamic hyperinflation and auto-PEEP, and can be aggravated by dehydration, sedatives and neuromuscular blocking agents. Arrhythmias, barotraumas, laryngospasm or even seizures have also characterized the post-intubation period [265,266]. Phenomena such as hypercapnia, hypoxemia and acidemia, as well as ventilatory lung injury and life threatening pneumotrauma (pneumothorax and pneumo-mediastinum), may also complicate the post-intubation period. Reasons for the aforementioned may be the severity and non-responsiveness of the disease, but may also be the result of inadequate sedation or patient–ventilator desynchrony. Wrong and harmful initial ventilator settings may also result in providing too little or too excessive minute ventilation, potentially deteriorating the already very fragile asthmatic patient [267].

Management of the asthmatic patient post intubation starts with ensuring adequate sedation in order to achieve the desirable patient–ventilator synchronization. Sedation and analgesia will also decrease the metabolic rate, oxygen consumption and carbon dioxide production. Dexmedetominide, propofol and remifentanyl are the appropriate drugs for sedation and analgesia. Their usage has been associated with shorter length of ICU stay, shorter duration of mechanical ventilation and improved long term neurocognitive outcomes when compared to benzodiazepines [266,268]. It is important to use agents that accomplish deep sedation, while at the same time allow rapid awakening, should the patient improve quickly, which is common in the asthma cases (Table 3).

Table 3. Sedation, analgesia and paralysis in patients with acute severe asthma exacerbation requiring intubation.

Medication	Dosing	Side Effects	References
Midazolam	0.03–0.1 mg/kg bolus iv infusion, followed by an infusion of 3–10 mg/h	Hypotension	[268,269]
Propofol	Infusion of 60–80 mg/min initially, up to 2 mg/kg. Continue with iv infusion of 5–10 mg/kg/h as needed, and for sedation on mechanical ventilation 1–4 mg/kg/h	Hypotension, seizures, hyperlipidemia	[262,268]
Fentanyl	50–100 μg/kg bolus iv infusion, followed by infusion of 50–100 μg/h	Bradycardia, histamine release	[268,269]
Remifentanyl	Initial dose of 1 μg/kg iv infusion, followed by an infusion of 0.25–0.5 μg/kg/min (up to 2 μg/kg/min)	Bradycardia, hypotension	[268,269]
Ketamine	1 mg/mL bolus iv infusion, followed by a maintenance infusion of 0.1–0.5 mg/min	Sympatheticomimetic effects, delirium	[250–252]
Dexmedetomidine	Initial loading dose of 1 μg/kg, iv over 10–30 min, followed by a maintenance infusion of 0.2–0.7 μg/kg/h	Hypotension, bradycardia	[68,269]
Cis-atracurium	0.1–0.2 mg/kg bolus iv infusion, followed by infusion in a rate of 3 μg/kg/min (up to 10 μg/mL/min)	Bronchospasm	[269,270]

Patients with severe asthma with persistently dangerous levels of hypercapnia and arterial hypoxemia, and extreme patient–ventilatory asynchrony may require paralysis in addition to sedation. The preferred paralytic, non-depolarizing agent is cis-atracurium, as it is eliminated by esterase degradation and spontaneous breakdown in the serum. Paralytic agents can be administered either intermittently through bolus injections, or by continuous intravascular infusion. Its duration must be as short as possible, because concomitant use of intravascular corticosteroids and paralytic neuromuscular agents increases the incidence of critical illness myopathy [269,270].

To avoid the hemodynamic effects of dynamic hyperinflation, once the patient is intubated, it is advised to perform a brief discontinuation (60–90 s) from the ventilation (apnea test), a slowly bagged ventilation and to administer fluids (1–2 L or more) and vasopressors. Although there is no clear evidence to support the volume-preset over the pressure-preset modes, the preferred ventilator modes for the asthmatic patient are the volume-limited ones [263]. Barotrauma seems to occur regardless of the mode of ventilation. Volume-limited modes of ventilation are usually used for near death asthmatic patients at their entrance in the ICU. It is essential to closely monitor the Peak inspiratory and Plateau pressures, to early detect any change in resistance and compliance, and this is easily achievable when using volume modes (Figure 8). Although high inspiratory flow rates of 80 L/min up to 100 L/min and square waveforms shorten inspiratory time and increase expiration time, thus reducing hyperinflation, it has been shown that this may not have a significant impact to the degree of hyperinflation once the minute ventilation has been limited by high peak inspiratory pressure [271]. Minute ventilation should be set at a level of less than 115 mL/kg/min (less than 10 L/min) with a respiratory rate of 10–12 breaths/min and a prolonged expiratory time by decreasing I:E ratio (1:3 or 1:4 up to 1:5) [263,266].

Tuxen and Lane showed a remarkable increase in hyperinflation when using higher levels of minute ventilation [120]. The fraction of inspired oxygen (FIO_2) should be titrated to maintain the pulse oxygen saturation (SpO_2) above 90% (up to 94%) or the arterial oxygen tension (PaO_2) above 60 mmHg. One should avoid SpO_2 > 96% due to oxygen toxicity (Table 4).

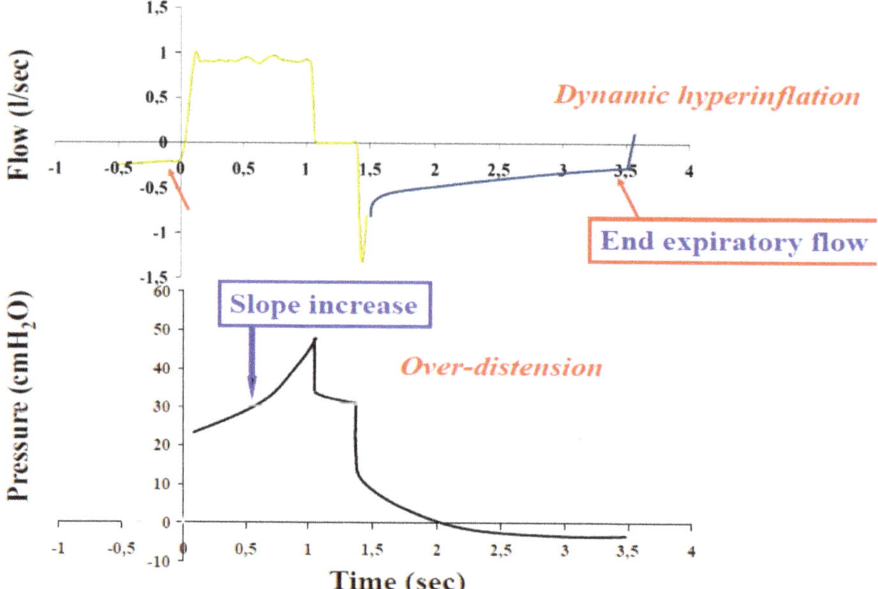

Figure 8. Flow time tracing of a patient with persistence of flow at the end of expiration which indicates dynamic hyperinflation and pressure time tracing with a slope increase indicative of over-distension.

Table 4. Initial ventilator settings in intubated patients with acute severe asthma exacerbation.

Mode	Settings
Tidal volume	6 mL/kg ideal bodyweight
Respiratory rate	8–10/min
Minute ventilation	<10 L/min
Inspiratory flow rate	60–80 L/min
Inspiratory to expiratory ratio	>1:3
Inspiratory wave form	Decelerated waveform
Expiratory time	4–5 s
Plateau pressure	<30 cm H_2O
PEEP	0 cm H_2O
FiO_2	100% initially and titrate to maintain SaO_2 > 90%

SaO_2: Oxygen saturation; Peep: positive end expiratory pressure.

Limited data exist about the use of external PEEP when ventilating a patient with severe asthma. The use of progressively higher external PEEP from 5 to 15 cmH_2O has been shown to have a deteriorating effect both in respiratory (deterioration of the end-inspiratory volume, the functional residual capacity and plateau pressure) and circulatory system (decrease of systolic arterial pressure and cardiac output) [271]. In one prospective study of patients undergoing control mode of ventilation, external PEEP worsened hyperinflation and had serious hemodynamic effects by worsening gas trapping [272]. On the other hand, other studies have shown that the application of external PEEP, may produce a paradoxical lung deflation by reducing lung volumes and airway pressures and increasing lung homogeneity [273]. In the case of assist mode of mechanical ventilation, the application of external PEEP at a value less than 80% of the intrinsic PEEP, or 5 cm H_2O if intrinsic PEEP is <10 cm H_2O can counterbalance the endogenous peep and reduce the work of breathing [274]. A trial of stepwise increase in PEEP can be used and terminated when indications of worsening of dynamic hyperinflation it is shown.

11.14. Permissive Hypercapnia

Hypercapnia is a common fact during mechanical ventilation of asthmatic patients. $PaCO_2$ levels up to 60 mmHg and pH values less than 7.20 are common on the first day of mechanical ventilation even with increased minute ventilation. The term permissive hypercapnia is a ventilating strategy that can be applied to mechanically ventilated asthma patients, that emphasizes on giving priority to the reduction of hyperinflation rather than normal minute ventilation. The reduction of minute ventilation through reduction of tidal volume and respiratory rate is used to decrease pulmonary hyperinflation. $PaCO_2$ levels should rise gradually during mechanical ventilation rather than rapidly, preferably at a rate of <10 mmHg per hour or even slower if the $PaCO_2$ exceeds 80 mmHg. Generally, a pH level of 7.20–7.25 is accepted, but the literature has failed to demonstrate a benefit from using alcalotic agents, such as bicarbonate infusion to accomplish that [274].

11.15. Additional and Unconventional Therapies for Acute Severe Asthma

11.15.1. Oxygen Delivery by High Flow Nasal Canula

Oxygen delivery via high flow nasal canula (HFNC) can be used to hypoxemic patients who are not expected to respond to conventional therapies. HFNC with flow up to 60 L/min of warmed and humidified oxygen, decreases inspiratory resistance, as well as the work of breathing, can wash out carbon dioxide, thus decreasing the anatomic dead space and may also produce a positive end expiratory pressure (up to 5 mmHg) by increasing the end expiratory lung volume. The role of HFNC in asthmatic adults is unknown. Studies in children have shown that its use reduces respiratory distress in moderate and severe asthma exacerbations and also reduces the need for intubation [275,276].

11.15.2. Extracorporeal Life Support (ECLS)

Extracorporeal membrane oxygenation (ECMO) is an invasive therapy, in which oxygenation and carbon dioxide removal are performed through an artificial membrane. Although evidence based on clinical trials for the use of ECMO in asthmatic patients is lacking [277,278], there is growing evidence on the subject, supporting the use of ECLS for patients receiving mechanical ventilation due to an asthmatic exacerbation. A 2009 review by Mikkelsen et al. has demonstrated that, when ECLS is used for status asthmaticus, it correlates with better outcomes in comparison to its use for other causes of respiratory failure [279]. In this study, they used data from the multicenter Extracorporeal Life Support Organization (ELSO), but included only a small number of patients. In 2017, there was another review of the same database, confirming that the use of ECMO is an acceptable option, and resulted in acceptable survival rates, although it is necessary to understand and reduce the ECMO related complications [280]. Di Lascio et al., using ECMO for asthmatic patients receiving IMV, showed that it could provide adjunctive pulmonary support for patients who remain severely acidotic and hypercapnic despite aggressive conventional therapy [281]. The writers conclude that ECMO should be considered as an early treatment in patients with status asthmaticus whose gas exchange is not satisfactory despite using conventional therapy, aiming to provide adequate gas change and to prevent ventilator induced lung injury.

A modified ECMO technique such as extracorporeal carbon dioxide removal ($ECCO_2R$) may also play an important role in severe asthmatic patient in mechanical ventilation. In a difficult to safely ventilate asthmatic patient, due to extremely high airway pressures, hypoventilation and persistent severe respiratory acidemia are common issues. The usage of $ECCO_2R$, considering the reversibility of the pathophysiology of asthma, provide the opportunity for more protective ventilation and more time for the bronchodilator agents to act and reverse inflammation and hyperinflation. There is no sufficient evidence to support a clear role of this technique in asthmatic patients, but there seems to be a growing interest on the subject [282,283]. Schneider et al. even presented a case where $ECCO_2R$ was used in an "awake" patient with a near fatal asthma attack, refractory to the use of pharmacological intervention and NIMV, resulting in avoidance of intubation [284]. However, more data are needed to establish an indication for this intervention in the context of an acute severe asthma exacerbation.

11.15.3. Anesthetic Agents

Some inhalational anesthetic agents such as halothane, isoflurane and sevoflurane act as bronchodilators, probably not only through a direct relaxation effect on airway smooth muscles but also by attenuating cholinergic tone [285,286]. This characteristic may have favorable effects in patients with refractory to conventional and optimized bronchodilatory therapy. Case report studies have indicated a positive effectiveness with halothane, but also with isoflurane and sevoflurane but with several limitations. Hypotension, myocardial depression, increased ventricular irritability especially in the presence of acidosis, beta-agonists and theophylline have been reported [287–289]. In addition, factors such as the expense of inhalational treatment, the need of a bedside anesthesiologist, the practical issues concerning the equipment for delivering the inhalational agents, the short time of duration of bronchodilation (immediate return of bronchoconstriction after discontinuation), and, finally, the absence of randomized trials to evaluate and confirm their efficacy in near-death adult asthmatic patients make the usage of anesthetic agents a last resort as a non- conventional bronchodilatory therapy for refractory near death asthma exacerbations [290,291].

11.15.4. Enoximone

Enoximone is an intravenous bronchodilatory agent that can be used in severe asthma exacerbation in adults. Enoximone, a selective phosphodiasterase inhibitor III, was tested in a study by Beute et al. on eight patients with status asthmaticus, six of whom had a respiratory arrest or hypercapnia [292]. The bronchodilatory effect was immediate. Even if the intravenous administration bypasses inhalation incapability in severe asthma, and no side-effects were observed in this study, phosphodiesterase inhibitors in general are associated with ventricular and atrial arrhythmias, hypotension, and hepatotoxicity. Further studies are needed to confirm enoximone efficacy and safety in patients with acute exacerbations of asthma that are refractory to conventional therapies.

12. Prognosis

Asthmatic patients who require mechanical ventilation, not only have increased hospital mortality (7%), but also long-term mortality [40,293]. Most of the long-term mortality is attributed to recurrent asthma [294]. Psychological disturbances such as depression and denial are also common features of asthmatic patients who survived a near fatal episode. Anxiety seems to be more common among close family members than the patients themselves [295]. Smoking cessation is one of the recognized factors that improves survival [151].

13. Prevention and Risk Reduction

GINA recommends that all adults and adolescents with asthma should receive ICS-containing controller treatment, either as-needed (in mild asthma) or daily, in order to reduce their risk of serious exacerbations and to control symptoms, [1] (Figure 9). Asthma treatment should be optimized in patients continuing having poor symptom control and/or exacerbations, even though Step 4 and Step 5 treatments and contributing factors should be assessed, in order to treat modifiable risk factors that compromise disease stability (smoking, environmental exposures, allergen exposure (if sensitized on skin prick testing or specific IgE), and medications such as beta-blockers and NSAIDs) (Table 5). It is imperative to optimize the inhaler technique and adherence to treatment, as well as overuse of SABAs, and medication side effects. Furthermore, comorbidities should be assessed including obesity,

GERD, chronic rhinosinusitis, obstructive sleep apnea, anxiety, depression, and social difficulties. Non-pharmacological interventions (e.g., smoking cessation, exercise, weight loss, mucus clearance, and influenza vaccination) should also be recommended where indicated.

If the problems continue after having optimized all the above parameters, patients should refer to a specialist center for phenotypic assessment and consideration of add-on therapy including biologics (Figure 10). The prevalence of severe, refractory asthma is generally estimated to be 5–10% of the total asthma population [77,151]. It is important to distinguish between asthma that is difficult to control and asthma that is truly severe. Severe asthma is defined by the joint European Respiratory Society/American Thoracic Society (ERS/ATS) guidelines according to the following criteria [151]:

- Requirement for treatment with high-dose inhaled corticosteroids (ICS) and a second controller (and/or systemic corticosteroids) to maintain control.
- Refractory to the treatment mentioned above.
- Incomplete management of comorbidities such as severe sinus disease or obesity.

The GINA 2019 guidelines for adolescents and adults with difficult-to-treat and severe asthma [77] recommend that assessment of the severe asthma phenotype should be done during high dose ICS treatment (or lowest possible dose of OCS), and biological treatment should be chosen accordingly (Figure 8). Where relevant, test for parasitic infection should precede and be treated if present, before commencing Type 2 targeted treatment. The currently approved add-on biological treatments for severe asthma include anti-IgE treatment for severe allergic asthma (omalizumab), anti-IL5 or anti-IL5R for severe eosinophilic (mepolizumab, benralizumab, and reslizumab), and anti-IL4R for severe eosinophilic/Type 2 asthma or patients requiring maintenance OCS asthma (dupilumab) (Table 6).

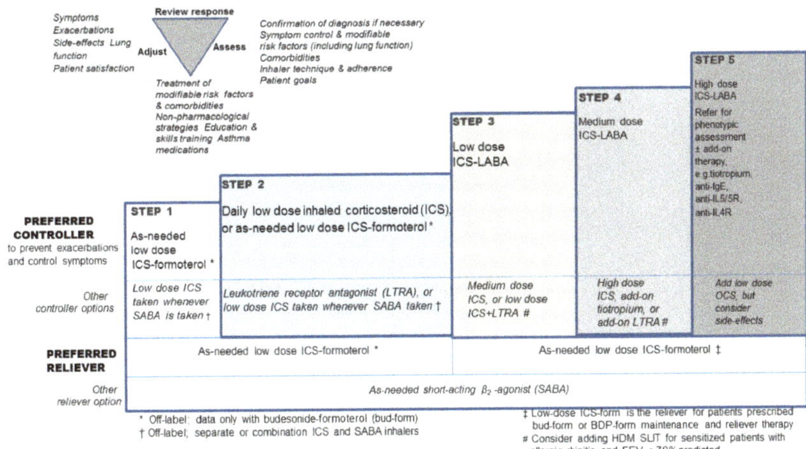

Figure 9. Personalized management for adults and adolescents to control symptoms and minimize future risk [1].

Table 5. Modifiable risk factors that have to be treated in order to reduce exacerbations.

Risk Factor	Treatment Strategy	Evidence
Any patient with 1 risk factor for exacerbations (including poor symptom control)	• Ensure patient is prescribed an ICS-containing controller	A
	• Ensure patient has a written action plan appropriate for their health literacy	A
	• Review patient more frequently than low-risk patients	A
	• Check inhaler technique and adherence frequently	A
≥1 severe exacerbation in last year	• Consider alternative controller regimens to reduce exacerbation risk, e.g., ICS-formoterol maintenance and reliever regimen	A
	• Consider stepping up treatment if no modifiable risk factors	A
	• Identify any avoidable triggers for exacerbations	C
Exposure to tobacco smoke	• Encourage smoking cessation by patient/family; provide advice and resources	A
	• Consider higher dose of ICS if asthma poorly-controlled	B
Low FEV_1, especially if <60% predicted	• Consider trial of 3 months of treatment with high-dose ICS and/or 2 weeks of OCS	B
	• Exclude other lung disease, e.g., COPD	D
	• Refer for expert advice if no improvement	D
Obesity	• Strategies for weight reduction	B
	• Distinguish asthma symptoms from symptoms due to deconditioning, mechanical restriction, and/or sleep apnoea	D
Major psychological problems	• Arrange mental health assessment	D
	• Help patient to distinguish between symptoms of anxiety and asthma; provide advice about management of panic attacks	D
Major socioeconomic problems	• Identify most cost-effective ICS-based regimen	D
Confirmed food allergy	• Appropriate food avoidance; injectable epinephrine	A
Allergen exposure if sensitized	• Consider trial of simple avoidance strategies; consider cost	C
	• Consider step up of controller treatment	D
	• Consider adding SLIT in symptomatic adult HDM-sensitive patients with allergic rhinitis despite ICS, provided FEV1 is >70% predicted	B
Allergen exposure if sensitized	• Increase ICS dose independent of level of symptom control	A

FEV_1, forced expiratory volume in 1 s; HDM, house dust mite; ICS, inhaled corticosteroids; OCS, oral corticosteroids; SLIT, sublingual immunotherapy.

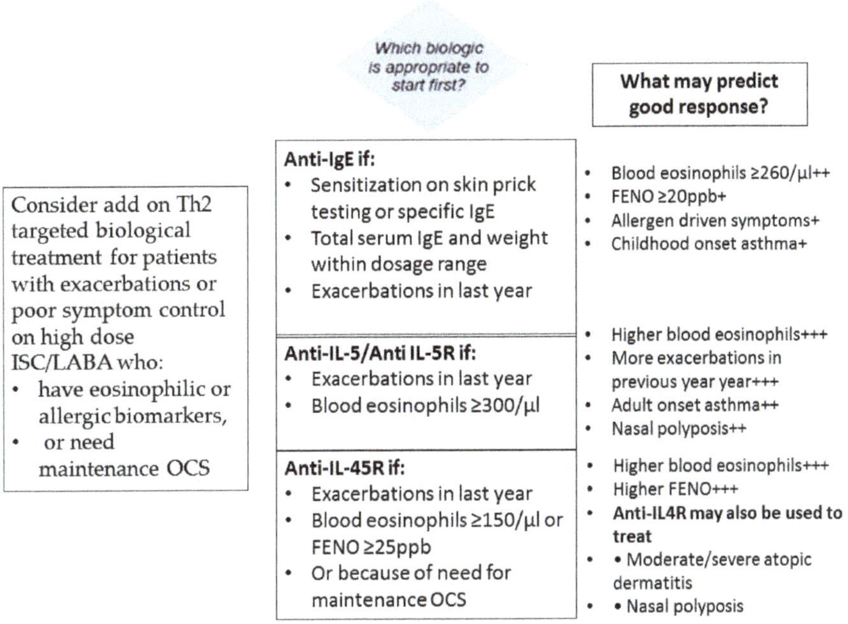

Which biologic is appropriate to start first?

What may predict good response?

Consider add on Th2 targeted biological treatment for patients with exacerbations or poor symptom control on high dose ISC/LABA who:
- have eosinophilic or allergic biomarkers,
- or need maintenance OCS

Anti-IgE if:
- Sensitization on skin prick testing or specific IgE
- Total serum IgE and weight within dosage range
- Exacerbations in last year

- Blood eosinophils ≥260/µl++
- FENO ≥20ppb+
- Allergen driven symptoms+
- Childhood onset asthma+

Anti-IL-5/Anti IL-5R if:
- Exacerbations in last year
- Blood eosinophils ≥300/µl

- Higher blood eosinophils+++
- More exacerbations in previous year year+++
- Adult onset asthma++
- Nasal polyposis++

Anti-IL-45R if:
- Exacerbations in last year
- Blood eosinophils ≥150/µl or FENO ≥25ppb
- Or because of need for maintenance OCS

- Higher blood eosinophils+++
- Higher FENO+++
- **Anti-IL4R may also be used to treat**
- • Moderate/severe atopic dermatitis
- • Nasal polyposis

Figure 10. Criteria for the choice of biologic as add on treatment in Th2 driven severe asthma.

Table 6. Currently available biologics: indications and adverse effects.

Medication	Use	Adverse Effects
Anti-IgE (omalizumab, SC, ≥6 years)	An add-on option for patients with severe allergic asthma uncontrolled on high dose ICS-LABA. elf-administration may be permitted	Reactions at the site of injection are common but minor. Anaphylaxis is rare.
Anti-IL5/anti-IL5R (anti-IL5 mepolizumab (SC, ≥12 or ≥6 years), reslizumab (IV, ≥18 years) or anti-IL5 receptor benralizumab (SC, ≥12 years))	Add-on options for patients with severe eosinophilic asthma uncontrolled on high dose ICS-LABA	Headache and reactions at injection site are common but minor.
Anti-IL4R (dupilumab, SC, ≥12 years)	An add-on option for patients with severe eosinophilic/Type 2 asthma uncontrolled on high dose ICS-LABA, or requiring maintenance OCS. It is also approved for treatment of moderate-severe atopic dermatitis. Self-administration may be permitted	Reactions at injection site are common but minor. Blood eosinophilia occurs in 4–13% of patients.

14. Conclusions

Severe asthma exacerbations are a major cause of disease morbidity, functional impairment, increased healthcare costs, and increased risk of mortality. Asthma patients experience exacerbations irrespective of underlying disease severity, phenotype, or despite optimal guideline-directed treatment, as a result of the ongoing inflammatory processes and loss of the disease control. Patients with frequent emergency department visits, patients requiring hospitalization, and, more importantly, patients intubated for an asthma exacerbation are at significantly increased risk for future severe exacerbations. It is evident that prevention of exacerbations remains a major unmet need in asthma management. The identification of patients at risk to have severe exacerbations is of paramount importance. Patient education and written plans of management, control of triggering/risk factors and co-morbid conditions, monitoring of asthma control and pulmonary function as well as optimal pharmacotherapy are needed to prevent and/or decrease exacerbations. A better understanding of the pathogenesis of asthma exacerbations will ultimately lead to better strategies and the development of novel treatments in the pursuit of preventing and treating severe asthma exacerbations.

Author Contributions: Conceptualization: N.R.; Literature search and data extraction: E.K. (Eirini Kostakou), E.K. (Evangelos Kaniaris), and N.R.; Writing—Original Draft Preparation: I.K., E.K. (Evangelos Kaniaris), and N.R.; Writing, Review and Editing: E.K. (Eirini Kostakou), E.K. (Evangelos Kaniaris), E.F., P.K., E.T., I.V., and N.R.; and Supervision: A.K., N.K, and N.R.

Conflicts of Interest: The authors declare no conflict of interest.

References

1. Global Initiative for Asthma (GINA). Global Strategy for Asthma Management and Prevention (2019 Update). Available online: http://search.ebscohost.com/login.aspx?direct=true&db=cin20&A.N.=118972966&site=ehost-live (accessed on 6 August 2019).
2. Teach, S.J.; Gill, M.A.; Togias, A.; Sorkness, C.A.; Arbes, S.J., Jr.; Calatroni, A.; Wildfire, J.J.; Gergen, P.J.; Cohen, R.T.; Pongracic, J.A.; et al. Preseasonal treatment with either omalizumab or an inhaled corticosteroid boost to prevent fall asthma exacerbations. *J. Allergy Clin. Immunol.* **2015**, *136*, 1476–1485. [CrossRef] [PubMed]
3. Trasande, L.; Thurston, G.D. The role of air pollution in asthma and other pediatric morbidities. *J. Allergy Clin. Immunol.* **2005**, *115*, 689–699. [CrossRef] [PubMed]
4. Rosser, F.; Brehm, J.M.; Forno, E.; Acosta-Pérez, E.; Kurland, K.; Canino, G.; Celedón, J.C. Proximity to a major road, vitamin D insufficiency, and severe asthma exacerbations in Puerto Rican children. *Am. J. Respir. Crit. Care Med.* **2014**, *190*, 1190–1193. [CrossRef] [PubMed]
5. Shmool, J.L.; Kubzansky, L.D.; Newman, O.D.; Spengler, J.; Shepard, P.; Clougherty, J.E. Social stressors and air pollution across New York City communities: A spatial approach for assessing correlations among multiple exposures. *Environ. Health* **2014**, *13*, 91. [CrossRef] [PubMed]
6. Johnston, S.L.; Pattemore, P.K.; Sanderson, G.; Smith, S.; Lampe, F.; Josephs, L.; Symington, P.; O'Toole, S.; Myint, S.H.; Tyrrell, D.A.J.; et al. Community study of role of viral infections in exacerbations of asthma in 9–11 year old children. *BMJ* **1995**, *310*, 1225–1229. [CrossRef] [PubMed]
7. Jackson, D.J.; Johnston, S.L. The role of viruses in acute exacerbations of asthma. *J. Allergy Clin. Immunol.* **2010**, *125*, 1178–1187. [CrossRef] [PubMed]
8. Jayasinghe, H.; Kopsaftis, Z.; Carson, K. Asthma Bronchiale and Exercise-Induced Bronchoconstriction. *Respiration* **2015**, *89*, 505–512. [CrossRef] [PubMed]
9. D'Amato, M.; Molino, A.; Calabrese, G.; Cecchi, L.; Annesi-Maesano, I.; D'Amato, G. The impact of cold on the respiratory tract and its consequences to respiratory health. *Clin. Transl. Allergy* **2018**, *8*, 20. [CrossRef]
10. Berns, S.H.; Halm, E.A.; Sampson, H.A.; Sicherer, S.H.; Busse, P.J.; Wisnivesky, J.P. Food allergy as a risk factor for asthma morbidity in adults. *J. Asthma* **2007**, *44*, 377–381. [CrossRef] [PubMed]
11. Vogel, N.M.; Katz, H.T.; Lopez, R.; Lang, D.M. Food allergy is associated with potentially fatal childhood asthma. *J. Asthma* **2008**, *45*, 862–866. [CrossRef]
12. Williams, W.R. Asthma exacerbation by aspirin and chemical additives: Use of a nucleotide template model to investigate potential mechanisms. *Gen. Physiol. Biophys.* **2018**, *37*, 461–468. [CrossRef] [PubMed]
13. Lee, H.Y.; Ye, Y.M.; Kim, S.H.; Ban, G.Y.; Kim, S.C.; Kim, J.H.; Shin, Y.S.; Park, H.S. Identification of phenotypic clusters of nonsteroidal anti-inflammatory drugs exacerbated respiratory disease. *Allergy* **2017**, *72*, 616–626. [CrossRef] [PubMed]
14. Ledford, D.K.; Wenzel, S.E.; Lockey, R.F. Aspirin or other nonsteroidal inflammatory agent exacerbated asthma. *J. Allergy Clin. Immunol. Pract.* **2014**, *2*, 653–657. [CrossRef] [PubMed]
15. Plourde, A.; Lavoie, K.L.; Raddatz, C.; Bacon, S.L. Effects of acute psychological stress induced in laboratory on physiological responses in asthma populations: A systematic review. *Respir. Med.* **2017**, *127*, 21–32. [CrossRef] [PubMed]
16. Lavoie, K.L.; Cartier, A.; Labrecque, M.; Bacon, S.L.; Lemière, C.; Malo, J.L.; Lacoste, G.; Barone, S.; Verrier, P.; Ditto, B. Are psychiatric disorders associated with worse asthma control and quality of life in asthma patients? *Respir. Med.* **2005**, *99*, 1249–1257. [CrossRef] [PubMed]
17. O'Byrne, P.M.; Inman, M.D. Bronchial hyperresponsiveness. *Chest* **2003**, *123*, 411S–416S. [CrossRef] [PubMed]

18. Wills-Karp, M. Immunologic basis of antigen-induced airway hyperresponsiveness. *Annu. Rev. Immunol.* **1999**, *17*, 255–281. [CrossRef] [PubMed]
19. Gauvreau, G.M.; El-Gammal, A.I.; O'Byrne, P.M. Allergen-induced airway responses. *Eur. Respir. J.* **2015**, *46*, 819–831. [CrossRef]
20. Laprise, C.; Laviolette, M.; Boutet, M.; Boulet, L.P. Asymptomatic airway hyperresponsiveness: Relationships with airway inflammation and remodelling. *Eur. Respir. J.* **1999**, *14*, 63–73. [CrossRef]
21. Leigh, R.; Ellis, R.; Wattie, J.; Southam, D.S.; De Hoogh, M.; Gauldie, J.; O'Byrne, P.M.; Inman, M.D. Dysfunction and remodeling of the mouse airway persist after resolution of acute allergen-induced airway inflammation. *Am. J. Respir. Cell Mol. Biol.* **2002**, *27*, 526–535. [CrossRef]
22. Southam, D.S.; Ellis, R.; Wattie, J.; Inman, M.D. Components of airway hyperresponsiveness and their associations with inflammation and remodeling in mice. *J. Allergy Clin. Immunol.* **2007**, *119*, 848–854. [CrossRef] [PubMed]
23. Leigh, R.; Ellis, R.; Wattie, J.N.; Hirota, J.A.; Matthaei, K.I.; Foster, P.S.; O'Byrne, P.M.; Inman, M.D. Type 2 cytokines in the pathogenesis of sustained airway dysfunction and airway remodeling in mice. *Am. J. Respir. Crit. Care Med.* **2004**, *169*, 860–867. [CrossRef] [PubMed]
24. Brożek, J.L.; Bousquet, J.; Agache, I.; Agarwal, A.; Bachert, C.; Bosnic-Anticevich, S.; Brignardello-Petersen, R.; Canonica, G.W.; Casale, T.; Chavannes, N.H.; et al. Allergic Rhinitis and its Impact on Asthma (ARIA) guidelines-2016 revision. *J. Allergy Clin. Immunol.* **2017**, *140*, 950–958. [CrossRef] [PubMed]
25. Dixon, A.E.; Kaminsky, D.A.; Holbrook, J.T.; Wise, R.A.; Shade, D.M.; Irvin, C.G. Allergic rhinitis and sinusitis in asthma: Differential effects on symptoms and pulmonary function. *Chest* **2006**, *130*, 429–435. [CrossRef] [PubMed]
26. Martínez-Rivera, C.; Crespo, A.; Pinedo-Sierra, C.; García-Rivero, J.L.; Pallarés-Sanmartín, A.; Marina-Malanda, N.; Pascual-Erquicia, S.; Padilla, A.; Mayoralas-Alises, S.; Plaza, V.; et al. Mucus hypersecretion in asthma is associated with rhinosinusitis, polyps and exacerbations. *Respir. Med.* **2018**, *135*, 22–28. [CrossRef] [PubMed]
27. Ayres, J.G.; Miles, J.F. Oesophageal reflux and asthma. *Eur. Respir. J.* **1996**, *9*, 1073–1078. [CrossRef] [PubMed]
28. Pereira Vega, A.; Sánchez Ramos, J.L.; Maldonado Pérez, J.A.; Alvarez Gutierrez, F.J.; Ignacio García, J.M.; Vázquez Oliva, R.; Romero, P.P.; Bravo, N.J.M.; Sánchez, R.I.; Gil, M.F. Variability in the prevalence of premenstrual asthma. *Eur. Respir. J.* **2010**, *35*, 980–986. [CrossRef] [PubMed]
29. Martinez-Moragón, E.; Plaza, V.; Serrano, J.; Picado, C.; Galdiz, J.B.; López-Viña, A.; Sanchis, J. Near-fatal asthma related to menstruation. *J. Allergy Clin. Immunol.* **2004**, *113*, 242–244. [CrossRef]
30. Cohen, J.M.; Bateman, B.T.; Huybrechts, K.F.; Mogun, H.; Yland, J.; Schatz, M.; Wurst, K.E.; Hernandez-Diaz, S. Poorly Controlled Asthma During Pregnancy Remains Common in the United States. *J. Allergy Clin. Immunol. Pract* **2019**. [CrossRef]
31. To, T.; Feldman, L.Y.; Zhu, J.; Gershon, A.S. Asthma health services utilisation before, during and after pregnancy: A population-based cohort study. *Eur. Respir. J.* **2018**, *51*, 1800209. [CrossRef]
32. British Thoracic Society; Scottish Intercollegiate Guidelines Network. *British Guideline on the Management of Asthma-QRG*; Royal College of Physicians: London, UK, 2003.
33. Reddel, H.K.; Taylor, D.R.; Bateman, E.D.; Boulet, L.; Boushey, H.A.; Busse, W.W.; Casale, T.B.; Chanez, P.; Enright, P.L.; Gibson, P.G.; et al. American Thoracic Society Documents an Official American Thoracic Society/European Respiratory Society Statement: Asthma Control and Exacerbations. *Am. J. Respir. Crit. Care Med.* **2009**, *180*, 59–99. [CrossRef] [PubMed]
34. Kenyon, N.; Zeki, A.; Albertson, T.E.; Louie, S. Definition of Critical Asthma Syndromes. *Clin. Rev. Allergy Immunol.* **2015**, *48*, 1–6. [CrossRef] [PubMed]
35. Bel, E.H.; Sousa, A.; Fleming, L.; Bush, A.; Chung, K.F.; Versnel, J.; Wagener, A.H.; Wagers, S.S.; Sterk, P.J.; Compton, C.H.; et al. Diagnosis and definition of severe refractory asthma: An international consensus statement from the Innovative Medicine Initiative (IMI). *Thorax* **2011**, *66*, 910–917. [CrossRef] [PubMed]
36. Shah, R.; Saltoun, C.A. Acute severe asthma (status asthmaticus). *Allergy Asthma Proc.* **2012**, *33*, 47–50. [CrossRef] [PubMed]
37. Soriano, J.B.; Abajobir, A.A.; Abate, K.H.; Abera, S.F.; Agrawal, A.; Ahmed, M.B. Global, regional, and national deaths, prevalence, disability-adjusted life years, and years lived with disability for chronic obstructive pulmonary disease and asthma, 1990–2015: A systematic analysis for the Global Burden of Disease Study 2015. *Lancet Respir. Med.* **2017**, *5*, 691–706. [CrossRef]

38. Eurostat (Version Dated November 2017). Available online: www.ec.europa.eu/Eurostat/web/health/health-care/data/database (accessed on 6 August 2019).
39. Vieira, E.; Alvaro, P.; Rodrigo, A.C.; Regina, A.; Fernandes, F.L.A.; Barreto, M.L.; Stelmach, R. Urbanization is associated with increased asthma morbidity and mortality in Brazil. *Clin. Respir. J.* **2018**, *12*, 410–417.
40. Krishnan, V.; Diette, G.B.; Rand, C.S.; Bilderback, A.L.; Merriman, B.; Hansel, N.N.; Krishnan, J.A. Mortality in Patients Hospitalized for Asthma Exacerbations in the United States. *Am. J. Respir. Crit. Care Med.* **2006**, *174*, 633–638. [CrossRef] [PubMed]
41. Zein, J.G.; Udeh, B.L.; Teague, W.G.; Koroukian, S.M.; Schlitz, N.K.; Bleecker, E.R.; Busse, W.B.; Calhoun, W.J.; Castro, M.; Count, S.A.; et al. Impact of Age and Sex on Outcomes and Hospital Cost of Acute Asthma in the United States, 2011–2012. *PLoS ONE* **2016**, *11*, e0157301. [CrossRef] [PubMed]
42. Sekiya, K.; Nakatani, E.; Fukutomi, Y.; Kaneda, H.; Iikura, M.; Yoshida, M.; Takahashi, K.; Tomii, K.; Nishikawa, M.; Kaneko, N.; et al. Severe or life-threatening asthma exacerbation: Patient heterogeneity identified by cluster analysis. *Clin. Exp. Allergy* **2016**, *46*, 1043–1055. [CrossRef] [PubMed]
43. Yii, A.; Tan, J.; Lapperre, T. Long-term future risk of severe exacerbations: Distinct 5-year trajectories of problematic asthma. *Allergy* **2017**, *72*, 1398–1405. [CrossRef] [PubMed]
44. Barr, R.G.; Woodruff, P.G.; Clark, S.; Camargo, C.A. Sudden-onset asthma exacerbations: Clinical features, response to therapy, and 2-week follow-up. *Eur. Respir. J.* **2000**, *15*, 266–273. [CrossRef] [PubMed]
45. Ramnath, V.R.; Clark, S.; Camargo, C.A.J. Multicenter Study of Clinical Features of Sudden-Onset Versus Slower-Onset Asthma Exacerbations Requiring Hospitalization. *Respir. Care* **2007**, *52*, 1013–1020. [PubMed]
46. Skobeloff, E.M.; Spivey, W.H.; St Clair, S.S.; Schoffstall, J.M. The influence of age and sex on asthma admissions. *JAMA* **1992**, *268*, 3437–3440. [CrossRef]
47. Tattersfield, A.E.; Postma, D.S.; Barnes, P.J.; Svensson, K.; Bauer, C.A.; O'Byrne, P.M.; Lofdahl, C.G.; Pauwels, R.A.; Ullman, A. Exacerbations of asthma: A descriptive study of 425 severe exacerbations. *Am. J. Respir. Crit. Care Med.* **1999**, *160*, 594–599. [CrossRef] [PubMed]
48. Borish, L.; Chipps, B.; Deniz, Y.; Gujrathi, S.; Zheng, B.; Dolan, C.M.; TENOR Study Group. Total serum IgE levels in a large cohort of patients with severe or difficult-to-treat asthma. *Ann. Allergy Asthma Immunol.* **2005**, *95*, 247–253. [CrossRef]
49. Leynaert, B.; Sunyer, J.; Garcia-Esteban, R.; Svanes, C.; Jarvis, D.; Cerveri, I.; Dratva, J.; Gislason, T.; Heinrich, J.; Janson, C.; et al. Gender differences in prevalence, diagnosis and incidence of allergic and nonallergic asthma: A population-based cohort. *Thorax* **2012**, *67*, 625–631. [CrossRef]
50. Redmond, A.M.; James, A.W.; Nolan, S.H.; Self, T.H. Premenstrual asthma: Emphasis on drug therapy options. *J. Asthma* **2004**, *41*, 687–693. [CrossRef]
51. Guy, E.S.; Kirumaki, A.; Hanania, N.A. Acute asthma in pregnancy. *Crit. Care Clin.* **2004**, *20*, 731–745. [CrossRef]
52. Moore, W.C.; Meyers, D.A.; Wenzel, S.E.; Teague, W.G.; Li, H.; Li, X.; D'Agostino, R., Jr.; Castro, M.; Curran-Everett, D.; Fitzpatrick, A.M.; et al. Identification of asthma phenotypes using cluster analysis in the Severe Asthma Research Program. *Am. J. Respir. Crit. Care Med.* **2010**, *181*, 315–323. [CrossRef]
53. Peters, U.; Dixon, A.E.; Forno, E. Obesity and asthma. *J. Allergy Clin. Immunol.* **2018**, *141*, 1169–1179. [CrossRef]
54. Eisner, M.D.; Katz, P.P.; Yelin, E.H.; Shiboski, S.C.; Blanc, P.D. Risk factors for hospitalization among adults with asthma: The influence of sociodemographic factors and asthma severity. *Respir. Res.* **2001**, *2*, 53–60. [CrossRef] [PubMed]
55. Griswold, S.K.; Nordstrom, C.R.; Clark, S.; Gaeta, T.J.; Price, M.L.; Camargo, C.A., Jr. Asthma exacerbations in North American adults: Who are the 'frequent fliers' in the emergency department? *Chest* **2005**, *127*, 1579–1586. [CrossRef] [PubMed]
56. Falsey, A.R.; Hennessey, P.A.; Formica, M.A.; Cox, C.; Walsh, E.E. Respiratory syncytial virus infection in elderly and high-risk adults. *N. Engl. J. Med.* **2005**, *352*, 1749–1759. [CrossRef] [PubMed]
57. Yoo, J.K.; Kim, T.S.; Hufford, M.M.; Braciale, T.J. Viral infection of the lung: Host response and sequelae. *J. Allergy Clin. Immunol.* **2013**, *132*, 1263–1276. [CrossRef] [PubMed]
58. Rumpel, J.A.; Ahmedani, B.K.; Peterson, E.L.; Wells, K.E.; Yang, M.; Levin, A.M.; Yang, J.J.; Kumar, R.; Burchard, E.G.; Williams, L.K. Genetic ancestry and its association with asthma exacerbations among African American subjects with asthma. *J. Allergy Clin. Immunol.* **2012**, *130*, 1302–1306. [CrossRef] [PubMed]

59. Reddel, H.; Ware, S.; Marks, G.; Salome, C.; Jenkins, C.; Woolcock, A. Differences between asthma exacerbations and poor asthma control. *Lancet* **1999**, *353*, 364–369. [CrossRef]
60. Pauwels, R.A.; Pedersen, S.; Busse, W.W.; Tan, W.C.; Chen, Y.Z.; Ohlsson, S.V.; Ullman, A.; Lamm, C.J.; O'Byrne, P.M.; START Investigators Group. Early intervention with budesonide in mild persistent asthma: A randomised, double-blind trial. *Lancet* **2003**, *361*, 1071–1076. [CrossRef]
61. Rodrigo, G.J. Anticholinergics for asthma. *Curr. Opin. Allergy Clin. Immunol.* **2018**, *18*, 38–43. [CrossRef]
62. Kirkland, S.; Vandenberghe, C.; Voaklander, B. Combined inhaled beta-agonist and anticholinergic agents for emergency management in adults with asthma (Review). *Cochrane Database Syst. Rev.* **2017**, *1*, CD001284.
63. Gottlieb, M.; Kuhns, M.J. Do Inhaled Anticholinergic Agents in Addition to β; -Agonists Improve Outcomes in Acute Asthma Exacerbations? *Ann. Emerg. Med.* **2017**, *70*, 421–422. [CrossRef]
64. Bobrovitz, N.; Heneghan, C.; Onakpoya, I.; Fletcher, B.; Collins, D.; Tompson, A.; Lee, J.; Nunan, D.; Fisher, R.; Scott, B.; et al. Medications that reduce emergency hospital admissions: An overview of systematic reviews and prioritisation of treatments. *BMC Med.* **2018**, *16*, 115. [CrossRef] [PubMed]
65. Suissa, S.; Ernst, P. Inhaled corticosteroids: Impact on asthma morbidity and mortality. *J. Allergy Clin. Immunol.* **2001**, *107*, 937–944. [CrossRef] [PubMed]
66. Miller, M.K.; Lee, J.H.; Miller, D.P.; Wenzel, S.E. Recent asthma exacerbations: A key predictor of future exacerbations. *Respir. Med.* **2007**, *101*, 481–489. [CrossRef] [PubMed]
67. Covar, R.A.; Szefler, S.J.; Zeiger, R.S.; Sorkness, C.A.; Moss, M.; Mauger, D.T.; Boehmer, S.J.; Strunk, R.C.; Martinez, F.D.; Taussig, L.M.; et al. Factors associated with asthma exacerbations during a long-term clinical trial of controller medications in children. *J. Allergy Clin. Immunol.* **2008**, *122*, 741–747. [CrossRef] [PubMed]
68. Haselkorn, T.; Fish, J.E.; Chipps, B.E.; Miller, D.P.; Chen, H.; Weiss, S.T. Effect of weight change on asthma related health outcomes in patients with severe or difficult-to-treat asthma. *Respir. Med.* **2009**, *103*, 274–283. [CrossRef] [PubMed]
69. Chipps, B.E.; Zeiger, R.S.; Borish, L.; Wenzel, S.E.; Yegin, A.; Hayden, M.L.; Miller, D.P.; Bleecker, E.R.; Simons, F.E.R.; Szefler, S.J.; et al. Key findings and clinical implications from The Epidemiology and Natural History of Asthma: Outcomes and Treatment and Treatment Regimens (TENOR) study. *J. Allergy Clin. Immunol.* **2012**, *130*, 332–342. [CrossRef]
70. Wenzel, S. Severe asthma: From characteristics to phenotypes to endotypes. *Clin. Exp. Allergy* **2012**, *42*, 650–658. [CrossRef] [PubMed]
71. Wenzel, S.E. Asthma phenotypes: The evolution from clinical to molecular approaches. *Nat. Med.* **2012**, *18*, 716–725. [CrossRef] [PubMed]
72. Killian, K.J.; Watson, R.; Otis, J.; St Amand, T.A.; O'Byrne, P.M. Symptom perception during acute bronchoconstriction. *Am. J. Respir. Crit. Care Med.* **2000**, *162*, 490–496. [CrossRef]
73. Magadle, R.; Berar-Yanay, N.; Weiner, P. The risk of hospitalization and near-fatal and fatal asthma in relation to the perception of dyspnea. *Chest* **2002**, *121*, 329–333. [CrossRef]
74. Hancox, R.J.; Cowan, J.O.; Flannery, E.M.; Herbison, G.P.; McLachlan, C.R.; Taylor, D.R. Bronchodilator tolerance and rebound bronchoconstriction during regular inhaled beta-agonist treatment. *Respir. Med.* **2000**, *94*, 767–771. [CrossRef] [PubMed]
75. Stanford, R.H.; Shah, M.B.; D'Souza, A.O.; Dhamane, A.D.; Schatz, M. Short-acting β-agonist use and its ability to predict future asthma related outcomes. *Ann. Allergy Asthma Immunol.* **2012**, *109*, 403–407. [CrossRef] [PubMed]
76. Suissa, S.; Ernst, P.; Benayoun, S.; Baltzan, M.; Cai, B. Low-dose inhaled corticosteroids and the prevention of death from asthma. *N. Engl. J. Med.* **2000**, *343*, 332–336. [CrossRef] [PubMed]
77. Adolescents and Adults with Difficult-to-Treat and Severe Asthma. Available online: http://search.ebscohost.com/login.aspx?direct=true&db=cin20&A.N.=118972966&site=ehost-live (accessed on 6 August 2019).
78. Alvarez, G.G.; FitzGerald, J.M. A systematic review of the psychological risk factors associated with near fatal asthma or fatal asthma. *Respiration* **2007**, *74*, 228–236. [CrossRef] [PubMed]
79. Foster, J.M.; McDonald, V.M.; Guo, M.; Reddel, H.K. "I have lost in every facet of my life": The hidden burden of severe asthma. *Eur. Respir. J.* **2017**, *50*, 1700765. [CrossRef] [PubMed]
80. Denlinger, L.C.; Phillips, B.R.; Ramratnam, S.; Ross, K.; Bhakta, N.R.; Cardet, J.C.; Castro, M.; Peters, S.P.; Phipatanakul, W.; Aujla, S.; et al. Inflammatory and Comorbid Features of Patients with Severe Asthma and Frequent Exacerbations. *Am. J. Respir. Crit. Care Med.* **2017**, *195*, 302–313. [CrossRef] [PubMed]

81. Grissell, T.V.; Powell, H.; Shafren, D.R.; Boyle, M.J.; Hensley, M.J.; Jones, P.D.; Whitehead, B.F.; Gibson, P.G. Interleukin-10 gene expression in acute virus-induced asthma. *Am. J. Respir. Crit. Care Med.* **2005**, *172*, 433–439. [CrossRef] [PubMed]
82. Libster, R.; Bugna, J.; Coviello, S.; Hijano, D.R.; Dunaiewsky, M.; Reynoso, N.; Cavalieri, M.L.; Guglielmo, M.C.; Areso, M.S.; Gilligan, T.; et al. Pediatric hospitalizations associated with **2009** pandemic influenza A (H1N1) in Argentina. *N. Engl. J. Med.* **2010**, *362*, 45–55. [CrossRef]
83. O'Riordan, S.; Barton, M.; Yau, Y.; Read, S.E.; Allen, U.; Tran, D. Risk factors and outcomes among children admitted to hospital with pandemic H1N1 influenza. *Cmaj* **2010**, *182*, 39–44. [CrossRef]
84. Winther, B.; Gwaltney, J.M.; Hendley, J.O. Respiratory virus infection of monolayer cultures of human nasal epithelial cells. *Am. Rev. Respir. Dis.* **1990**, *141*, 839–845. [CrossRef]
85. Unger, B.L.; Ganesan, S.; Comstock, A.T.; Faris, A.N.; Hershenson, M.B.; Sajjan, U.S. Nod-like receptor X-1 is required for rhinovirus-induced barrier dysfunction in airway epithelial cells. *J. Virol.* **2014**, *88*, 3705–3718. [CrossRef] [PubMed]
86. Jacobs, S.E.; Lamson, D.M.; St George, K.; Walsh, T.J. Human rhinoviruses. *Clin. Microbiol. Rev.* **2013**, *26*, 135–162. [CrossRef] [PubMed]
87. Ritchie, A.I.; Jackson, D.J.; Edwards, M.R.; Johnston, S.L. Airway epithelial orchestration of innate immune function in response to virus infection. A focus on asthma. *Ann. Am. Thorac. Soc.* **2016**, *13*, S55–S63. [PubMed]
88. Fensterl, V.; Sen, G.C. Interferons and viral infections. *Biofactors* **2009**, *35*, 14–20. [CrossRef] [PubMed]
89. Makris, S.; Johnston, S. Recent advances in understanding rhinovirus immunity. *F1000Research* **2018**, *21*, 7. [CrossRef] [PubMed]
90. Miller, E.K.; Hernandez, J.Z.; Wimmenauer, V.; Shepherd, B.E.; Hijano, D.; Libster, R.; Serra, M.E.; Bhat, N.; Batalle, J.P.; Mohamed, Y.; et al. A mechanistic role for type, III IFN-_1 in asthma exacerbations mediated by human rhinoviruses. *Am. J. Respir. Crit. Care Med.* **2012**, *185*, 508–516. [CrossRef] [PubMed]
91. Jones, A.C.; Anderson, D.; Galbraith, S.; Fantino, E.; Gutierrez Cardenas, D.; Read, J.F.; Serralha, M.; Holt, B.J.; Strickland, D.H.; Sly, P.D.; et al. Personalised transcriptomics reveals heterogeneous immunophenotypes in children with viral bronchiolitis. *Am. J. Respir. Crit. Care Med.* **2019**, *199*, 1537–1549. [CrossRef] [PubMed]
92. Khoo, S.K.; Read, J.; Franks, K.; Zhang, G.; Bizzintino, J.; Coleman, L.; McCrae, C.; Öberg, L.; Troy, N.M.; Prastanti, F.; et al. Upper airway cell transcriptomics identify a major new immune, logical phenotype with strong clinical correlates in young children with acute wheezing. *J. Immunol.* **2019**, *202*, 1845–1858. [CrossRef] [PubMed]
93. Turi, K.N.; Shankar, J.; Anderson, L.J.; Rajan, D.; Gaston, K.; Gebretsadik, T.; Das, S.R.; Stone, C.; Larkin, E.K.; Rosas-Salazar, C.; et al. Infant viral respiratory infection nasal immune-response patterns and their association with subsequent childhood recurrent wheeze. *Am. J. Respir. Crit. Care Med.* **2018**, *198*, 1064–1073. [CrossRef] [PubMed]
94. Fedele, G.; Schiavoni, I.; Nenna, R.; Pierangeli, A.; Frassanito, A.; Leone, P.; Petrarca, L.; Scagnolari, C.; Midulla, F. Analysis of the immune response in infants hospitalized with viral bronchiolitis shows different Th1/Th2 profiles associated with respiratory syncytial virus and human rhinovirus. *Pediatr. Allergy Immunol.* **2018**, *29*, 555–557. [CrossRef] [PubMed]
95. Oliver, B.G.; Lim, S.; Wark, P.; Laza-Stanca, V.; King, N.; Black, J.L.; Roth, M.; Johnston, S.L. Rhinovirus exposure impairs immune responses to bacterial products in human alveolar macrophages. *Thorax* **2008**, *63*, 519–525. [CrossRef] [PubMed]
96. Harford, C.G.; Leidler, V.; Hara, M. Effect of the lesion due to influenza virus on the resistance of mice to inhaled pneumococci. *J. Exp. Med.* **1949**, *89*, 53–68. [CrossRef] [PubMed]
97. Kloepfer, K.M.; Lee, W.M.; Pappas, T.E.; Kang, T.J.; Vrtis, R.F.; Evans, M.D.; Gangnon, R.E.; Bochkov, Y.A.; Jackson, D.J.; Lemanske, R.F., Jr.; et al. Detection of pathogenic bacteria during rhinovirus infection is associated with increased respiratory symptoms and asthma exacerbations. *J. Allergy Clin. Immunol.* **2014**, *133*, 1301–1307. [CrossRef] [PubMed]
98. Papadopoulos, N.G.; Stanciu, L.A.; Papi, A.; Holgate, S.T.; Johnston, S.L. Rhinovirus-induced alterations on peripheral blood mononuclear cell phenotype and costimulatory molecule expression in normal and atopic asthmatic subjects. *Clin. Exp. Allergy* **2002**, *32*, 537–542. [CrossRef] [PubMed]

99. Jackson, D.J.; Makrinioti, H.; Rana, B.M.; Shamji, B.W.; Trujillo-Torralbo, M.B.; Footitt, J.; Del-Rosario, J.; Telcian, A.G.; Nikonova, A.; Zhu, J.; et al. IL-33-dependent type 2 inflammation during rhinovirus-induced asthma exacerbations in vivo. *Am. J. Respir. Crit. Care Med.* **2014**, *190*, 1373–1382. [CrossRef] [PubMed]
100. Beale, J.; Jayaraman, A.; Jackson, D.J.; Macintyre, J.D.R.; Edwards, M.R.; Walton, R.P.; Zhu, J.; Ching, Y.M.; Shamji, B.; Edwards, M.; et al. Rhinovirus-induced, IL-25 in asthma exacerbation drives type 2 immunity and allergic pulmonary inflammation. *Sci. Transl. Med.* **2014**, *6*, 256ra134. [CrossRef]
101. Hong, J.Y.; Bentley, J.K.; Chung, Y.; Lei, J.; Steenrod, J.M.; Chen, Q.; Sajjan, U.S.; Hershenson, M.B. Neonatal rhinovirus induces mucous metaplasia and airways hyperresponsiveness through, IL-25 and type 2 innate lymphoid cells. *J. Allergy Clin. Immunol.* **2014**, *134*, 429–439. [CrossRef]
102. Shariff, S.; Shelfoon, C.; Holden, N.S.; Traves, S.L.; Wiehler, S.; Kooi, C.; Proud, D.; Leigh, R. Human rhinovirus infection of epithelial cells modulates airway smooth muscle migration. *Am. J. Respir. Cell Mol. Biol.* **2017**, *56*, 796–803. [CrossRef]
103. Leigh, R.; Oyelusi, W.; Wiehler, S.; Koetzler, R.; Zaheer, R.S.; Newton, R.; Proud, D. Human rhinovirus infection enhances airway epithelial cell production of growth factors involved in airway remodeling. *J. Allergy Clin. Immunol.* **2008**, *121*, 1238–1245. [CrossRef]
104. Djukanovic, R.; Harrison, T.; Johnston, S.L.; Gabbay, F.; Wark, P.; Thomson, N.C.; Niven, R.; Singh, D.; Reddel, H.K.; Davies, D.E.; et al. The effect of inhaled, I.F.N-beta on worsening of asthma symptoms caused by viral infections. A randomized trial. *Am. J. Respir. Crit. Care Med.* **2014**, *190*, 145–154. [CrossRef]
105. Sporik, R.; Holgate, S.T.; Platts-Mills, T.A.; Cogswell, J.J. Exposure to house-dust mite allergen (Der p I) and the development of asthma in childhood. A prospective study. *N. Engl. J. Med.* **1990**, *323*, 502–507. [CrossRef] [PubMed]
106. Zureik, M.; Neukirch, C.; Leynaert, B.; Liard, R.; Bousquet, J.; Neukirch, F. Sensitisation to airborne moulds and severity of asthma: Cross sectional study from European Community respiratory health survey. *BMJ* **2002**, *325*, 411–414. [CrossRef] [PubMed]
107. Message, S.D.; Laza-Stanca, V.; Mallia, P.; Parker, H.L.; Zhu, J.; Kebadze, T.; Contoli, M.; Sanderson, G.; Kon, O.M.; Papi, A.; et al. Rhinovirus-induced lower respiratory illness is increased in asthma and related to virus load and Th1/2 cytokine and, IL-10 production. *Proc. Natl. Acad. Sci. USA* **2008**, *105*, 13562–13567. [CrossRef] [PubMed]
108. Rosas, I.; McCartney, H.A.; Payne, R.W.; Calderon, C.; Lacey, J.; Chapela, R.; Ruiz-Velazco, S. Analysis of the relationships between environmental factors (aeroallergens, air pollution, and weather) and asthma emergency admissions to a hospital in Mexico City. *Allergy* **1998**, *53*, 394–401. [CrossRef] [PubMed]
109. Downs, S.H.; Mitakakis, T.Z.; Marks, G.B.; Car, N.G.; Belousova, E.G.; Leuppi, J.D.; Xuan, W.; Downie, S.R.; Tobias, A.; Peat, J.K.; et al. Clinical importance of Alternaria exposure in children. *Am. J. Respir. Crit. Care Med.* **2001**, *164*, 455–459. [CrossRef] [PubMed]
110. Donohue, K.M.; Al-alem, V.; Perzanowshi, M.S.; Chew, G.L.; Johnson, A.; Divjan, A.; Kelvin, E.A.; Hoepner, L.A.; Perera, F.P.; Miller, R.L. Anti-cockroach and anti-mouse IgE are associated with early wheeze and atopy inan inner-city birth cohort. *J. Allergy Clin. Immunol.* **2008**, *122*, 914–920. [CrossRef] [PubMed]
111. Kim, J.S.; Ouyang, F.X.; Pongracic, J.A.; Fang, Y.P.; Wang, B.Y.; Liu, X.; Xing, H.; Caruso, D.; Liu, X.; Zhang, S.; et al. Dissociation between the prevalence of atopy and allergic disease in rural China among children and adults. *J. Allergy Clin. Immunol.* **2008**, *122*, 929–935. [CrossRef] [PubMed]
112. Salo, P.M.; Arbes, S.J.; Crockett, P.W.; Thorne, P.S.; Cohn, R.D.; Zeldin, D.C. Exposure to multiple indoor allergens in, U.S. homes and its relationship to asthma. *J. Allergy Clin. Immunol.* **2008**, *121*, 678–684. [CrossRef]
113. Kanchongkittiphon, W.; Mendell, M.J.; Gaffin, J.M.; Wang, G.; Phipatanakul, W. Indoor environmental exposures and exacerbation of asthma: An update to the 2000 review by the Institute of Medicine. *Environ. Health Perspect.* **2015**, *123*, 6–20. [CrossRef]
114. Matsui, E.C. Environmental exposures and asthma morbidity in children living in urban neighborhoods. *Allergy* **2014**, *69*, 553–558. [CrossRef]
115. Yang, J.J.; Burchard, E.G.; Choudhry, S.; Johnson, C.C.; Ownby, D.R.; Favro, D.; Chen, J.; Akana, M.; Ha, C.; Kwok, P.-Y.; et al. Differences in allergic sensitization by self-reported race and genetic ancestry. *J. Allergy Clin. Immunol.* **2008**, *122*, 820–827. [CrossRef] [PubMed]
116. Thomson, N.C.; Chaudhuri, R.; Livingston, E. Asthma and cigarette smoking. *Eur. Respir. J.* **2004**, *24*, 822–833. [CrossRef] [PubMed]

117. Polosa, R.; Knoke, J.D.; Russo, C.; Piccillo, G.; Caponnetto, P.; Sarva, M.; Proietti, L.; Al-Delaimy, W.K. Cigarette smoking is associated with a greater risk of incident asthma in allergic rhinitis. *J. Allergy Clin. Immunol.* **2008**, *121*, 1428–1434. [CrossRef] [PubMed]
118. Quinto, K.B.; Kit, B.K.; Lukacs, S.L.; Akinbami, L.J. Environmental tobacco smoke exposure in children aged 3–19 years with and without asthma in the United States, 1999–2010. *NCHS Data Brief* **2013**, *126*, 1–8.
119. McCarville, M.; Sohn, M.W.; Oh, E.; Weiss, K.; Gupta, R. Environmental tobacco smoke and asthma exacerbations and severity: The difference between measured and reported exposure. *Arch. Dis. Child.* **2013**, *98*, 510–514. [CrossRef]
120. Vargas, P.A.; Brenner, B.; Clark, S.; Boudreaux, E.D.; Camargo, C.A., Jr. Exposure to environmental tobacco smoke among children presenting to the emergency department with acute asthma: A multicenter study. *Pediatr. Pulmonol.* **2007**, *42*, 646–655. [CrossRef] [PubMed]
121. Hassanzad, M.; Khalilzadeh, S.; Eslampanah Nobari, S.; Bloursaz, M.; Sharifi, H.; Mohajerani, S.A.; Nejad, S.T.; Velayati, A.A. Cotinine level is associated with asthma severity in passive smoker children. *Iran. J. Allergy Asthma Immunol.* **2015**, *14*, 67–73.
122. Ferrante, G.; Simoni, M.; Cibella, F.; Liotta, G.; Malizia, V.; Corsello, G.; Viegi, G.; La Grutta, S. Third-hand smoke exposure and health hazards in children. *Monaldi Arch. Chest Dis.* **2013**, *79*, 38–43. [CrossRef]
123. Samoli, E.; Nastos, P.T.; Paliatsos, A.G.; Katsouyanni, K.; Priftis, K.N. Acute effects of air pollution on pediatric asthma exacerbation: Evidence of association and effect modification. *Environ. Res.* **2011**, *111*, 418–424. [CrossRef]
124. Gasana, J.; Dillikar, D.; Mendy, A.; Forno, E.; Ramos Vieira, E. Motor vehicle air pollution and asthma in children: A meta-analysis. *Environ. Res.* **2012**, *117*, 36–45. [CrossRef]
125. Delfino, R.J.; Wu, J.; Tjoa, T.; Gullesserian, S.K.; Nickerson, B.; Gillen, D.L. Asthma morbidity and ambient air pollution: Effect modification by residential traffic-related air pollution. *Epidemiology* **2014**, *25*, 48–57. [CrossRef] [PubMed]
126. Moffatt, M.F.; Kabesch, M.; Liang, L.; Dixon, A.L.; Strachan, D.; Heath, S.; Depner, M.; von Berg, A.; Bufe, A.; Rietschel, E.; et al. Genetic variants regulating, ORMDL3 expression contribute to the risk of childhood asthma. *Nature* **2007**, *448*, 470–473. [CrossRef] [PubMed]
127. Portelli, M.A.; Hodge, E.; Sayers, I. Genetic risk factors for the development of allergic disease identified by genome-wide association. *Clin. Exp. Allergy* **2015**, *45*, 21–31. [CrossRef] [PubMed]
128. Du, R.; Litonjua, A.A.; Tantisira, K.G.; Lasky-Su, J.; Sunyaev, S.R.; Klanderman, B.J.; Celedon, J.C.; Avila, L.; Soto-Quiros, M.E.; Weiss, S.T.; et al. Genome-wide association study reveals class I M.H.C-restricted T cell-associated molecule gene (CRTAM) variants interact with vitamin D levels to affect asthma exacerbations. *J. Allergy Clin. Immunol.* **2012**, *129*, 368–373. [CrossRef] [PubMed]
129. Tavendale, R.; Macgregor, D.F.; Mukhopadhyay, S.; Palmer, C.N. A polymorphism controlling, ORMDL3 expression is associated with asthma that is poorly controlled by current medications. *J. Allergy Clin. Immunol.* **2008**, *121*, 860–863. [CrossRef] [PubMed]
130. Tantisira, K.G.; Silverman, E.S.; Mariani, T.J.; Xu, J.; Richter, B.G.; Klanderman, B.J.; Litonjua, A.A.; Lazarus, R.; Rosenwasser, L.J.; Fuhlbrigge, A.L.; et al. FCER2: A pharmacogenetics basis for severe exacerbations in children with asthma. *J. Allergy Clin. Immunol.* **2007**, *120*, 1285–1291. [CrossRef] [PubMed]
131. Chupp, G.L.; Lee, C.G.; Jarjour, N.; Shim, Y.M.; Holm, C.T.; He, S.; Dziura, J.D.; Reed, J.; Coyle, A.J.; Kiener, P.; et al. A chitinase-like protein in the lung and circulation of patients with severe asthma. *N. Engl. J. Med.* **2007**, *357*, 2016–2027. [CrossRef] [PubMed]
132. Cunningham, J.; Basu, K.; Tavendale, R.; Palmer, C.N.; Smith, H.; Mukhopadhyay, S. The CHI3L1 rs4950928 poly morphism is associated with asthma-related hospital admissions in children and young adults. *Ann. Allergy Asthma Immunol.* **2011**, *106*, 381–386. [CrossRef] [PubMed]
133. Lee, C.G.; Hartl, D.; Lee, G.R.; Koller, B.; Matsuura, H.; Da Silva, C.A.; Sohn, M.H.; Cohn, L.; Homer, R.J.; Kozhich, A.A.; et al. Role of breast regression protein 39 (BRP-39)/chitinase 3-like-1 in Th2 and, IL-13-induced tissue responses and apoptosis. *J. Exp. Med.* **2009**, *206*, 1149–1166. [CrossRef] [PubMed]
134. Tang, H.; Sun, Y.; Shi, Z.; Huang, H.; Fang, Z.; Chen, J.; Xiu, Q.; Li, B. YKL-40 induces, IL-8 expression from bronchial epithelium via, MAPK. (JNK and, ERK) and, NF-kB pathways, causing bronchial smooth muscle proliferation and migration. *J. Immunol.* **2013**, *190*, 438–446. [CrossRef] [PubMed]
135. Russell, R.J.; Brightling, C. Pathogenesis of asthma: Implications for precision medicine. *Clin. Sci.* **2017**, *131*, 1723–1735. [CrossRef] [PubMed]

136. Rovina, N.; Baraldo, S.; Saetta, M. Severe asthma: Inflammation. *Pneumon* **2011**, *24*, 306–313.
137. Robinson, D.; Humbert, M.; Buhl, R.; Cruz, A.A.; Inoue, H.; Korom, S.; Hanania, N.A.; Nair, P. Revisiting Type 2-high and Type 2-low airway inflammation in asthma: Current knowledge and therapeutic implications. *Clin. Exp. Allergy* **2017**, *47*, 161–175. [CrossRef] [PubMed]
138. Santus, P.; Saad, M.; Damiani, G.; Patella, V.; Radovanovic, D. Current and future targeted therapies for severe asthma: Managing treatment with biologics based on phenotypes and biomarkers. *Pharmacol. Res.* **2019**, *146*, 104296. [CrossRef] [PubMed]
139. Kulkarni, N.S.; Hollins, F.; Sutcliffe, A.; Saunders, R.; Shah, S.; Siddiqui, S.; Gupta, S.; Haldar, P.; Green, R.; Pavord, I.; et al. Eosinophil protein in airway macrophages: A novel biomarker of eosinophilic inflammation in patients with asthma. *J. Allergy Clin. Immunol.* **2010**, *126*, 61–69. [CrossRef] [PubMed]
140. Papi, A.; Brightling, C.; Pedersen, S.E.; Reddel, H.K. Asthma. *Lancet* **2017**, *391*, 783–800. [CrossRef]
141. Lambrecht, B.N.; Hammad, H. The immunology of asthma. *Nat. Immunol.* **2015**, *16*, 45–56. [CrossRef] [PubMed]
142. Xue, L.; Gyles, S.L.; Wettey, F.R.; Gazi, L.; Townsend, E.; Hunter, M.G.; Pettipher, R. Prostaglandin D2 causes preferential induction of proinflammatory Th2 cytokine production through an action on chemoattractant receptor-like molecule expressed on Th2 cells. *J. Immunol.* **2005**, *175*, 6531–6536. [CrossRef] [PubMed]
143. Doherty, T.A.; Broide, D.H. Group 2 innate lymphoid cells: New players in human allergic diseases. *J. Investig. Allergol. ClinImmunol.* **2015**, *25*, 1–11.
144. Aron, J.L.; Akbari, O. Regulatory T cells and type 2 innate lymphoid cell-dependent asthma. *Allergy* **2017**, *72*, 1148–1155. [CrossRef] [PubMed]
145. Sokolowska, M.; Chen, L.Y.; Liu, Y.; Martinez-Anton, A.; Logun, C.; Alsaaty, S.; Cuento, R.A.; Cai, R.; Sun, J.; Quehenberger, O.; et al. Dysregulation of lipidomic profile and antiviral immunity in response to hyaluronan in patients with severe asthma. *J. Allergy Clin. Immunol.* **2017**, *139*, 1379–1383. [CrossRef] [PubMed]
146. Chen, R.; Smith, S.G.; Salter, B.; El-Gammal, A.; Oliveria, J.P.; Obminski, C.; Watson, R.; O'Byrne, P.M.; Gauvreau, G.M.; Sehmi, R.; et al. Allergen-induced Increases in Sputum Levels of Group 2 Innate Lymphoid Cells in Subjects with Asthma. *Am. J. Respir. Crit. Care Med.* **2017**, *196*, 700–712. [CrossRef] [PubMed]
147. Sugita, K.; Steer, C.A.; Martinez-Gonzalez, I.; Altunbulakli, C.; Morita, H.; Castro-Giner, F.; Kubo, T.; Wawrzyniak, P.; Ruckert, B.; Sudo, K.; et al. Type 2 innate lymphoid cells disrupt bronchial epithelial barrier integrity by targeting tight junctions through, IL-13 in asthmatic patients. *J. Allergy Clin. Immunol.* **2018**, *141*, 300–310. [CrossRef] [PubMed]
148. Wawrzyniak, P.; Wawrzyniak, M.; Wanke, K.; Sokolowska, M.; Bendelja, K.; Ruckert, B.; Globinska, A.; Jakiela, B.; Kast, J.I.; Idzko, M.; et al. Regulation of bronchial epithelial barrier integrity by type 2 cytokines and histone deacetylases in asthmatic patients. *J. Allergy Clin. Immunol.* **2017**, *139*, 93–103. [CrossRef] [PubMed]
149. Pascual, R.M.; Peters, S.P. Airway remodeling contributes to the progressive loss of lung function in asthma: An overview. *J. Allergy Clin. Immunol.* **2005**, *116*, 477–486. [CrossRef] [PubMed]
150. Doherty, T.; Broide, D. Cytokines and growth factors in airway remodeling in asthma. *Curr. Opin. Immunol.* **2007**, *19*, 676–680. [CrossRef] [PubMed]
151. Chung, K.F.; Wenzel, S.E.; Brozek, J.L.; Bush, A.; Castro, M.; Sterk, P.J.; Adcock, I.M.; Bateman, E.D.; Bel, E.H.; Bleecker, E.R.; et al. International, ERS/ATS guidelines on definition, evaluation and treatment of severe asthma. *Eur. Respir. J.* **2014**, *43*, 343–373. [CrossRef] [PubMed]
152. Strickland, D.H.; Holt, P.G. T regulatory cells in childhood asthma. *Trends Immunol.* **2011**, *32*, 420–427. [CrossRef] [PubMed]
153. Josefowicz, S.Z.; Niec, R.E.; Kim, H.Y.; Treuting, P.; Chinen, T.; Zheng, Y.; Umetsu, D.T.; Rudensky, A.Y. Extrathymically generated regulatory T cells control mucosal, TH2 inflammation. *Nature* **2012**, *482*, 395–399. [CrossRef] [PubMed]
154. Hartl, D.; Koller, B.; Mehlhorn, A.T.; Reinhardt, D.; Nicolai, T.; Schendel, D.J.; Griese, M.; Krauss-Etschmann, S. Quantitative and functional impairment of pulmonary, C.D.4+C.D.25hi regulatory T cells in pediatric asthma. *J. Allergy Clin. Immunol.* **2007**, *119*, 1258–1266. [CrossRef] [PubMed]
155. Smyth, L.J.; Eustace, A.; Kolsum, U.; Blaikely, J.; Singh, D. Increased airway T reg-ulatory cells in asthmatic subjects. *Chest* **2010**, *138*, 905–912. [CrossRef] [PubMed]

156. Ling, E.M.; Smith, T.; Nguyen, X.D.; Pridgeon, C.; Dallman, M.; Arbery, J.; Carr, V.A.; Robinson, D.S. Relation of, CD4+CD25+ regulatory T-cell suppression of allergen-driven T-cell activation to atopic status and expression of allergic disease. *Lancet* **2004**, *363*, 608–615. [CrossRef]
157. Nguyen, K.D.; Vanichsarn, C.; Fohner, A.; Nadeau, K.C. Selective deregulation in chemokine signaling pathways of, CD4+CD25(hi)C.D.127(lo)/(-) regulatory T cells in human allergic asthma. *J. Allergy Clin. Immunol.* **2009**, *123*, 933–939. [CrossRef] [PubMed]
158. Akdis, C.A.; Akdis, M. Mechanisms and treatment of allergic disease in the big picture of regulatory T cells. *J. Allergy Clin. Immunol.* **2009**, *123*, 735–746. [CrossRef] [PubMed]
159. Kearley, J.; Barker, J.E.; Robinson, D.S.; Lloyd, C.M. Resolution of airway inflam-mation and hyperreactivity after in vivo transfer of, CD4+CD25+ regulatory T cells is interleukin 10 dependent. *J. Exp. Med.* **2005**, *202*, 1539–1547. [CrossRef]
160. Xu, W.; Lan, Q.; Chen, M.; Chen, H.; Zhu, N.; Zhou, X.; Wang, J.; Fan, H.; Yan, C.-S.; Kuang, J.-L.; et al. Adoptive transfer of induced-Treg cells effectively attenuates murine airway allergic inflammation. *PLoS ONE* **2012**, *7*, e40314. [CrossRef] [PubMed]
161. Kearley, J.; Robinson, D.S.; Lloyd, C.M. CD4+CD25+ regulatory T cells reverse established allergic airway inflammation and prevent airway remodeling. *J. Allergy Clin. Immunol.* **2008**, *122*, 617–624. [CrossRef]
162. Bobolea, I.; Barranco, P.; Del Pozo, V.; Romero, D.; Sanz, V.; Lopez-Carrasco, V.; Canabal, J.; Villasante, C.; Quirce, S. Sputum periostin in patients with different severe asthma phenotypes. *Allergy* **2015**, *70*, 540–546. [CrossRef]
163. Wu, W.; Bleecker, E.; Moore, W.; Busse, W.W.; Castro, M.; Chung, K.F.; Calhoun, W.J.; Erzurum, S.; Gaston, B.; Israel, E.; et al. Unsupervised phenotyping of Severe Asthma Research Program participants using expanded lung data. *J. Allergy Clin. Immunol.* **2014**, *133*, 1280–1288. [CrossRef]
164. Moore, W.C.; Hastie, A.T.; Li, X.; Li, H.; Busse, W.W.; Jarjour, N.N.; Wenzel, S.E.; Peters, S.P.; Meyers, D.A.; Bleecker, E.R.; et al. Sputum neutrophil counts are associated with more severe asthma phenotypes using cluster analysis. *J. Allergy Clin. Immunol.* **2014**, *133*, 1557–1563. [CrossRef]
165. Shaw, D.E.; Berry, M.A.; Hargadon, B.; McKenna, S.; Shelley, M.J.; Green, R.H.; Brightling, C.E.; Wardlaw, A.J.; Pavord, I.D. Association between neutrophilic airway inflammation and airflow limitation in adults with asthma. *Chest* **2007**, *6*, 1871–1875. [CrossRef] [PubMed]
166. Douwes, J.; Gibson, P.; Pekkanen, J.; Pearce, N. Non-eosinophilic asthma: Importance and possible mechanisms. *Thorax* **2002**, *57*, 643–648. [CrossRef] [PubMed]
167. Berry, M.; Morgan, A.; Shaw, D.E.; Parker, D.; Green, R.; Brightling, C.; Bradding, P.; Wardlaw, A.J.; Pavord, I.D. Pathological features and inhaled corticosteroid response of eosinophilic and non-eosinophilic sthma. *Thorax* **2007**, *62*, 1043–1049. [CrossRef] [PubMed]
168. Bullens, D.M.; Truyen, E.; Coteur, L.; Dilissen, E.; Hellings, P.W.; Dupont, L.J.; Ceuppens, J.L. IL-17 mRNA in sputum of asthmatic patients: Linking T cell driven inflammation and granulo cytic influx? *Respir. Res.* **2006**, *7*, 135. [CrossRef] [PubMed]
169. Manni, M.L.; Trudeau, J.B.; Scheller, E.V.; Mandalapu, S.; Elloso, M.M.; Kolls, J.K.; Wenzel, S.E.; Alcorn, J.F. The complex relationship between inflammation and lung function in severe asthma. *Mucosal Immunol.* **2014**, *7*, 1186–1198. [CrossRef] [PubMed]
170. Besnard, A.G.; Togbe, D.; Couillin, I.; Tan, Z.; Zheng, S.G.; Erard, F.; Le Bert, M.; Quesniaux, V.; Ryffel, B. Inflammasome-IL-1-Th17 response in allergic lung inflammation. *J. Mol. Cell Biol.* **2012**, *4*, 3–10. [CrossRef] [PubMed]
171. Krishnaswamy, J.K.; Chu, T.; Eisenbarth, S.C. Beyond pattern recognition:NOD-like receptors in dendritic cells. *Trends Immunol.* **2013**, *34*, 224–233. [CrossRef]
172. Bruijnzeel, P.L.; Uddin, M.; Koenderman, L. Targeting neutrophilic inflammation in severe neutrophilic asthma: Can we target the disease-relevant neutrophil phenotype? *J. Leukoc. Biol.* **2015**, *4*, 549–556. [CrossRef]
173. Simpson, J.L.; Grissell, T.V.; Douwes, J.; Scott, R.J.; Boyle, M.J.; Gibson, P.G. Innate immune activation in neutrophilic asthma and bronchiectasis. *Thorax* **2007**, *3*, 211–218. [CrossRef]
174. Petsky, H.L.; Cates, C.J.; Lasserson, T.J.; Li, A.M.; Turner, C.; Kynaston, J.A.; Chang, A.B. A systematic review and meta-analysis: Tailoring asthma treatment on eosinophilic markers (exhaled nitric oxide or sputum eosinophils). *Thorax* **2012**, *67*, 199–208. [CrossRef]

175. Gaillard, E.A.; McNamara, P.S.; Murray, C.S.; Pavord, I.D.; Shields, M.D. Blood eosinophils as a marker of likely corticosteroid response in children with preschool wheeze: Time for an eosinophil guided clinical trial? *Clin. Exp. Allergy* **2015**, *45*, 1384–1395. [CrossRef] [PubMed]
176. Bleecker, E.R.; FitzGerald, J.M.; Chanez, P.; Papi, A.; Weinstein, S.F.; Barker, P.; Sproule, S.; Gilmartin, G.; Aurivillius, M.; Werkstrom, V.; et al. Efficacy and safety of benralizumab for patients with severe asthma uncontrolled with high-dosage inhaled corticosteroids and long-acting beta2-agonists (SIROCCO): A randomised, multicentre, placebo-controlled phase 3 trial. *Lancet* **2016**, *388*, 2115–2127. [CrossRef]
177. Ortega, H.G.; Liu, M.C.; Pavord, I.D.; Brusselle, G.G.; FitzGerald, J.M.; Chetta, A.; Humbert, M.; Katz, L.E.; Keene, O.N.; Yancey, S.W.; et al. Mepolizumab treatment in patients with severe eosinophilic asthma. *N. Engl. J. Med.* **2014**, *371*, 1198–1207. [CrossRef] [PubMed]
178. Ortega, H.G.; Yancey, S.W.; Mayer, B.; Gunsoy, N.B.; Keene, O.N.; Bleecker, E.R.; Brightling, C.E.; Pavord, I.D. Severe eosinophilic asthma treated with mepolizumab stratified by baseline eosinophil thresholds: A secondary analysis of the DREAM and MENSA studies. *Lancet Respir. Med.* **2016**, *4*, 549–556. [CrossRef]
179. Katz, L.E.; Gleich, G.J.; Hartley, B.F.; Yancey, S.W.; Ortega, H.G. Blood eosinophil count is a useful biomarker to identify patients with severe eosinophilic asthma. *Ann. Am. Thorac. Soc.* **2014**, *11*, 531–536. [CrossRef] [PubMed]
180. Price, D.B.; Rigazio, A.; Campbell, J.D.; Bleecker, E.R.; Corrigan, C.J.; Thomas, M.; Wenzel, S.E.; Wilson, A.M.; Small, M.B.; Gopalan, G.; et al. Blood eosinophil count and prospective annual asthma disease burden: A UK cohort study. *Lancet Respir. Med.* **2015**, *3*, 849–858. [CrossRef]
181. Zeiger, R.S.; Schatz, M.; Dalal, A.A.; Chen, W.; Sadikova, E.; Suruki, R.Y.; Kawatkar, A.A.; Qian, L. Blood eosinophil count and outcomes in severe uncontrolled asthma: A prospective study. *J. Allergy Clin. Immunol. Pract.* **2017**, *5*, 144–153. [CrossRef] [PubMed]
182. Woodruff, P.G.; Modrek, B.; Choy, D.F.; Jia, G.; Abbas, A.R.; Ellwanger, A.; Koth, L.L.; Arron, J.R.; Fahy, J.V. T-helper type 2-driven inflammation defines major subphenotypes of asthma. *Am. J. Respir. Crit. Care Med.* **2009**, *180*, 388–395. [CrossRef] [PubMed]
183. FitzGerald, J.M.; Bleecker, E.R.; Nair, P.; Korn, S.; Ohta, K.; Lommatzsch, M.; Ferguson, G.T.; Busse, W.W.; Barker, P.; Sproule, S.; et al. Benralizumab, an anti-interleukin-5 receptor α monoclonal antibody, as add-on treatment for patients with severe, uncontrolled, eosinophilic asthma (CALIMA): A randomised, double-blind, placebo-controlled phase 3 trial. *Lancet* **2016**, *388*, 2128–2141. [CrossRef]
184. Hanania, N.A.; Wenzel, S.; Rosen, K.; Hsieh, H.J.; Mosesova, S.; Choy, D.F.; Lal, P.; Arron, J.R.; Harris, J.M.; Busse, W. Exploring the effects of omalizumab in allergic asthma: An analysis of biomarkers in the EXTRA study. *Am. J. Respir. Crit. Care Med.* **2013**, *187*, 804–811. [CrossRef]
185. Bjermer, L.; Alving, K.; Diamant, Z.; Magnussen, H.; Pavord, I.; Piacentini, G.; Price, D.; Roche, N.; Sastre, J.; Thomas, M.; et al. Current evidence and future research needs for FeNO measurement in respiratory diseases. *Respir. Med.* **2014**, *108*, 830–841. [CrossRef] [PubMed]
186. Dweik, R.A.; Sorkness, R.L.; Wenzel, S.; Hammel, J.; Curran-Everett, D.; Comhair, S.A.; Bleecker, E.; Busse, W.; Calhoun, W.J.; Castro, M.; et al. National Heart, Lung, and Blood Institute Severe Asthma Research Program. Use of exhaled nitric oxide measurement to identify a reactive, at-risk phenotype among patients with asthma. *Am. J. Respir. Crit. Care Med.* **2010**, *181*, 1033–1041. [CrossRef] [PubMed]
187. Gemicioglu, B.; Musellim, B.; Dogan, I.; Guven, K. Fractional exhaled nitric oxide (FeNo) in different asthma phenotypes. *Allergy Rhinol.* **2014**, *5*, 157–161. [CrossRef] [PubMed]
188. Sippel, J.M.; Holden, W.E.; Tilles, S.A.; O'Hollaren, M.; Cook, J.; Thukkani, N.; Priest, J.; Nelson, B.; Osborne, M.L. Exhaled nitric oxide levels correlate with measures of disease control in asthma. *J. Allergy Clin. Immunol.* **2000**, *106*, 645–650. [CrossRef] [PubMed]
189. van Veen, I.H.; Ten Brinke, A.; Sterk, P.J.; Sont, J.K.; Gauw, S.A.; Rabe, K.F.; Bel, E.H. Exhaled nitric oxide predicts lung function decline in difficult-to-treat asthma. *Eur. Respir. J.* **2008**, *32*, 344–349. [CrossRef] [PubMed]
190. Jones, S.L.; Kittelson, J.; Cowan, J.O.; Flannery, E.M.; Hancox, R.J.; McLachlan, C.R.; Taylor, D.R. The predictive value of exhaled nitric oxide measurements in assessing changes in asthma control. *Am. J. Respir. Crit. Care Med.* **2001**, *164*, 738–743. [CrossRef] [PubMed]
191. Van Vliet, D.; Alonso, A.; Rijkers, G.; Heynens, J.; Rosias, P.; Muris, J.; Jobsis, Q.; Dompeling, E. Prediction of asthma exacerbations in children by innovative exhaled inflammatory markers: Results of a longitudinal study. *PLoS ONE* **2015**, *10*, e0119434. [CrossRef] [PubMed]

192. Van der Valk, R.J.; Baraldi, E.; Stern, G.; Frey, U.; de Jongste, J.C. Daily exhaled nitric oxide measurements and asthma exacerbations in children. *Allergy* **2012**, *67*, 265–271. [CrossRef] [PubMed]
193. Robroeks, C.M.; van Vliet, D.; Jobsis, Q.; Braekers, R.; Rijkers, G.T.; Wodzig, W.K.; Bast, A.; Zimmermann, L.; Dompeling, E. Prediction of asthma exacerbations in children: Results of a one-year prospective study. *Clin. Exp. Allergy* **2012**, *42*, 792–798. [CrossRef] [PubMed]
194. Song, J.S.; You, J.S.; Jeong, S.I.; Yang, S.; Hwang, I.T.; Im, Y.G.; Baek, H.S.; Kim, H.Y.; Suh, D.I.; Lee, H.B.; et al. Serum periostin levels correlate with airway hyper-responsiveness to methacholine and mannitol in children with asthma. *Allergy* **2015**, *70*, 674–681. [CrossRef] [PubMed]
195. Wedes, S.H.; Wu, W.; Comhair, S.A.; McDowell, K.M.; DiDonato, J.A.; Erzurum, S.C.; Hazen, S.L. Urinary bromotyrosine measures asthma control and predicts asthma exacerbations in children. *J. Pediatr.* **2011**, *159*, 248–255. [CrossRef] [PubMed]
196. Kimura, H.; Suzuki, M.; Konno, S.; Nishimura, M.; Bobolea, I.; Barranco, P.; Del Pozo, V.; Romero, D.; Sanz, V.; López-Carrasco, V.; et al. Sputum periostin in patients with different severe asthma phenotypes. *Allergy* **2015**, *70*, 884–885. [CrossRef] [PubMed]
197. Hoshino, M.; Ohtawa, J.; Akitsu, K. Association of airway wall thickness with serum periostin in steroid-naive asthma. *Allergy Asthma Proc.* **2016**, *37*, 225–230. [CrossRef] [PubMed]
198. Sabiner, U.; Birben, E.; Erzurum, S. Oxidative Stress in Asthma: Part of the puzzle. *Pediatr. Allergy Immunol.* **2018**, *29*, 789–800. [CrossRef] [PubMed]
199. Rodriguez-Roisin, R. Acute severe asthma: Pathophysiology and pathobiology of gas exchange abnormalities. *Eur. Respir. J.* **1997**, *10*, 1359–1371. [CrossRef] [PubMed]
200. Brochard, L. Intrinsic (or auto-) PEEP. during controlled mechanical ventilation. *Intensive Care Med.* **2012**, *28*, 1376–1378. [CrossRef] [PubMed]
201. Adams, J.Y.; Sutter, M.E.; Albertson, T.E. The patient with asthma in the emergency department. *Clin. Rev. Allergy Immunol.* **2012**, *43*, 14–29. [CrossRef] [PubMed]
202. Pepe, P.E.; Marini, J.J. Occult Positive End-Expiratory Pressure in Mechanically Ventilated, PA tients with Airflow Obstruction. *Am. Rev. Respir. Dis.* **1982**, *126*, 166–170. [PubMed]
203. Brenner, B.; Corbridge, T.; Kazzi, A. Intubation and mechanical ventilation of the asthmatic patient in respiratory failure. *J. Emerg. Med.* **2009**, *37*, S23–S34. [CrossRef] [PubMed]
204. Alvarez, G.G.; Schulzer, M.; Jung, D.; Fitzgerald, J. A systematic review of risk factors associated with near-fatal and fatal asthma. *Can. Respir. J.* **2005**, *12*, 265–270. [CrossRef] [PubMed]
205. Suissa, S.; Blais, L.; Ernst, P. Patterns of increasing beta-agonist use and the risk of fatal or near-fatal asthma. *Eur. Respir. J.* **1994**, *7*, 1602–1609. [CrossRef] [PubMed]
206. FitzGerald, J.M.; Tavakoli, H.; Lynd, L.D.; Al Efraij, K.; Sadatsafavi, M. The impact of inappropriate use of short acting beta agonists in asthma. *Respir. Med.* **2017**, *131*, 135–140. [CrossRef] [PubMed]
207. Hodder, R.; Lougheed, M.D.; Rowe, B.H.; FitzGerald, J.M.; Kaplan, A.G.; McIvor, R.A. Management of acute asthma in adults in the emergency department: Nonventilatory management. *CMAJ* **2010**, *182*, E55–E67. [CrossRef] [PubMed]
208. Fergeson, J.E.; Patel, S.S.; Lockey, R.F. Acute asthma, prognosis, and treatment. *J. Allergy Clin. Immunol.* **2017**, *139*, 438–447. [CrossRef] [PubMed]
209. Lockey, R.F.; Ledford, D.K. *Asthma: Comorbidities, Coexisting Conditions, and Differential Diagnosis*; Oxford University Press: Oxford, UK, 2014; pp. 231–367.
210. Fretzayas, A.; Moustaki, M.; Loukou, I.; Douros, K. Differentiating vocal cord dysfunction from asthma. *J. Asthma Allergy* **2017**, *10*, 277–283. [CrossRef] [PubMed]
211. Keeley, D.; Osman, L. Dysfunctional breathing and asthma. It is important to tell the difference. *BMJ* **2001**, *322*, 1075–1076. [CrossRef]
212. Carruthers, D.M.; Harrison, B.D. Arterial blood gas analysis or oxygen saturation in the assessment of acute asthma? *Thorax* **1995**, *50*, 186–188. [CrossRef] [PubMed]
213. Vasileiadis, I.; Alevrakis, E.; Ampelioti, S.; Vagionas, D.; Rovina, N.; Koutsoukou, A. Acid-Base Disturbances in Patients with Asthma: A Literature Review and Comments on Their Pathophysiology. *J. Clin. Med.* **2019**, *8*, 563. [CrossRef]
214. Cates, C.; Welsh, E.; Rowe, B. Holding chambers (spacers) versus nebulisers for beta-agonist treatment of acute asthma (Review). *Cochrane Database Syst. Rev.* **2013**, *13*, CD000052.

215. Rodrigo, G.J.; Rodrigo, C. Continuous vs intermittent beta-agonists in the treatment of acute adult asthma: A systematic review with meta-analysis. *Chest* **2002**, *122*, 160–165. [CrossRef]
216. Camargo, C.J.; Spooner, C.; Rowe, B. Continuous versus intermittent beta-agonists for acute asthma (Review). *Cochrane Database Syst. Rev.* **2003**, *4*, CD001115.
217. Wilkinson, M.; Bulloch, B.; Garcia-Filion, P.; Keahey, L. Efficacy of racemic albuterol versus levalbuterol used as a continuous nebulization for the treatment of acute asthma exacerbations: A randomized, double-blind, clinical trial. *J. Asthma* **2011**, *48*, 188–193. [CrossRef] [PubMed]
218. Nowak, R.; Emerman, C.; Hanrahan, J.P.; Parsey, M.V.; Hanania, N.A.; Claus, R.; Schaefer, K.; Baumgartner, R.A.; XOPENEX Acute Severe Asthma Study Group. A comparison of levalbuterol with racemic albuterol in the treatment of acute severe asthma exacerbations in adults. *Am. J. Emerg. Med.* **2006**, *24*, 259–267. [CrossRef] [PubMed]
219. Tobin, A. Intravenous salbutamol: Too Much of a Good Thing? *Crit. Care Resusc.* **2005**, *7*, 119–127. [PubMed]
220. Travers, A.H.; Milan, S.J.; Jones, A.P.; Camargo, C.A., Jr.; Rowe, B.H. Addition of intravenous β_2 -agonists to inhaled β_2 -agonists for acute asthma. *Cochrane Database Syst. Rev.* **2012**, *12*, CD010179. [CrossRef] [PubMed]
221. Jones, G.H.; Scott, S.J. Continuous infusions of terbutaline in asthma—A review. *J. Asthma* **2011**, *48*, 753–756. [CrossRef] [PubMed]
222. Rodrigo, G.J.; Nannini, L.J. Comparison between nebulized adrenaline and β2 agonists for the treatment of acute asthma. A meta-analysis of randomized trials. *Am. J. Emerg. Med.* **2006**, *24*, 217–222. [CrossRef]
223. Gosens, R.; Gross, N. The mode of action of anticholinergics in asthma. *Eur. Respir. J.* **2018**, *52*, 1701247. [CrossRef]
224. Vogelberg, C. Anticholinergics in asthma: Are we utilizing asthma therapies effectively? *Ther Clin Risk Manag.* **2019**, *15*, 405–408. [CrossRef]
225. Edmonds, M.; Milan, S.; Camargo, C.A., Jr.; Pollack, C.V.; Rowe, B.H. Early use of inhaled corticosteroids in the emergency department treatment of acute asthma (Review). *Cochrane Database Syst. Rev.* **2012**, *12*, CD002308.
226. Rowe, B.H.; Vethanayagam, D. The role of inhaled corticosteroids in the management of acute asthma. *Eur. Respir. J.* **2007**, *30*, 1035–1037. [CrossRef] [PubMed]
227. Craig, S.; Kuan, W.S.; Kelly, A.M.; Van Meer, O.; Motiejunaite, J.; Keijzers, G.; Jones, P.; Body, R.; Karamercan, M.A.; Klim, S.; et al. Treatment and outcome of adult patients with acute asthma in emergency departments in Australasia, South East Asia and Europe: Are guidelines followed? AANZDEM/EuroDEM study. *Emerg. Med. Australas.* **2019**. (Epub ahead of print). [CrossRef] [PubMed]
228. Rowe, B.H.; Edmonds, M.L.; Spooner, C.H.; Diner, B.; Camargo, C.A. Corticosteroid therapy for acute asthma. *Respir. Med.* **2004**, *98*, 275–284. [CrossRef] [PubMed]
229. Fulco, P.P.; Lone, A.A.; Pugh, C.B. Intravenous versus oral corticosteroids for treatment of acute asthma exacerbations. *Ann. Pharmacother.* **2002**, *36*, 565–570. [CrossRef] [PubMed]
230. Kirkland, S.; Campbell, S.; Villa-Roel, C.; Rowe, B. Intramuscular versus oral corticosteroids to reduce relapses following discharge from the emergency department for acute asthma (Review). *Cochrane Database Syst. Rev.* **2018**, *2018*, CD012629.
231. Normansell, R.; Kew, K.; Mansour, G. Different oral corticosteroid regimens for acute asthma (Review). *Cochrane Database Syst. Rev.* **2016**, *5*, CD011801.
232. Rowe, B.; Bretzlaff, J.; Bourdon, C.; Bota, G.; Blitz, S.; Camargo, C.A., Jr. Magnesium sulfate for treating exacerbations of acute asthma in the emergency department. *Cochrane Database Syst. Rev.* **2000**, *2*, CD001490.
233. Kew, K.; Kirtchuk, L.; Michell, C. Intravenous magnesium sulfate for treating adults with acute asthma in the emergency department (Review). *Cochrane Database Syst. Rev.* **2014**, *5*, CD010909. [CrossRef]
234. Green, R.H. Asthma in adults (acute): Magnesium sulfate treatment. *BMJ Clin. Evid.* **2016**, *1*, 1513.
235. Knightly, R.; Milan, S.; Hughes, R.; Knopp-sihota, J.; Rowe, B.; Normansell, R.; Powell, C. Inhaled magnesium sulfate in the treatment of acute asthma (Review). *Cochrane Database Syst. Rev.* **2017**, *11*, CD003898.
236. Javor, E.; Grle, S.P. Limitations of the results from randomized clinical trials involving intravenous and nebulised magnesium sulphate in adulta with severe acute asthma. *Pulm. Pharmacol. Ther.* **2019**, *55*, 31–37. [CrossRef] [PubMed]
237. Goodacre, S.; Cohen, J.; Bradburn, M.; Stevens, J.; Gray, A.; Benger, J.; Coats, T.; 3Mg Research Team. The 3Mg trial: A randomised controlled trial of intravenous or nebulised magnesium sulphate versus placebo in adults with acute severe asthma. *Health Technol. Assess.* **2014**, *18*, 1–168. [CrossRef] [PubMed]

238. Nair, P.; Milan, S.; Rowe, B. Addition of intravenous aminophylline to inhaled β_2—Agonists in adults with acute asthma (Review). *Cochrane Database Syst. Rev.* **2012**, *12*, CD002742. [PubMed]
239. Mahemuti, G.; Zhang, H.; Li, J. Efficacy and side effects of intravenous theophylline in acute asthma: A systematic review and meta-analysis. *Drug Des. Dev. Ther.* **2018**, *12*, 99–120. [CrossRef] [PubMed]
240. Silverman, R.A.; Chen, Y.; Bonuccelli, C.M.; Simonson, S.G. Zafirlukast improves emergency department outcomes after an acute asthma episode. *Ann. Emerg. Med.* **1999**, *34*, S1. [CrossRef]
241. Camargo, C.A.J.; Smithline, H.A.; Malice, M.-P.; Green, S.A.; Reiss, T.F. A randomized controlled trial of intravenous montelukast in acute asthma. *Am. J. Respir. Crit. Care Med.* **2003**, *167*, 528–533. [CrossRef]
242. Watts, K.; Chavasse, R. Leukotriene receptor antagonists in addition to usual care for acute asthma in adults and children (Review). *Cochrane Database Syst. Rev.* **2012**, *5*, CD006100.
243. Perrin, K.; Wijesinghe, M.; Healy, B.; Wadsworth, K.; Bowditch, R.; Bibby, S.; Baker, T.; Weatherall, M.; Beasley, R. Randomised controlled trial of high concentration versus titrated oxygen therapy in severe exacerbations of asthma. *Thorax* **2011**, *66*, 937–941. [CrossRef]
244. Rodrigo, G.J.; Verde, M.R.; Peregalli, V. Effects of Short-term 28% and 100% Oxygen on Pa, CO_2 and Peak Expiratory Flow Rate in Acute Asthma—A randomized trial. *Chest* **2003**, *124*, 1312–1317. [CrossRef]
245. Inwald, D.; Roland, M.; Kuitert, L.; Mckenzie, S.A.; Petros, A.; Inwald, D. Oxygen treatment for acute severe asthma. *BMJ* **2001**, *323*, 98–100. [CrossRef]
246. Rodrigo, G.J.; Castro-Rodriguez, J.A. Heliox-driven β_2 -agonists nebulization for children and adults with acute asthma: A systematic review with meta-analysis. *Ann. Allergy Asthma Immunol.* **2014**, *112*, 29–34. [CrossRef] [PubMed]
247. Rodrigo, G.J.; Rodrigo, C.; Pollack, C.V.; Rowe, B.; Em, C. Use of Helium-Oxygen Mixtures in the Treatment of Acute Asthma a Systematic Review. *Chest* **2003**, *123*, 891–896. [CrossRef] [PubMed]
248. El-Khatib, M.; Jamaleddine, G.; Kanj, N. Effect of Heliox- and Air-Driven Nebulized Bronchodilator Therapy on Lung Function in Patients with Asthma. *Lung* **2014**, *192*, 377–383. [CrossRef] [PubMed]
249. L'Hommedieu, C.S.; Arens, J.J. The use of ketamine for the emergency intubation of patients with status asthmaticus. *Ann. Emerg. Med.* **1987**, *16*, 568–571. [CrossRef]
250. Goyal, S.; Agrawal, A. Ketamine in status asthmaticus: A review. *Indian J. Crit. Care Med.* **2013**, *17*, 154–161. [PubMed]
251. Esmailian, M.; Esfahani, M.K.; Heydari, F. The Effect of Low-Dose Ketamine in Treating Acute Asthma Attack; A Randomized Clinical Trial. *Emergency* **2018**, *6*, e21. [PubMed]
252. Stefan, M.S.; Shieh, M.S.; Spitzer, K.A.; Pekow, P.S.; Krishnan, J.A.; Au, D.H.; Lindenauer, P.K. Association of Antibiotic Treatment with Outcomes in Patients Hospitalized for an Asthma Exacerbation Treated with Systemic Corticosteroids. *JAMA Intern. Med.* **2019**, *179*, 333–339. [CrossRef] [PubMed]
253. Lindenauer, P.K.; Stefan, M.S.; Feemster, L.C. Use of antibiotics among patients hospitalized for exacerbations of asthma. *JAMA Intern. Med.* **2016**, *176*, 1397–1400. [CrossRef] [PubMed]
254. Stefan, M.S.; Nathanson, B.H.; Lagu, T.; Priya, A.; Pekow, P.S.; Steingrub, J.S.; Hill, N.S.; Goldberg, R.J.; Kent, D.M.; Lindenauer, P.K. Outcomes of Noninvasive and Invasive Veltilation in Patients Hospitalized with Asthma Exacerbation. *Ann. Am. Thorac. Soc.* **2016**, *13*, 1096–1104. [CrossRef]
255. Pallin, M.; Naughton, M.T. Noninvasive ventilation in acute asthma. *J. Crit. Care* **2014**, *29*, 586–593. [CrossRef]
256. Burns, K.E.A.; Meade, M.O.; Premji, A. Noninvasive ventilation as a weaning strategy for mechanical ventilation in adults with respiratory failure: A Cochrane systematic review. *CMAJ* **2014**, *186*, E112–E122. [CrossRef] [PubMed]
257. Wu, R.S.C.; Wu, K.C.; Wong, T.K.M.; Tsai, Y.H.; Cheng, R.K.S.; Bishop, M.J.; Tan, P.P. Effects of fenoterol and ipratropium on respiratory resistance of asthmatics after tracheal intubation. *Br. J. Anaesth.* **2000**, *84*, 358–362. [CrossRef] [PubMed]
258. Davidson, C.; Banham, S.; Elliott, M. BTS/ICS Guideline for the Ventilatory Management of Acute Hypercapnic Respiratory Failure in Adults. *Thorax* **2016**, *71*, ii1–ii35. [CrossRef] [PubMed]
259. Davidson, C.; Banham, S.; Elliott, M.; Kennedy, D.; Gelder, C.; Glossop, A.; Church, A.C.; Creagh-Brown, B.; Dodd, J.W.; Felton, T.; et al. Guideline for the ventilatory management of acute hypercapnic respiratory failure in adults. *BMJ Open Respir Res.* **2016**, *14*, e000133.
260. Davis, D.P.; Hwang, J.Q.; Dunford, J.V. Rate of decline in oxygen saturation at various pulse oximetry values with prehospital rapid sequence intubation. *Prehosp. Emerg. Care* **2008**, *12*, 46–51. [CrossRef] [PubMed]

261. Eames, W.; Rooke, G.; Wu, R.; Bishop, M. Comparison of the effects of Etomidate, Propofol, and Thiopental on respiratory resistance asther tracheal intubation. *Anesthesiology* **1996**, *84*, 1307–1311. [CrossRef] [PubMed]
262. Laher, A.; Buchanan, S. Mechanically Ventilating the Severe Asthmatic Mechanically Ventilating the Severe Asthmatic. *J. Intensive Care Med.* **2018**, *33*, 491–501. [CrossRef] [PubMed]
263. Laghi, F.; Goyal, A. Auto-PEEP in respiratory failure. *Minerva Anestesiol.* **2012**, *78*, 201–221. [PubMed]
264. Williams, T.J.; Tuxen, D.; Scheinkestel, C.D.; Czarny, D.; Bowes, G. Risk Factors for Morbidity in Mechanically Ventilated Patients with Acute Severe Asthma 1, 2. *Am. Rev. Respir. Dis.* **1992**, *146*, 607–615. [CrossRef] [PubMed]
265. Leatherman, J. Mechanical ventilation for severe asthma. *Chest* **2015**, *147*, 1671–1680. [CrossRef]
266. Kollef, M.H. Lung hyperinflation caused by inappropriate ventilation resulting in electromechanical dissociation: A case report. *Heart Lung* **1992**, *21*, 74–77.
267. Riker, R.R.; Shehabi, Y.; Bokesch, P.M.; Ceraso, D.; Wisemandle, W.; Whitten, P.; Margolis, B.D.; Byrne, D.W.; Ely, E.W.; Rocha, M.G.; et al. Dexmedetomidine vs Midazolam for Sedation of Critically Ill Patients. *JAMA* **2009**, *301*, 489–499. [CrossRef] [PubMed]
268. Burburan, S.M.; Xisto, D.G.; Rocco, P.R.M. Anaesthetic management in asthma. *Minerva Anestesiol.* **2007**, *73*, 357–365. [PubMed]
269. Behbehani, N.A.; Al-Mane, F.; D'yachkova, Y.; Pare, P.; FitzGerald, J.M. Myopathy following mechanical ventilation for acute severe asthma: The role of muscle relaxants and corticosteroids. *Chest* **1999**, *115*, 1627–1631. [CrossRef] [PubMed]
270. Tuxen, D.; Lane, S. The Effects of Ventilatory Pattern on Hyperinflation, Airway Pressures, and Circulation in Mechanical Ventilation of Patients with Severe Air-Flow. *Am. Rev. Respir. Dis.* **1987**, *136*, 872–879. [CrossRef] [PubMed]
271. Tuxen, D.V. Detrimental Effects of Positive End-expiratory Pressure during Controlled Mechanical Ventilation of Patients with Severe Airflow Obstruction. *Am. Rev.* **1989**, *140*, 5–9. [CrossRef] [PubMed]
272. Caramez, M.; Borges, J.; Tucci, M.; Okamoto, V. Paradoxical responses to positive end-expiratory pressure in patients with airway obstruction during controlled ventilation. *Crit. Care Med.* **2005**, *33*, 1519–1528. [CrossRef] [PubMed]
273. Stather, D.R.; Stewart, T.E. Clinical review: Mechanical ventilation in severe asthma. *Crit. Care* **2005**, *9*, 581–587. [CrossRef]
274. Baudin, F.; Buisson, A.; Vanel, B.; Massenavette, B.; Pouyau, R.; Javouhey, E. Nasal high flow in management of children with status asthmaticus: A retrospective observational study. *Ann. Intensive Care* **2017**, *7*, 55. [CrossRef]
275. Pilar, J.; Modesto, I.; Alapont, V.; Lopez-Fernandez, Y.M.; Lopez-Macias, O.; Garcia-Urabayen, D.; Amores-Hernandez, I. High-flow nasal cannula therapy versus non-invasive ventilation in children with severe acute asthma exacerbation: An observational cohort study. *Med. Intensiva* **2017**, *41*, 418–424. [CrossRef]
276. Chang, C.L.; Yates, D.H. Use of Early Extra-Corporeal Membrane Oxygenation (E.C.M.O.) for Severe Refractory Status Asthmaticus. *J. Med. Cases* **2011**, *2*, 124–126.
277. Alzeer, A.H.; Otair, H.A.A.; Khurshid, S.M.; Badrawy, S.E.; Bakir, B.M. Case Report A case of near fatal asthma: The role of ECMO as rescue therapy. *Ann. Thorac. Med.* **2015**, *10*, 89–91. [CrossRef] [PubMed]
278. Mikkelsen, M.E.; Woo, Y.J.; Sager, J.S.; Fuchs, B.D.; Christie, J.D. Outcomes using extracorporeal life support for adult respiratory failure due to status asthmaticus. *ASAIO J.* **2009**, *55*, 47. [CrossRef] [PubMed]
279. Yeo, H.J.; Kim, D.; Jeon, D.; Kim, Y.S.; Rycus, P.; Cho, W.H. Extracorporeal membrane oxygenation for life-threatening asthma refractory to mechanical ventilation: Analysis of the Extracorporeal Life Support Organization registry. *Crit. Care* **2017**, *21*, 297. [CrossRef] [PubMed]
280. Di Lascio, G.; Prifti, E.; Messai, E.; Peris, A.; Harmelin, G.; Xhaxho, R.; Fico, A.; Sani, G.; Bonacchi, M. Extracorporeal membrane oxygenation support for life-threatening acute severe status asthmaticus. *Perfusion* **2017**, *32*, 157. [CrossRef] [PubMed]
281. Lobaz, S.; Carey, M. Case reports Rescue of acute refractory hypercapnia and acidosis secondary to life-threatening asthma with extracorporeal carbon dioxide removal (ECCO2R) Case report. *J. Intensive Care Soc.* **2011**, *12*, 140–142. [CrossRef]
282. Brenner, K.; Abrams, D.C.; Agerstrand, C.L.; Brodie, D. Extracorporeal carbon dioxide removal for refractory status asthmaticus: Experience in distinct exacerbation phenotypes. *Perfusion* **2014**, *29*, 26–28. [CrossRef]

283. Schneider, T.; Bence, T.; Brettner, F. "Awake" ECCO2R superseded intubation in a near-fatal asthma attack. *J. Intensive Care* **2017**, *5*, 53. [CrossRef]
284. Tobias, J.D. Inhalational Anesthesia: Basic Pharmacology, End Organ Effects, and Applications in the Treatment of Status Asthmaticus. *J. Intensive Care Med.* **2009**, *24*, 361–371. [CrossRef]
285. Vaschetto, R.; Bellotti, E.; Turucz, E.; Gregoretti, C.; Corte, F.D.; Navalesi, P. Inhalational Anesthetics in Acute Severe Asthma. *Curr. Drug Targets* **2009**, *10*, 826–832. [CrossRef]
286. Rosseel, P.; Lauwers, L.F.; Baute, L.; Care, I.; Stuivenberg, A.Z. Halothane treatment in life-threatening asthma. *Intensive Care Med.* **1985**, *11*, 241–246. [CrossRef]
287. Bierman, M.; Brown, M.; Muren, O. Prolonged isoflurane anesthesia in status asthmaticus. *Crit. Care Med.* **1986**, *14*, 832–833. [CrossRef] [PubMed]
288. Schutte, D.; Zwitserloot, A.M.; Houmes, R.; Hoog, M.D.; Draaisma, J.M.; Lemson, J. Sevoflurane therapy for life-threatening asthma in children. *Br. J. Anaesth.* **2013**, *111*, 967–970. [CrossRef] [PubMed]
289. Ng, E.; Fahimi, J.; Hern, H. Sevoflurane administration initiated out of the, ED for life-threatening status asthmaticus. *Am. J. Emerg. Med.* **2015**, *33*, e3–e6. [CrossRef] [PubMed]
290. Ruszkai, Z.; Bokretas, G.; Bartha, P. Sevoflurane therapy for life-threatening acute severe asthma: A case report. *Can. J. Anesth.* **2014**, *61*, 943–950. [CrossRef] [PubMed]
291. Beute, J. Emergency treatment of status asthmaticus with enoximone. *Br. J. Anaesth.* **2014**, *112*, 1105–1108. [CrossRef] [PubMed]
292. Nanchal, R.; Kumar, G.; Majumdar, T.; Taneja, A.; Patel, J.; Dagar, G.; Jacobs, E.R.; Whittle, J. Utilization of mechanical ventilation for asthma exacerbations: Analysis of a national database. *Respir. Care* **2014**, *59*, 644–653. [CrossRef]
293. Marquette, C.H.; Saulnier, F.; Leroy, O.; Wallaert, B.; Chopin, C.; Demarcq, J.M.; Durocher, A.; Tonnel, A.B. Long-term prognosis of near-fatal asthma. A 6-year follow-up study of 145 asthmatic patients who underwent mechanical ventilation for a near-fatal attack of asthma. *Am. Rev. Respir. Dis.* **1992**, *146*, 76–81. [CrossRef]
294. Yellowlees, P.M.; Ruffin, R.E. Psychological defenses and coping styles in patients following a life-threatening attack of asthma. *Chest* **1989**, *95*, 1298–1303. [CrossRef]
295. Lemmetyinen, R.E.; Karjalainen, J.V.; But, A.; Renkonen, R.L.O.; Pekkanen, J.R.; Toppila-Salmi, S.K.; Haukka, J.K. Higher mortality of adults with asthma: A 15-year follow-up of a population-based cohort. *Allergy* **2018**, *73*, 1479–1488. [CrossRef]

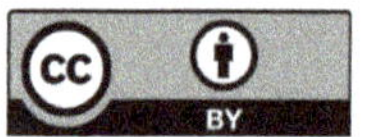

www.ingramcontent.com/pod-product-compliance
Lightning Source LLC
LaVergne TN
LVHW070153170726
843515LV00007B/1912

* 9 7 8 3 0 3 9 4 3 8 5 9 4 *

MDPI
St. Alban-Anlage 66
4052 Basel
Switzerland
Tel. +41 61 683 77 34
Fax +41 61 302 89 18
www.mdpi.com

Journal of Clinical Medicine Editorial Office
E-mail: jcm@mdpi.com
www.mdpi.com/journal/jcm